Management of Diabetes Mellitus

Edited by

Rubin Bressler

David G. Johnson

John Wright • PSG Inc

Boston   Bristol   London

1982

Library of Congress Cataloging in Publication Data

Main entry under title:

Management of diabetes mellitus.

   Bibliography: p.
   Includes index.
   1.   Diabetes.   I.   Bressler, Rubin.
  [DNLM: 1.   Diabetes mellitus–Therapy.
  WK815 M265]
  RC660.M33   616.4′62   80-10866
  ISBN 0-88416-259-1

Published by:
John Wright • PSG Inc, 545 Great Road, Littleton,
Massachusetts 01460, U.S.A.
John Wright & Sons Ltd, 42–44 Triangle West,
Bristol BS8 1EX, England

Medicine is an ever-changing science. As new research and clinical experience broaden our knowledge, changes in treatment and drug therapy are required. The editors and the publisher of this work have made every effort to ensure that the treatment and drug dosage schedules herein are accurate and in accord with the standards accepted at the time of publication. Readers are advised, however, to check the product information sheet included in the package of each drug they plan to administer to be certain that changes have not been made in the recommended dose or in the indications and contraindications for administrations. This recommendation is of particular importance in regard to new or infrequently used drugs.

Printed in the United States of America.

International Standard Book Number: 0-88416-259-1

Library of Congress Catalog Card Number: 80-10866

CONTRIBUTORS

Stanton G. Axline, MD
Associate Professor of Medicine
Section of Infectious Disease
University of Arizona
  Health Sciences Center
Tucson

Thomas W. Boyden, MD
Assistant Professor of
  Internal Medicine
Section of Endocrinology
University of Arizona
  Health Sciences Center
Tucson

Rubin Bressler, MD
Professor and Head
Department of Internal Medicine
University of Arizona
  Health Sciences Center
Tucson

David L. Earnest, MD
Associate Professor of Internal
  Medicine
Section of Gastroenterology
University of Arizona
  Health Sciences Center
Tucson

John A. Galloway, MD
Senior Clinical Pharmacologist
Lilly Laboratory for Clinical
  Research
William N. Wishard Memorial
  Hospital
Indianapolis, Indiana

David G. Johnson, MD
Associate Professor of Internal
  Medicine
Section of Endocrinology
University of Arizona
  Health Sciences Center
Tucson

James D. Kingham, MD
Assistant Professor of Surgery
Section of Ophthalmology
University of Arizona
  Health Sciences Center
Tucson

Stanley M. Lee, MB
Assistant Professor of
  Internal Medicine
Renal Section
University of Arizona
  Health Sciences Center
Tucson

Ian L. MacGregor, MD
Associate Professor of
  Internal Medicine
University of Arizona
  Health Sciences Center
Tucson

Charles A. Nugent, MD
Professor of Internal
  Medicine
Section of Endocrinology
University of Arizona
  Health Sciences Center
Tucson

William A. Sibley, MD
Professor and Head
Department of Neurology
University of Arizona
  Health Sciences Center
Tucson

Jay W. Smith, MD
Professor of Internal Medicine
Section of General Medicine
University of Arizona
  Health Sciences Center
Tucson

CONTENTS

INTRODUCTION

Major advances in understanding of the physiologic chemistry and pathophysiology of diabetes mellitus have occurred in the past twenty years. These insights have been translated in part into the therapeutic armamentarium of the practicing physician. However, many problems, both practical and conceptual, remain unresolved in the therapy of diabetes mellitus. This book addresses some of the therapeutic issues that confront the physician caring for patients with diabetes mellitus. It is not intended to be an encyclopedic textbook of diabetes mellitus. It was written for the primary care physician engaged in the practice of medicine. A number of selected areas of therapy will be discussed from the vantage points of pathophysiology and clinical pharmacology.

The diagnosis of diabetes mellitus is itself an issue of some controversy. Is there some level of fasting or postprandial blood glucose that can definitely be called abnormal? Is this a function of age? Is the glucose tolerance test of value in the diganosis of diabetes mellitus?

In recent years the weight of clinical and experimental evidence has supported the value of better blood glucose control in slowing or preventing the development of diabetic microangiopathy and nephropathy. This is an important issue in light of the potential hazards of hypoglycemia. An important question relates to whether degrees of blood glucose control result in degrees of protection from diabetic complications.

Underlying the problem of diabetic control is the recognition that the assessment of longitudinal blood glucose control is difficult. Rapid glycemic fluctuations are common in the insulin-dependent diabetic patient. The use of hemoglobin A_{1C} measurements may alleviate this important problem.

Diabetes mellitus has been classified in a number of ways based on therapy, obesity, genetics, age of onset and infectious-immunologic aspects. However, in spite of the variety of "types" of diabetes, hyperglycemia appears to be the common feature that characterizes these disease states. Most if not all types of diabetic patients appear to be at risk for developing microangiopathy, nephropathy and neuropathy.

The complications of diabetes mellitus are thought to depend in some way on blood glucose control, duration of the disease, and hereditary factors. Diabetic patients who once died of ketoacidosis, infections, hypertensive complications, cardiovascular disease or chronic renal failure now live longer because of insulin, antibiotics, antihypertensive drugs, renal dialysis, and renal transplantation. The resultant increase in life span contributes to the increased volume of chronic diabetic complications seen by the practicing physician. The mainstays of good blood glucose control are diet, regular physical activity, and insulin (or oral sulfonylureas for certain selected patients).

The chapters that follow focus primarily on diagnostic and treatment problems encountered by physicians involved in longitudinal care of diabetic patients. A number of important therapeutic issues are discussed. These include:

- The aims of a "diabetic" diet. In addition to the necessity for normalizing body weight, what other aspects of diet are important (dietary fat, fiber, complex carbohydrates)?
- Clinical pharmacology of insulin and the oral sulfonylureas.
- Therapy of diabetic ketoacidosis and hyperosmolar coma.

The complications of diabetes are widespread and result in great morbidity and mortality. The ubiquitous nature of the pathology makes examination of specific organ systems essential.

Diabetes frequently causes pathologic changes in the eye. Severe retinal disease can result in blindness and the frequent occurrence of cataracts impairs vision. The therapy of these conditions in recent years has been encouraging. Diabetic nephropathy is the leading cause of death in the younger patient, but it is a frequent complication that results in morbidity and mortality in all age groups. Diabetic neuropathy is an annoying condition characterized by pain, paresthesias, dysesthesias, gastrointestinal disturbances, and impotence. The non-fatal complications have an unclear etiology and somewhat unpredictable natural history. Both diabetic gastrointestinal and primary myocardial diseases are still in phases of being characterized.

Infection in the diabetic patient can be a serious problem. Diabetes mellitus has been considered to render the patient more susceptible to infection and less capable of combating it. The infectious agent, site of infection, status of the patient's blood glucose control, and therapy of the infection may all play roles in the outcome.

The selection of topics in this book was based partly on the interests and expertise of the authors, all but one of whom are members of the faculty at the Arizona Health Sciences Center in Tucson Arizona, and partly on our sense of what was important.

Rubin Bressler, MD
David G. Johnson, MD

1 Pathophysiology of Diabetes Mellitus

David G. Johnson, MD

Diabetes mellitus is recognized as a clinical disorder by the presence of hyperglycemia and glycosuria. Rather than defining a single disease or group of diseases this emphasis on glucose regulation draws attention to the most apparent pathophysiologic abnormality shared by patients with this condition. The term diabetes mellitus is also used in a more specific sense to designate a group of primary diseases characterized not only by hyperglycemia but many other pathophysiologic features. Central to this "definition" of diabetes mellitus is the recognition that most of the metabolic consequences are due, at least in part, to a deficiency in the actions of insulin on its target tissues. The apparent deficiency in the action of insulin can be the result of inadequate secretion of insulin from the pancreas or a poor response to endogenous insulin in the major target tissues (liver, adipose tissue, and muscle). Both mechanisms — inadequate secretion and defective tissue response — are present in many patients.

Concepts regarding the pathogenesis of diabetes have changed considerably during the past two decades. The actual cause for most cases of diabetes mellitus is still unknown. However, new information from many areas of scientific investigation has challenged previous ideas regarding the pathogenesis of diabetes and suggested new avenues for future study. The success of Minkowski and Von Mering (in 1886) in producing diabetes mellitus in dogs by total pancreatectomy suggested to early workers that diabetes mellitus was the result of a degenerative process involving the pancreatic β-cells. The important influence of heredity supported the notion that diabetes was an inborn disorder leading to abnormal degeneration of pancreatic β-cells. Occasional reports suggested that acute viral infections such as mumps could also produce diabetes.[1] Recent study has directed attention to many pathologic processes, including infectious etiologies,[2] autoimmune phenomena,[3-4] and target tissue defects.[5] At the present time, it appears likely that the condition known as diabetes mellitus can be produced by nearly all of the commonly recognized pathologic processes — infections, toxins, immune reactions, inflammatory necrosis of the pancreas, genetic defects of the "one gene one protein" type, and, rarely, neoplastic phenomena (eg, glucagonoma).

HETEROGENEITY OF DIABETES MELLITUS

It has been recognized for many years that diabetes mellitus occurs in more than one typical syndrome. Based on his studies in the 1930s Himsworth noted that patients with diabetes could be separated into two groups depending on their sensitivity to insulin.[6] Whereas patients prone to ketosis were usually sensitive to insulin, Himsworth found that the older individuals with nonketotic diabetes tended to be insensitive to exogenous injections of insulin.[7]

Using a bioassay to estimate plasma insulin activity, Bornstein and Trewhella found that untreated patients with diabetes could be divided into two groups based on the presence or absence of plasma insulin activity.[8] It was noted that the patients with weight loss and ketosis had no detectable insulin activity whereas obese, nonketotic diabetics had essentially normal insulin activity.[9] However, it was not until the development of radioimmunoassay techniques to measure insulin in the early 1960s that fundamental differences between juvenile-onset and adult-onset diabetes mellitus were recognized.[10] When plasma insulin concentrations were measured, it became clear that most adult-onset diabetics have considerable amounts of circulating insulin. Obese individuals without diabetes were found to have higher than average plasma insulin concentrations.[11,12] Since most patients with adult-onset diabetes are obese, the concept developed that there is a resistance of target tissues to the action of insulin in obesity and adult-onset diabetes mellitus.[13,14] In people with adult-onset diabetes this resistance is not adequately compensated by augmented insulin secretion, resulting in hyperglycemia and other metabolic alterations characteristic of the diabetic state.

The antibodies against insulin that develop in insulin-dependent (juvenile-onset) diabetes interfere with the radioimmunoassay determination of insulin levels. However, measurement of plasma C-peptide levels is a reliable index of release of endogenous insulin, since this fragment of proinsulin is secreted in equimolar amounts with insulin.[15] Studies of C-peptide in juvenile-onset diabetics after several years of disease indicate that endogenous secretion of insulin is usually deficient or absent, in contrast to patients with adult-onset diabetes.[16]

INFECTIONS AND AUTOIMMUNITY

Recent advances in immunology have led to the important recognition that juvenile-onset (ie, insulin-dependent) diabetics have islet-cell antibodies in their circulation that can mediate both humoral and cellular immune responses that injure or destroy pancreatic β-cells.[3,4,17-20] Titers of these antibodies are highest in the earliest stages of clinical disease, suggesting that an inciting agent, such as a chemical toxin or a virus, may damage the β-cell or elicit an immune response that leads to later loss of β-cells and development of insulin-dependent diabetes mellitus. Several animal models using viruses as inciting agents to provoke diabetes mellitus have already been developed. Epidemiologic data have drawn attention to the association of mumps, infectious mononucleosis, hepatitis, rubella, or coxsackievirus B4 with the onset of human diabetes mellitus.[2] A variant of coxsackievirus B4 has recently been isolated from the pancreas of a patient with newly diagnosed diabetes.[21] This virus attacks cultured mouse pancreatic cells. It also appears that toxic chemical agents can damage pancreatic β-cells, leading to the formation of islet cell antibodies and the development of diabetes mellitus in a manner similar to viral infections.[22,23]

Additional evidence linking insulin-dependent diabetes mellitus to abnormal immunologic responses comes from study of HLA genotypes.[24,25] Several HLA genotypes occur with greater-than-normal frequency in patients with juvenile-onset diabetes, including HLA B8, B18 (Southern Europeans), BW15 (Northern Europeans), BW22 (Japanese), DW3 and DW4. The overall incidence of these genotypes among juvenile diabetics is not high, suggesting that the genes conferring susceptibility to diabetes are not identical with or very closely adjacent to the HLA genes. In addition there does not appear to be any increased incidence of diabetes in people who are homozygous for any of the HLA

4

genotypes vs heterozygotes (no "double-dosing" effect). However, the incidence of juvenile-onset diabetes is increased in people with both B8 and BW15 or both DW3 and DW4, suggesting that there could be several genes located near different HLA loci that each contribute to the predisposition to diabetes.[24] Recently it has been shown that an unusual genetic type (BfF1) of properdin factor B, is present in 22.6% of patients with insulin-dependent diabetes mellitus compared to 1.9% of the general population.[26] The genetic locus for properdin factor B (Bf) is closely linked to the HLA genes. Although the susceptibility to develop adult-onset diabetes is inherited to an even greater extent than juvenile-onset diabetes, no correspondence with any HLA genotypes has been found.

RESISTANCE OF TARGET ORGANS TO INSULIN

The resistance to the actions of insulin seen in patients with adult-onset diabetes mellitus can be explained in some cases by a decrease in insulin binding to target cells.[5,27] This "down regulation" of receptors may be the consequence of higher circulating levels of insulin, since similar changes in other hormonal receptors occur in response to increasing concentrations of hormone.[5,28] In a few patients with diabetes mellitus and acanthosis nigricans the presence of antibodies directed against the insulin receptor has been demonstrated.[5,29] Another group of young female patients with acanthosis nigricans and diabetes were found to have decreased numbers of insulin receptors. Bar et al have also reported a case of a woman with diabetes and acanthosis nigricans who had normal insulin receptors but was resistant to insulin due to an apparent "postreceptor defect."[30]

Recently Tager and co-workers have described a patient with adult-onset diabetes, who had a normal sensitivity to exogenous insulin, and high circulating insulin levels.[31] Analysis of this patient's insulin revealed a substitution of leucine for phenylalanine at position B-23 or B-24. These observations emphasize that multiple pathogenetic mechanisms can also produce the clinical syndrome of adult-onset diabetes mellitus. It is likely that more causes of adult-onset diabetes mellitus will be discovered in the future.

VARIANTS OF ADULT-ONSET DIABETES MELLITUS

It has long been recognized that typical juvenile-onset diabetes mellitus can appear at any age. The work of Fajans and his colleagues has drawn attention to the occurrence of typical adult or maturity-onset diabetes mellitus among children.[32] In at least some of these cases, the genetic predisposition appears to be inherited as an autosomal dominant with a high degree of penetrance.

SECONDARY TYPES OF DIABETES MELLITUS

Diabetes mellitus can be caused by any pathologic process that destroys pancreatic tissue, such as pancreatitis or hemochromatosis. Diseases that produce excessive secretion of counterregulatory hormones can also lead to diabetes. These include acromegaly, hyperthyroidism, hyperadrenocorticism, pheochromocytoma, and glucagonomas. Exogenous administration of hormones, such as progestins (birth control pills) and glucocorticoids can produce or exacerbate a diabetic state. Numerous other drugs, including thiazides, diazoxide, furosemide, phenytoin (diphenylhydantoin), and catecholamines can inhibit insulin release, leading to hyperglycemia and glucosuria. Usually drug-induced diabetes is not severe enough to cause ketoacidosis and does not continue long enough to produce the characteristic chronic complications of diabetes. Uremia commonly results in impaired glucose tolerance and a pseudodiabetic condition that seldom requires special treatment.

INSULIN SECRETION IN DIABETES

Patients with established insulin-dependent diabetes mellitus have decreased numbers of β-cells in the pancreas. The secretion of insulin from the remaining β-cells can be estimated by measuring the concentration of C-peptide in peripheral blood.[15] Numerous studies have shown that this secretion of insulin by residual β-cells is depressed or absent in insulin-dependent diabetics and responds poorly to normal stimuli.[16]

Function of β-cells is also abnormal in adult-onset diabetes mellitus. Although circulating levels of insulin can be low, normal, or high in this condition, certain pathologic alterations in β-cell secretion are usually demonstrable. One characteristic abnormality is a loss of the acute release of insulin ("first phase") seen in diabetic subjects when the fasting blood sugar exceeds 115 mg/dl.[33,34] Another characteristic of β-cell secretion in diabetes is that glucose is a poor stimulator of insulin release, whereas the response to other stimulating agents, such as secretin[35] or isoproterenol[36] may be quite normal. Some of the abnormality of β-cell secretion seen in adult-onset diabetes mellitus may be conditioned by the changes in secretion of other hormones, such as gastric inhibitory polypeptide (GIP), that have been demonstrated in diabetic subjects.[37-39]

GLUCAGON SECRETION IN DIABETES

In both juvenile-onset (insulin-dependent) and adult-onset diabetes mellitus there are associated abnormalities in glucagon secretion from the pancreatic α-cells.[40,41] This altered function of the α-cell may be secondary to impaired β-cell function, but direct confirmation of this hypothesis has not been obtained. Three characteristic abnormalities of pancreatic α-cell secretion in diabetes are: 1) hyperglucagonemia during hyperglycemia,[41] 2) decreased or absent release of glucagon in response to hypoglycemia,[42] and 3) greatly enhanced sensitivity to the stimulating action of catecholamines.[43-44]

Unger and associates have stressed the importance of excessive glucagon secretion in contributing to the abnormal metabolism of diabetic patients.[40,41] They have advanced the concept of the insulin:glucagon ratio as the final determinant of the metabolic disposition of energy substrates, particularly in the liver.

The demonstration by Gerich and co-workers that infusion of somatostatin, which inhibits release of glucagon, can partially block the development of ketoacidosis in insulin-dependent diabetics deprived of insulin suggests that abnormal glucagon secretion is an important contributory factor in producing the metabolic abnormalities seen in diabetes.[45]

PATHOPHYSIOLOGIC CONSEQUENCES OF DIABETES

Regardless of its etiology, diabetes mellitus represents a condition of inadequate insulin action in target tissues. Since insulin is the major hormone for promoting storage of body nutrients, a deficiency leads to inadequate disposal of ingested food and excessive consumption of endogenous metabolic fuels. The effects of insulin in responsive tissues involve multiple aspects of the metabolism of glucose, amino acids, lipids, and nucleic acids. If the action of insulin is insufficient, predictable abnormalities in the disposition of affected substrates occur (Table 1-1).

In patients with minimal deficiency the most apparent abnormality is an impaired ability to dispose of ingested carbohydrate and protein. Clinically this is reflected in decreased glucose tolerance and glycosuria. Glucose and amino acid uptake into muscle and fat cells is impaired. Abnormal disposition of ingested and endogenously derived lipids (triglyceride and cholesterol) can also occur under conditions of relatively mild insulin deficiency, chiefly as a consequence of inadequate lipoprotein lipase activity.[46] This leads to elevated circulating concentrations of plasma lipoproteins and chylomicrons.

Table 1-1
Major Effects of Insulin on Important Target Tissues

Effect	Liver	Muscle	Adipose Tissue
Anabolic	Increased glycogen synthesis	Increased uptake of glucose and amino acids	Increase uptake of glucose and amino acids
	Increased synthesis of RNA and protein	Increased synthesis of glycogen and protein	Increased synthesis of glycerol, fatty acids, and triglyceride
	Increased synthesis of fatty acids and triglyceride		
Anticatabolic	Decreased glycogenolysis and gluconeogenesis	Decreased protein catabolism and amino acid output	Decreased lipolysis
	Decreased fatty acid oxidation and ketogenesis		

More severe deficiency of insulin causes further impairment in uptake of glucose and amino acids. Synthesis of glycogen, protein, fat, DNA, RNA, and ATP are all diminished. Conversely, glycogenolysis and protein catabolism, with release of amino acids from peripheral tissues, are enhanced.[47] This is evident clinically by stunted growth in children and weight loss, protein wasting, and chronic fatigue in adults. Without the effect of insulin to oppose it, hormone-sensitive lipase is activated, liberating free fatty acids from adipocytes. If these catabolic processes causing break down of glycogen, protein, and fat in peripheral tissues are not checked, the patient will develop ketoacidosis or die of inanition. A detailed analysis of the metabolic derangements in ketoacidosis is included in Chapter 8.

ABNORMALITIES OF HEPATIC METABOLISM IN DIABETES

Hepatic extraction of glucose from the portal blood is decreased in diabetes. In normal subjects about 60% of ingested glucose is retained by the liver.[48] In patients with adult-onset diabetes the hepatic extraction of ingested glucose is half that amount. It must be emphasized that this abnormally low uptake of glucose by the liver occurs despite hyperglycemia and hyperinsulinemia. This has led one group of investigators to conclude that there may be a deficiency of a gastrointestinal mediator of insulin action on the liver in adult-onset diabetics.[49]

8

Lack of insulin leads to abnormally low levels of several of the enzymes responsible for glycolysis in the liver, including glucokinase, phosphofructokinase, and pyruvate kinase. Metabolism of glucose via the phosphogluconate pathway is also reduced by insulin deficiency. Conversely lack of insulin stimulates gluconeogenetic pathways leading to increased hepatic synthesis of glucose. Finally, glycogen synthesis is dependent on sufficient insulin action, resulting in depletion of glycogen stores in the liver in uncontrolled diabetes. The end result of all these changes is a large increase in glucose output from the liver (Figure 1-1).

In addition to the derangements of glucose metabolism in the liver that occur in diabetes there are important changes in the pathways of lipid metabolism. The elevated levels of circulating free fatty acids that occur in insulin insufficiency are taken up and metabolized in the liver to ketone bodies (beta-hydroxybutyrate, acetoacetate, and acetone). During conditions of insulin lack and high plasma glucagon levels, as seen in uncontrolled diabetes, the hepatic metabolism of free fatty acids is shifted from synthesis of triglycerides and phospholipids to fatty acid oxidation and ketone body formation (Figure 1-2).[50] This shift is due at least partially to increased stores of carnitine in the liver.[51] The ketone bodies formed in the liver are released into the circulation. This process can outstrip the ability of peripheral tissues to metabolize the ketone bodies, leading to ketoacidosis. Conversely, when glucose and insulin are present in high concentration, hepatic synthesis of fatty acids and triglyceride are stimulated, and fatty acid oxidation is diminished. Malonyl CoA is the first committed intermediate in the conversion of glucose to triglyceride. McGarry and associates have shown that malonyl CoA inhibits hepatic carnitine acyltransferase I, thus decreasing the mitochondrial oxidation of fatty acids during periods of insulin-promoted glucose metabolism.[52]

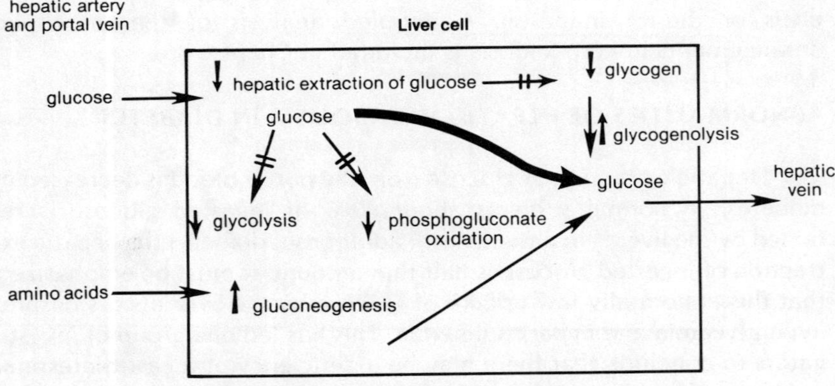

Figure 1-1   Derangements of glucose metabolism in the liver.

PERIPHERAL LIPID METABOLISM

Deficiency of insulin decreases the activity of lipoprotein lipase in peripheral tissues, interfering with the peripheral metabolism of plasma lipoproteins.[46,53] This can lead to accumulation of lipoproteins in the plasma, particularly very-low-density lipoproteins (VLDL) and chylomicrons. In severe cases, the high concentration of circulating lipoproteins can cause eruptive xanthomata and pancreatitis.

Recently increased attention has been focused on the importance of high-density lipoproteins (HDL) in the regulation of body lipids. This is due in large measure to the observation that low plasma concentrations of HDL are associated with increased atherosclerotic disease, whereas high HDL concentrations are associated with a lower incidence of atherosclerotic disease.[54] Studies in patients with diabetes have yielded conflicting data regarding HDL concentrations. Negative correlations between HDL concentration and serum glucose[55] or hemoglobin A_{1c}[56] have been reported. Another study found low HDL levels in maturity-onset diabetics but normal levels in juvenile-onset diabetics.[57] Other investigators have not found lower plasma HDL concentrations in diabetics.[58] In fact, Nikkila et al have reported higher than average HDL concentrations in diabetic patients treated with insulin.[59] Reckless et al studied the correlation between HDL, LDL, and vascular disease in a large group of diabetic patients.[60] In general, the positive association between LDL and vascular disease was seen more consistently in all diabetic groups than the negative association between HDL and vascular disease. Patients with diabetes mellitus are predisposed to the early development of atherosclerosis. To what extent this is due to the abnormalities cited above in lipid metabolism is still unclear.

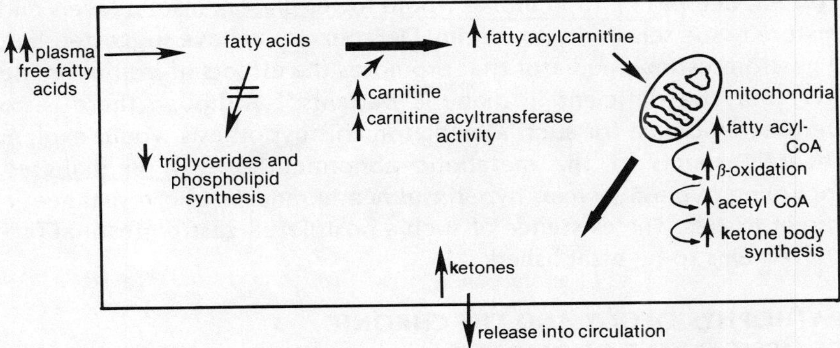

Figure 1-2 Changes in the pathways of lipid metabolism.

DEFECTIVE INSULIN SECRETION VS INSULIN-RESISTANCE — THE HORSE AND CART OF ADULT-ONSET DIABETES

The vast majority of patients with diabetes mellitus have the adult-onset form of the disease. Although a few cases may be due to unusual causes, such as insulin-receptor antibodies or biologically less effective forms of insulin, most patients with adult-onset diabetes mellitus do not exhibit these identifiable abnormalities to explain the autoregulatory paradox of hyperglycemia despite coexistent hyperinsulinemia. Since many of these patients are obese, and obesity is known to produce resistance to insulin, it is tempting to speculate that the primary defect resides in the abnormal insulin receptor responses produced by the obese state. By this reasoning, the difference between normal obese persons and obese diabetics is determined by the limited ability of the pancreas to increase its release of insulin in the diabetic group. Evidence to support this mechanism is the reversibility of hyperglycemia and glycosuria in many adult-onset diabetics that occurs when they sharply curtail their caloric intake. Insulin responses to glucose challenge have been shown to improve following a period of weight reduction.[61] Czech[62] and Olefsky[63] have found evidence for a postreceptor defect to explain some of the insulin insensitivity of large adipocytes. In the case of obese patients with diabetes the obesity could lead to a postreceptor defect that interferes with the effects of insulin on target tissues. This would result in increased insulin secretion and down-regulation of insulin receptors.

Against the hypothesis of a primary target tissue defect in adult-onset diabetes is the observation that some patients with adult-onset diabetes are not obese. It is also possible that the insulin receptor changes noted in obesity and adult-onset diabetes are both secondary to increased levels of circulating insulin released by either ingested stimulants or endogenous hormones, such as gastric inhibitory polypeptide released in response to meals. If this alternative explanation is correct, decreasing food intake would lower plasma insulin levels and restore tissue sensitivity to insulin. DeFronzo et al have suggested that a gastrointestinal mediator that promotes the effects of insulin on the liver may be deficient in diabetic patients.[49] Although there is no definite evidence for such a mediator, this hypothesis would explain several aspects of the metabolic abnormalities seen in diabetes, including hyperglycemia, hyperinsulinemia, and insulin resistance in target tissues. The existence of such a postulated gastrointestinal factor remains to be established.

PATHOPHYSIOLOGY AND THE CHRONIC COMPLICATIONS OF DIABETES

The pathophysiologic mechanisms that lead to the chronic lesions of diabetes—retinopathy, nephropathy, neuropathy, and increased thickening of capillary basement membranes are not yet understood. As discussed in Chapter 7, increasing evidence suggests that the late pathologic complications of diabetes are related to the alterations in metabolism of glucose, fat, and amino acids outlined above. The fact that the late pathologic complications of diabetes can develop in patients with diverse genetic predispositions and with diabetes as a result of many different pathophysiologic mechanisms is compelling evidence that the metabolic consequences of defective insulin action are responsible for the long-term effects of diabetes as well. The association of the metabolic abnormalities and the chronic lesions of diabetes does not appear to be the coincident result of a more basic underlying defect. It is the only known relationship shared in common by patients with a large variety of diseases due to different causes and pathophysiologic mechanisms.

REFERENCES

1. Harris, H.F. A case of diabetes mellitus quickly following mumps. *Bost Med Surg J.* 140:465–469, 1899.

2. Notkins, A.L. Virus-induced diabetes mellitus. *Arch Virol* 54:1–17, 1977.

3. Nerup, J., Andersen, O., Christy, M. et al. HLA, autoimmunity, virus and the pathogenesis of juvenile diabetes mellitus. *Acta Endocrinol* 83(suppl 205): 167–175, 1976.

4. Maclaren N.K. Viral and immunological bases of beta cell failure in insulin-dependent diabetes. *Am J Dis Child.* 131:1149–1154, 1977.

5. Flier, J.S., Kahn, C.R., and Roth J. Receptors, antireceptor antibodies and mechanisms of insulin resistance. *N Engl J Med.* 300:413–419, 1979.

6. Himsworth, H.P. Diabetes mellitus, its differentiation into insulin-sensitive and insulin-insensitive types. *Lancet* 1:127–130, 1936.

7. Himsworth, H.P. The syndrome of diabetes mellitus and its causes. *Lancet* 1:465–473, 1949.

8. Bornstein, J., and Trewhella, P. Plasma insulin levels in diabetes mellitus in man. *Aust J Exp Biol Med Sci.* 28:569–572, 1950.

9. Bornstein, J., and Lawrence, D.D. Plasma insulin in human diabetes mellitus. *Br Med J.* 2:1541–1544, 1951.

10. Yalow, R.S., and Berson, S.A. Immunoassay of endogenous plasma insulin in man. *J Clin Invest.* 39:1157–1175, 1960.

11. Karam, J.H., Grodsky, G.M., and Forsham, P.H. Excessive insulin response to glucose in obese subjects as measured by immunochemical assay. *Diabetes* 12:197–204, 1963.

12. Bagdade, J.D., Bierman, E.L., and Porte, D., Jr. The significance of basal insulin levels in the evaluation of the insulin response to glucose in diabetic and non-diabetic subjects. *J Clin Invest.* 46:1549–1557, 1967.

13. Karam, J.H., Pavlatos, F.C., Grodsky, G.M. et al. Obesity in maturity-onset diabetes and growth hormone in acromegaly. *Lancet* 1:286–289, 1965.

14. Reaven, G.M., and Olefsky, J.M. The role of insulin resistance in the pathogenesis of diabetes mellitus. *Med Clin North Am.* 62:313–331, 1978.

15. Horwitz, D.L., Rubenstein, A.H., and Steiner, D.F. Proinsulin and C-peptide in diabetes. *Med Clin North Am.* 62:723–733, 1978.

16. Madsbad, S., Faber, O.K., Binder, C. et al. Prevalence of residual beta-cell function in insulin-dependent diabetics in relation to age at onset and duration of diabetes. *Diabetes* 27(suppl 1):262–264, 1978.

17. Lendrum, R, Walker, G., and Gamble, D.R. Islet-cell antibodies in juvenile diabetes mellitus of recent onset. *Lancet* 1:880–883, 1975.

18. Irvine, W.J., Al-Khateeb, S.F., Dimario, V. et al. Soluble immune complexes in the sera of newly diagnosed insulin-dependent diabetics and in treated diabetics. *Clin Exp Immunol.* 30:16–21, 1977.

19. Bottazzo, G.F., Mann, J.J., Thorogood, M. et al. Autoimmunity in juvenile diabetics and their families. *Br Med J.* 2:165–168, 1978.

20. Lernmark, A., Freedman, Z.R., Hofmann, C. et al. Islet-cell-surface antibodies in juvenile diabetes mellitus. *N Engl J Med.* 229:375–380, 1978.

21. Yoon, J.W., Austin, M., Onodera, T. et al. Virus-induced diabetes mellitus: isolation of a virus from the pancreas of a child with diabetic ketoacidosis. *N Engl J Med.* 300:1173–1179, 1979.

22. Prosser, P.R., and Karam, J.H. Diabetes mellitus following rodenticide ingestion in man. *JAMA.* 239:1148–1150, 1978.

23. Karam, J.H., Prosser, P.R., and LeWitt, D.A. Islet-cell surface antibodies in a patient with diabetes mellitus after rodenticide ingestion. *N Engl J Med.* 299:1191, 1978.

24. Nerup, J. HLA studies in diabetes mellitus: a review. *Adv Metab Disord.* 9:263–281, 1978.

25. Ganda, O.P., and Soeldner, S.S. Genetic, acquired, and related factors in the etiology of diabetes mellitus. *Arch Intern Med.* 137:461–469, 1977.

26. Raum, D., Alper, C.A., Stein, R. et al. Genetic marker for insulin-dependent diabetes mellitus. *Lancet* 1:1208, 1979.

27. Olefsky, J.M., and Reaven, G.M. Decreased insulin binding to lymphocytes from diabetic subjects. *J Clin Invest.* 54:1323–1328, 1974.

28. Kahn, C.R., Meghesi, K., Bar, R.S. et al. Receptors for peptide hormones. *Am Intern Med.* 86:205–219, 1977.

29. Bar, R.S., and Roth, J. Insulin receptor status in disease states of man. *Arch Intern Med.* 137:474–481, 1977.

30. Bar, R.S., Muggeo, M., Roth, J. et al. Insulin resistance, acanthosis nigricans, and normal insulin receptors in a young woman: evidence for a postreceptor defect. *J Clin Endocrinol Metab.* 47:620–625, 1978.

31. Tager, H., Given, B., Mako, M. et al. Characterization of an abnormal insulin from a patient with diabetes. *Clin Res.* 27:378A, 1979.

32. Fajans, S.S., Cloutier, M.C., and Crowther, R.L. Clinical and etiologic heterogeneity of idiopathic diabetes mellitus. *Diabetes* 27:1112–1125, 1978.

33. Seltzer, H.S., Allen, E.W., Herron, A.L., Jr. et al. Insulin secretion in response to the glycemic stimulus: relation of the delayed initial release to carbohydrate tolerance in mild diabetes. *J Clin Invest.* 46:323–335, 1967.

34. Simpson, R.G., Benedetti, A., Grodsky, G.M. et al. Early phase of insulin release. *Diabetes* 17:684–692, 1968.

35. Lerner, R.L., and Porte, D., Jr. Studies of secretion-stimulated insulin responses in man. *J Clin Invest.* 51:2205–2210, 1972.

36. Robertson, R.P., and Porte, D., Jr. The glucose receptor. A defective mechanism in diabetes mellitus distinct from the beta adrenergic receptor. *J Clin Invest.* 52:870–876, 1973.

37. Crockett, S.E., Mazzaferri, L., and Cataland, S. Gastric inhibitory polypeptide (GIP) in maturity-onset diabetes mellitus. *Diabetes* 25:931–935, 1976.

38. Ross, S.A., Brown, J.C., and Dupre, J. Hypersecretion of gastric in-

hibitory polypeptide following oral glucose in diabetes mellitus. *Diabetes* 26:525–529, 1977.

39. May, J.M., and Williams, R.H. The effect of endogenous gastric in-hibitory polypeptide following oral glucose in diabetes mellitus. *Diabetes* 26:525–529, 1977.

40. Unger, R.H., and Orci, L. Role of glucagon in diabetes. *Arch Intern Med.* 137:482–491, 1977.

41. Unger, R.H., and Orci, L. The role of glucagon in the endogenous hyperglycemia of diabetes mellitus. *Annu Rev Med.* 28:119–130, 1977.

42. Gerich, J.E., Langlois, M., Noacco, C. et al. Lack of glucagon response to hyperglycemia in diabetes: evidence for an intrinsic pancreatic alpha cell defect. *Science* 182:171–173, 1973.

43. Gerich, J.E., Lorenzi, M., Tsalikian, E. et al. Studies on the mechanism of epinephrine-induced hyperglycemia in man: evidence for participation of pancreatic glucagon secretion. *Diabetes* 25:65–71, 1976.

44. Benson, J.W., Johnson, D.G., Palmer, J.P. et al. Glucagon and catecholamine secretion during hypoglycemia in normal and diabetic man. *J Clin Endocrinol Metab.* 44:459–464, 1977.

45. Gerich, J.E., Lorenzi, M., Bier, D.M. et al. Prevention of human diabetic ketoacidosis by somatostatin. Evidence for an essential role of glucagon. *N Engl J Med.* 292:985–989, 1975.

46. Eckel, R.H., Fujimoto, W.Y., and Brunzell, J.D. Insulin regulation of lipoprotein lipase in cultured 3T3-L1 cells. *Biochem Biophys Res Commun.* 84:1069–1075, 1978.

47. Felig, P., Wahren, J., Sherwin, R. et al. Amino acid and protein metabo-lism in diabetes mellitus. *Arch Intern Med.* 137:507–513, 1977.

48. Sherwin, R., and Felig, P. Pathophysiology of diabetes mellitus. *Med Clin North Am.* 62:695–711, 1978.

49. DeFronzo, R., Ferrannini, E., Wahren, J. et al. Lack of gastrointestinal mediator of insulin action in maturity-onset diabetes. *Lancet* 2:1077–1079, 1978.

50. McGarry, J.D., and Foster, D.W. Hormonal control of ketogenesis. *Arch Intern Med.* 137:495–501, 1977.

51. McGarry, J.D., Robles-Valdes, C., and Foster, D.W. The role of carnitine in hepatic ketogenesis. *Proc Natl Acad Sci USA.* 72:4385–4388, 1975.

52. McGarry, J.D., Leatherman, F.G., and Foster, D.W. Carnitine palmitoyl-transferase. I. The site of inhibition of hepatic fatty acid oxidation by malonyl-CoA. *J Biol Chem.* 253:4128–4136, 1978.

53. Bagdade, J.D., Porte, D., Jr., and Bierman, E.L. Diabetic lipemia a form of acquired fat-induced lipemia. *N Engl J Med.* 276:427–433, 1967.

54. Miller, G.J., and Miller, N.E. Plasma-high-density-lipoprotein concen-tration and development of ischaemic heart-disease. *Lancet* 1:16–19, 1975.

55. Lopes-Virella, M.F., Stone, P.G., and Colwell, J.A. Serum and high den-sity lipoprotein in diabetic patients. *Diabetologia* 13:285–291, 1977.

56. Calvert, G.D., Graham, J.J., Mannik, T. et al. Effects of therapy on plasma-high-density-lipoprotein-cholesterol concentration in diabetes mellitus. *Lancet* 2:66–68, 1978.

57. Kennedy, A.L., Lappin, T.R., Lavery, T.D. et al. Relation of high-density lipoprotein cholesterol concentration to type of diabetes and its control. *Br Med J.* 2:1191–1194, 1978.

58. Elkeles, R.S., Wu, J., and Hambley, J. Hemoglobin A$_1$, blood glucose, and high-density lipoprotein cholesterol in insulin-requiring diabetics. *Lancet* 2:547–549, 1978.

59. Nikkila, E.A., Hormilla, P., and Huttunen, J.K. Increase of high density

lipoprotein levels and of post-heparin plasma lipoprotein lipase activity in insulin-treated diabetics. *Circulation* 56:23, 1977 (abstract).

60. Reckless, J.P., Betteridge, D.J., Wu, P. et al. High-density and low-density lipoproteins and prevalence of vascular disease in diabetes mellitus. *Br Med J.* 1:883–886, 1978.

61. Stanik, S., and Marcus, R. Insulin deficiency in obese patients with severe diabetes improves after weight loss. *Clin Res.* 27:51A, 1979.

62. Czech, M.P. Cellular basis of insulin insensitivity in large rat adipocytes. *J Clin Invest.* 57:1523–1532, 1976.

63. Olefsky, J.M. The insulin receptor: its role in insulin resistance of obesity and diabetes. *Diabetes* 25:1154–1165, 1976.

2 Diagnosing Diabetes and Monitoring Insulin Therapy

Thomas W. Boyden, MD

It is not difficult to diagnose overt diabetes mellitus, but detecting the disease before obvious clinical signs and symptoms appear is not easy or precise. All people with hyperglycemia do not have diabetes, nor do all persons with signs of diabetes show glucose intolerance. Presently we are limited in our ability to return glucose intolerance to or towards normal. Because of this limitation the benefit of early identification of diabetes mellitus has been questioned.[1] The debate over the advantages of loose or tight glucose control will probably not be resolved until practical methods of achieving better glucose control are developed. Until that goal is reached we are left with the vagaries of blood and urine glucose measurements or indirect indices such as glycosylated hemoglobin, to monitor the conventional therapy of diabetes.

This chapter will first examine the tests used to diagnose diabetes mellitus with emphasis on their specificity, reliability, and predictive value. The discussion then turns to the tests that are used to monitor insulin therapy.

DIAGNOSING DIABETES MELLITUS

Most individuals with diabetes have abnormal carbohydrate tolerance, which is the basis for the traditional laboratory tests to diagnose the disease. There are also many reasons for abnormal carbohydrate tolerance that are not related to diabetes. Making this distinction is important because erroneous diagnosis of diabetes may adversely affect a person's job, insurance, and psychologic status. The risk of inappropriate treatment being given to an individual misdiagnosed as having diabetes is also a serious hazard.

Evaluation of Glucose Tolerance

Patients who develop diabetic ketoacidosis, or patients with retinopathy, neuropathy, or dermopathy with hyperglycemia and persistent glucosuria do not require additional tests to establish the diagnosis of diabetes mellitus. In fact, nearly all insulin-deficient diabetics have an obvious onset to their disease. Persistent fasting hyperglycemia is another criterion used to establish the diagnosis of diabetes. The use of glucose tolerance testing has been primarily used to identify individuals with inconspicuous insulin-resistant diabetes who are at risk for developing the microvascular and macrovascular lesions of diabetes. Implicit in this identification procedure is the notion that the tests are accurate and that some benefit will accrue to the patient.

For years physicians have relied on a nonstandard oral glucose tolerance test (OGTT) (it is performed differently in different clinics and countries). The test has multiple sets of criteria for abnormality, is poorly reproducible, altered by many drugs and clinical settings, and is a poor predictor of the disease for which it was designed. An exhaustive examination of the OGTT by Siperstein[2] concluded that this test is a pitfall in establishing the diagnosis of diabetes mellitus.

The OGTT is usually performed by analyzing blood glucose in the fasting state, administering 100 gm of glucose orally, and measuring blood glucose one, two, and three hours after the challenge. Frequently, only the one and two hour values are examined. At least five different sets of OGTT criteria have been suggested as indicative of diabetes. If each of these sets of criteria are applied to the same OGTTs of 746 first-degree relatives of individuals with diabetes the results indicate that between 12.7% and 28.6% of these subjects would be classified as having diabetes.[3] Not only do the percentages of abnormal tests vary greatly, but the different methods of evaluation do not identify the same subjects as having diabetes. There is no universally accepted set of OGTT criteria to reliably identify diabetes. A committee on statistics of the American Diabetes Association (ADA) established a plasma glucose of 185 mg/dl at one hour and 140 mg/dl at two hours as another criterion constituting an abnormal OGTT.[4] Even the ADA statistics committee suggested analyzing each OGTT result by two sets of criteria.

A good diagnostic test must be reproducible; the OGTT is not. Examination of 400 institutionalized men every two months for a year with repeated OGTTs indicated that the average blood glucose for the group remained stable.[5] But there was considerable variability of single tests for a given individual. None of the subjects were known to have diabetes, yet some of the tests were clearly abnormal some of the time. This percentage varied with the criteria used for interpretation, but in no subject were all six OGTTs abnormal by any criteria.

Still another requirement of a good test is validity under most testing circumstances. Nearly all biologic tests have false-positive or false-negative results under certain conditions. But the OGTT is altered under many conditions, including increasing age, obesity, inactivity, drugs (thiazide diuretics, phenytoin, phenylephrine, estrogens, progestogens, glucocorticoids), surgery, viral or bacterial infection, prior diet, and afternoon testing.[2]

A single abnormal OGTT in an asymptomatic individual is not predictive of overt diabetes. A study of 200 subjects found to have an abnormal OGTT and then reexamined after five to ten years, showed that only 20% had developed overt diabetes.[6] Twenty-five percent had reverted to a normal OGTT. In a similar study of 352 women with abnormal OGTTs follow-up studies showed that only 27.3% had developed overt diabetes.[7] From these data it may be concluded that if a single OGTT is abnormal there is a 70% to 80% chance that it is a false-positive indicator of future diabetes during a five to ten year period. Kobberling and his co-workers[8] performed OGTTs on 488 first-degree relatives of diabetic individuals and retested them five years later. Of those subjects with a normal first test, retesting showed that 17.6% had deterioration of their glucose tolerance to "subclinical diabetes" and 1.3% were found to have overt diabetes. Of those subjects with subclinical diabetes on the first OGTT, 35.6% reverted to normal glucose tolerance whereas only 13.6% progressed to overt diabetes. More interesting are the 17 subjects whose first OGTT demonstrated overt diabetes. Three of the 17 reverted to subclinical diabetes and an additional three retested as normal.

An offshoot of the misinformation concerning the predictive value of the OGTT has been the mass screening programs for early detection of diabetes. The results of a program in Cleveland have been recently reviewed.[9,10] Screening was performed by administering 75 gm of glucose orally and measuring blood glucose two hours later. Rescreening was performed three and five years later. In the original group with a positive test the relative risk for diabetes five years later was 22 times greater than those persons whose original test was negative. However, about half of the original subjects with positive findings had negative findings upon retesting five years later. On the basis of initial screening, 12% of the group subsequently shown to have a normal test had already been treated with oral hypoglycemic drugs. The value of mass screening programs has been questioned because of the tests' nonspecificity and the possibility that therapy will be given to subjects who may not have diabetes.

For years postprandial hypoglycemia has been proposed as an early manifestation of diabetes. This syndrome was thought to be distinct from idiopathic reactive hypoglycemia since the OGTT was supposed to show blood glucose values obviously diagnostic of diabetes during the first two hours of the test. Seltzer et al[11] provided some of the earliest data on this syndrome when they reported a six-year follow-up on 110 patients with a diabetic OGTT (by their criteria) and a blood glucose ≤ 50 mg/dl three to five hours after glucose ingestion. Ninety-three percent of their subjects had a normal fasting blood glucose. The hypoglycemic part of the OGTT was not found in any subject with a fasting blood glucose > 130 mg/dl.

O'Sullivan and Mahan[7] have reported that 66% of subjects with an abnormal OGTT by the Seltzer et al criteria do not develop overt diabetes. Moreover, it has been shown that 23% of normal individuals and 25% of individuals whose parents both have diabetes have at least one blood glucose value < 50 mg/dl during a five hour OGTT.[12] Others have found that at least 33% of normal subjects will have a blood glucose ≤ 50 mg/dl during an OGTT.[13] The finding of chemical hypoglycemia during an OGTT does not increase the likelihood of diabetes.

Widely differing opinions of normal and abnormal fasting and two-hour postprandial glucose concentrations were received from a survey of diabetologists.[14] Criteria given for the highest fasting plasma glucose considered to be normal ranged from 105 to 120 mg/dl, and for the lowest fasting value considered abnormal from 120 to 160 mg/dl. Corresponding ranges of values given for a two-hour postprandial plasma glucose were 105 to 180 mg/dl for highest normal values and 120 to 200 mg/dl for the lowest abnormal values. The problem of defining blood glucose criteria increases with the age of the population tested, since mean blood glucose concentrations increase with age in most industrialized populations. Although the frequency distributions of glucose levels in white populations are continuous and unimodal,[15-17] there is increasing epidemiologic evidence that the risk of specific diabetic complications becomes important in those individuals with a plasma glucose greater than 200 mg/dl two hours after a glucose load.[18-23]

It would appear that conservative criteria such as persistent fasting plasma glucose above 120 mg/dl or a plasma glucose greater than 200 mg/dl two hours after a glucose load are the best discriminators of "diabetes." In the five-year prospective Bedford survey[18] nearly all of the diabetic retinopathy was confined to those people with a baseline capillary whole-blood-glucose concentration exceeding 200 mg/dl two hours after a 50-gm oral glucose load. Even those individuals with initial glucose tolerance that worsened over 10 years have not developed significant retinopathy. Jarrett and colleagues[18,19] have also prospectively studied 204 male civil servants, all of whom had abnormal glucose tolerance, but whose blood glucose values did not exceed 200 mg/dl two hours after a glucose load. After six to eight years none of the subjects developed diabetic retinopathy by ophthalmoscopy even though 13% worsened to overt diabetes.

In contrast to white populations the Pima Indians in Arizona and the Nauruans in Micronesia show a distinct bimodal distribution of glucose tolerance that can be used to divide the populations into normal and hyperglycemic groups.[20,21] The plasma glucose concentrations of the Pima Indians were measured at both one and two hours after 75 gm of oral glucose. By examining the one- and two-hour bimodality there is mathematical rationale for preferring the two-hour level.[22] Misclassification of a normal as hyperglycemic is almost twice as common if the one-hour plasma glucose level is used. The two-hour hyperglycemic group is mainly in excess of 200 mg/dl. (A venous plasma glucose concentration two hours after a 75 gm oral glucose load is roughly equivalent to the capillary whole-blood-glucose concentration two hours after a 50 gm glucose load used by Jarrett and Keen.[18]) Most interesting is that the incidence of diabetic retinopathy and nephropathy is virtually confined to the group with a two-hour plasma glucose concentration exceeding 200 mg/dl.[23] The tendency toward development of hypoinsulinemia in the Pima Indians also occurs at two-hour glucose concentrations between 200 and 239 mg/dl.[24] If the definition of diabetes includes the likelihood of developing specific microvascular disease, these studies suggest that a value 200≥ mg/dl two hours after glucose ingestion would be necessary to diagnose diabetes from the plasma glucose response to an oral glucose load. This is in contrast to the lower conventional range.

The plasma glucose value of 200 mg/dl two hours after a glucose load roughly corresponds to an overnight fasting plasma glucose of 110 mg/dl.[18] In the Pima Indians, mean fasting plasma glucose was 114 mg/dl in those with two hour concentrations between 225 and 244 mg/dl.[25] At two-hour values greater than this the fasting plasma glucose was considerably greater, suggesting that fasting glucose homeostasis is intact in subjects with a two hour post–glucose-load value up to about 250 mg/dl. This would tend to validate the idea that persistent fasting hyperglycemia is a relatively late manifestation of diabetes and occurs at a point when hypoinsulinemia, rather than hyperinsulinemia, is seen.[24]

It has been proposed that measuring the insulin response during an OGTT may be a more accurate predictor of those destined to develop definite diabetes (retinopathy or persistent elevations of fasting blood glucose).[26] During an examination of subjects with an abnormal OGTT followed for three months to eight years, definite diabetes occurred exclusively in the low insulin-responder group (ie, insulin/blood glucose less than 0.5 30 minutes after a glucose load), although many individuals with a low insulin response did not develop definite diabetes.

The National Diabetes Data Group has recently published its recommendations for the diagnosis of non–insulin-dependent diabetes mellitus. Nonpregnant adults can be diagnosed as having diabetes mellitus if they have 1) overt symptoms of diabetes with unequivocal hyperglycemia, 2) persistent fasting glucose concentrations in excess of 140 mg/dl, or 3) a plasma glucose concentration greater than 200 mg/dl two hours after a 75 gm oral carbohydrate load and a plasma glucose concentration in excess of 200 mg/dl at some other point between time zero and two hours. These diagnostic criteria are applicable to adults of all ages.[27]

CONCLUSIONS

1. In the absence of overt signs or symptoms of diabetes the diagnosis of diabetes mellitus, based on tests of glucose tolerance, should be made cautiously.

2. Persistent elevations of fasting plasma glucose ($>$ 140 mg/dl) or plasma glucose concentrations $\geq$ 200 mg/dl two hours after a glucose load are potent predictors of future overt diabetes and its sequelae.

3. The OGTT should be reserved for clinical investigations and establishing the diagnosis of "diabetes of pregnancy" because of its limited usefulness in the practical diagnosis of diabetes mellitus.

4. The finding of chemical hypoglycemia during an OGTT does not increase the likelihood of developing diabetes mellitus.

5. Plasma insulin response during the OGTT, as a practical tool to diagnose diabetes, needs further investigation before it can be recommended for routine use.

MONITORING THE INSULIN THERAPY
OF DIABETES MELLITUS

Most patients with insulin-resistent (adult-onset) diabetes mellitus do not require drug therapy for control of their hyperglycemia. Monitoring the biochemical aspects of their disease can be accomplished by occasional measurements of fasting plasma glucose concentrations and by having the patient test for glucosuria at home. Day-to-day adjustments of treatment are not necessary in this group of patients whose main therapy is usually directed toward weight reduction. For the occasional individual judged to be a candidate to receive one of the sulfonylureas these simple tests of glucose tolerance will also suffice.

Insulin-deficient patients, who must match exogenous insulin administration to meals, activity, and illness, must have their glycemic changes monitored more frequently and with greater accuracy in order that rational therapeutic changes can be made. The discussion that follows is an examination of the blood and urine tests that are routinely used to follow insulin-dependent patients.

Blood Glucose as an Index of Control

In the past it has been common to obtain frequent fasting blood glucose (FBG) measurements on patients who require insulin. This practice rarely yields the useful information that it is assumed to provide. An examination of how FBG relates to 24-hour glycemic changes in insulin-dependent persons with diabetes should help to clarify this point.

Service et al[28] studied subjects by continuous blood glucose analysis during 48-hour periods while the subjects were free to walk and to eat in an ambulatory fashion. Three normal subjects and eleven subjects with insulin-dependent diabetes were studied. As expected, the mean amplitude of glycemic excursions (MAGE), a measure of diabetic instability, for the normal subjects was small (22 to 60 mg/dl). Subjects with diabetes judged to be clinically stable had MAGE 67 to 82 mg/dl, while those with clinically unstable diabetes had MAGE from 119 to 200 mg/dl. An attempt to improve glucose control in the unstable group by injecting additional amounts of short-acting insulin resulted in no change in MAGE but did significantly increase the number of hypoglycemic episodes.

By examining the tracings of the continuously measured blood glucose it is readily apparent that in an individual patient a slight change in the time at which a FBG is determined may give greatly varying results. For example, in Figure 2-1, if the blood sample for the FBG is drawn at 6 AM (as might be done in a hospitalized patient) the value on one day is 240 mg/dl. In contrast, a blood sample obtained at 7:15 AM of the same day would yield a FBG of 115 mg/dl. Traditionally, each of these results would be interpreted as reflecting poor and good glucose control, respectively. Yet neither result predicts the tremendous variability seen throughout the remainder of the day. The higher FBG value might suggest that additional insulin is needed, but increasing the insulin dose might also result in a reduction of blood glucose near 6 PM sufficient to cause frank hypoglycemia. On the other hand, the FBG of 115 mg/dl might suggest that the amount of injected insulin is quite satisfactory, although many physicians would consider the three blood glucose values of 300 mg/dl during the rest of the day as poor control.

In another study,[29] the same group of Mayo Clinic investigators found few clues to between-day blood glucose variability in individual subjects with diabetes by examining day-to-day changes in discrete blood glucose measurements. Stated another way, the blood glucose curve depicted in Figure2-1 may be quite dissimilar to the next day's curve from the same patient.

Knowing that a discrete blood glucose measurement is an inaccurate reflection of the many glycemic changes that occur during the same day should limit the number of decisions to change insulin

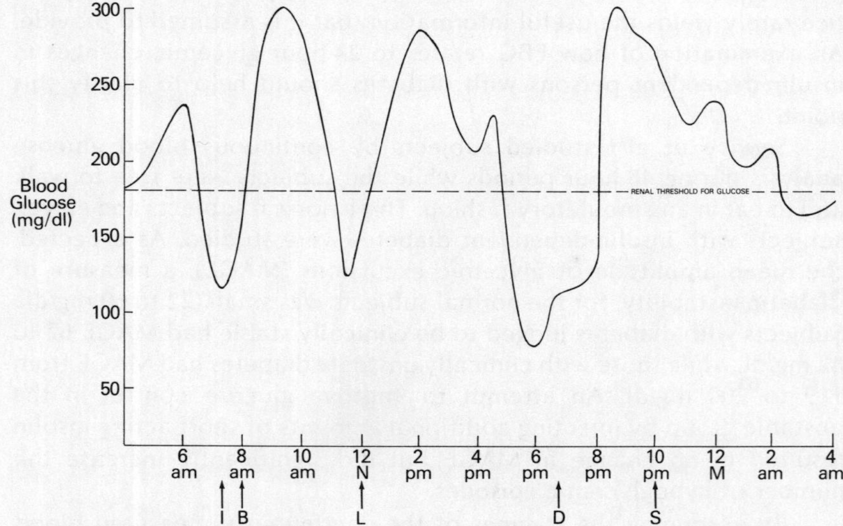

Figure 2-1 Representative blood glucose curve obtained during 24 hours of continuous blood glucose analysis. I = single injection of intermediate-acting insulin, B = breakfast, L = lunch, D = dinner, S = snack.

dosage that are based solely on FBG determination. Use of FBG can help in making decisions in the treatment of insulin-dependent patients but it should be recognized that the information is limited.

Measurements of Urinary Glucose

The ease of repeated collection and testing of urine for its glucose content makes this method of monitoring insulin therapy attractive to both patient and physician. All of the testing materials give a qualitative indication of blood glucose averaged over some minutes prior to urine collection. In Figure 2-2 the same blood glucose curve as in Figure 2-1 is presented with the approximate duration of renal glucose exposure, as might be reflected by a qualitative urine test for glucose, shown in the shaded areas. It can be seen that some of the high and low glycemic changes may fall into a single urine-sample period and therefore be expressed in the urine test as an averaged value for that time period. One of the first things that is apparent from this figure is an explanation for the common clinical misuse of the terminology "renal threshold for glucose."

There is a renal threshold, or tubular maximum, for glucose that can be determined by simultaneous ureteral and peripheral venous catheterization. At a time when the urine sample from the catheter in

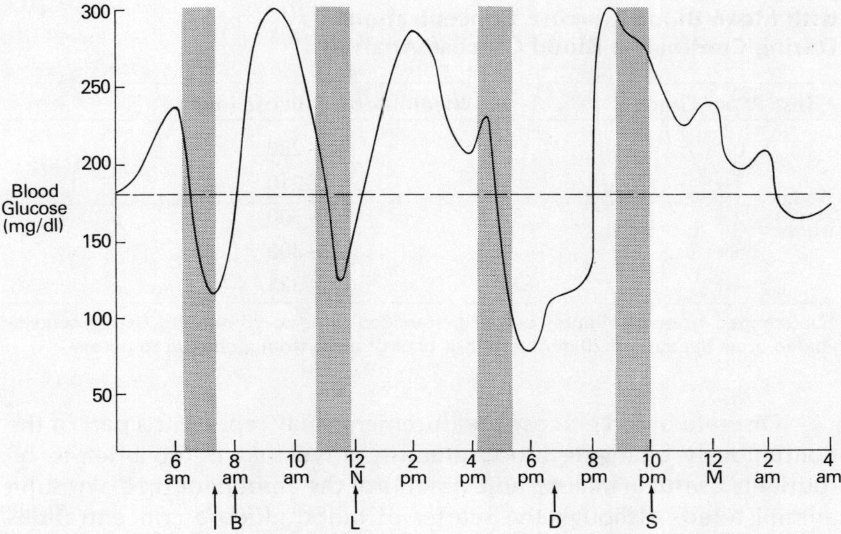

Figure 2-2 The same blood glucose curve and abbreviations as in Figure 2-1. Shaded areas represent approximate duration of renal blood glucose exposure as reflected by a qualitative test for urine glucose.

the ureter first contains measurable glucose a simultaneous blood glucose concentration must be determined. In the majority of normal subjects and subjects with diabetes (but without renal disease) this threshold occurs at a blood glucose of 160 to 180 mg/dl. Usually the renal handling of glucose is significantly altered only in pregnancy, chronic renal failure, and the uncommon diseases of renal glucosuria. The case illustrated in Figure 2-2 could easily be misinterpreted by comparing the FBG of 240 mg/dl (measured at 6 AM) to the first test for urine glucose of 0% to ⅛%. This would erroneously be called a high renal threshold for glucose. Likewise if the FBG of 115 mg/dl (measured at 7:15 AM) was measured and the first urine tested at ⅛% glucose, a low renal threshold would be suspected. In fact, neither statement is correct.

Although there is a highly significant correlation between blood glucose and the qualitative second-voided urinary glucose determination the overlap in measured blood glucose, during continuous blood glucose analysis, between sequential test-paper (Tes-Tape) grades is considerable (Table 2-1).[30] One reason for some of the blood glucose determinations being lower than the test paper grade would have estimated might be that the blood glucose was rapidly falling immediately prior to the collection of the second-voided urine specimen.

Table 2-1
Comparison of Urinary Tes-Tape Results
with Mean Blood Glucose Concentrations
During Continuous Blood Glucose Analysis

Test Paper Grade	Mean Blood Glucose (mg/dl)*
0	25–280
1+	50–210
2+	100–300
3+	25–300
4+	175–325

*Determined from 20 minutes before first-voided urine to 20 minutes before second-voided urine because of 20-minute transit time of urine from glomeruli to ureters.

Discrete blood glucose measurements may represent a part of the continuously changing blood glucose curve that is too brief to be routinely useful in making adjustments of the amount or type of insulin administered. Although the scatter of blood glucose concentrations measured at each urine test grade is great, the overall correlation of blood glucose with both first- and second-voided urine specimens is quite good.[31] It is the *pattern* of glycemic response reflected in the urinary glucose determinations that is most useful in assessing glucose control.

For instance, patients who are glucosuric throughout the day, but who usually have negative urinary tests for glucose on the first daily urine specimen might be suspected of having nocturnal hypoglycemia. Likewise, patients who routinely are aglucosuric before lunch but have glucosuria at other times may be identified as transient responders to insulin (see Chapter 4). In both cases an alteration in the amount or type of insulin may make the average pattern of glycemic response more acceptable.

The other benefit derived from having patients routinely monitor their own glucosuria is to help them identify stressful circumstances (ie, inactivity, infection) and respond by either changing the amount of injected insulin or seeking professional help. Patients who become heavily glucosuric, or symptomatic from their diabetes may also test their urine for ketone bodies to identify situations that require the attention of their physician.

There are four popular preparations used for the estimation of urinary glucose content: Clinitest tablets, Clinistix, Diastix, and Tes-Tape. The Clinitest tablet color change results from cupric acid being reduced to cuprous oxide. This reaction can occur with any reducing agent. The other three preparations employ glucose oxidase methods and will not react with other reducing substances. Tes-Tape is the most sensitive method, detecting 100% of aglucosuric urine fortified to 0.05% glucose.[32] Clinistix is the least sensitive method, giving no positive results in the same test. In a comparison test of the four urinary testing preparations 389 urine specimens fortified to 0.5% glucose revealed 85 falsely low and 172 falsely high readings.[32] Of the false-negative readings Clinistix was responsible for 19%, Diastix for 25%, both Clinistix and Diastix for 56%, and none were from either Clinitest or Tes-Tape. Ascorbic acid or aspirin ingestion was felt to be responsible in half of the false-negative tests. Sixty-five percent of the false-positive tests were Clinitest readings. Dilute urine caused false over-reading by any method, but was particularly troublesome with Clinitest.

Many drugs interfere with all of the urinary tests for glucose and for ketone bodies. Table 2-2 lists the most common drug interactions.

First- and second-voided urine specimens tested for glucose content are in agreement about two thirds of the time.[31] However, when the two specimens differ, the second-voided specimen usually moves the result from higher concentrations of urinary glucose to lower levels. The mean plasma glucose concentration predicted by either the first- or second-voided urine specimens is not statistically different, even when the two urine tests differ.

Table 2-2
Common Drugs that May Affect the Outcome of Urine Testing for Glucose and/or Ketones*

	Clinitest	Clinistix	Tes-Tape	Ketostix	Acetest
Ascorbic acid	+	−	−		
Cephalosporins	+				
Chloramphenicol	+				
Levodopa	+	−	−	+	+
Methyldopa	+		−		
Nalidixic acid	+				
Probenecid	+				
Salicylates	+	−	−	+	+
Sulfonamides	+				
Tetracyclines	+				

* + = false-positive; − = false-negative

Hemoglobin A_{1c}

At present the clinical estimation of diabetes control relies on patient history, daily measurement of glucosuria, and determinations of FBG during clinic visits. All methods have severe limitations. A better marker of the chronic, ambient levels of glucose may be one of the naturally occurring minor hemoglobins, hemoglobin A_{1c} (HbA_{1c}).

Hemoglobin A_{1c} is produced by postsynthetic glycosylation of hemoglobin A.[33] This addition of carbohydrate to hemoglobin is slow and presumably a nonenzymatic process, which occurs continuously throughout the 120-day life span of the human erythrocyte. This glycosylated hemoglobin, which constitutes 3% to 6% of the total hemoglobin in normal persons, is often increased to 6% to 12% of the total hemoglobin in patients with diabetes mellitus.[34,35]

In a study of five hospitalized patients with diabetes, there was a highly significant correlation of FBG and HbA_{1c} levels.[36] Before adequate control the mean FBG was 343 mg/dl and the HbA_{1c} concentration 9.8%. After instituting therapy to reduce the mean FBG to 84 mg/dl the concentration of HbA_{1c} fell to 5.8%. The concentration of HbA_{1c} in the blood appears to reflect the carbohydrate status of the patient during the preceding weeks or months.

Application of HbA_{1c} measurements to an outpatient population with diabetes has shown similar results.[37] Seventy-two patients with diabetes were rated by their physicians, both on their general degree of control and on their FBG concentrations. Both of these variables had significantly positive correlations with HbA_{1c} levels. In an outpatient pediatric population with diabetes a similar positive correlation existed between HbA_{1c} concentration and the 24-hour urinary glucose excretion, current FBG, mean FBG and the physician assessment of diabetic control.[38]

As a biologic method, the measurement of HbA_{1c} appears to integrate the concentrations of blood glucose over time, and may provide a means to relate the degree of blood glucose control to the development of the long-term sequelae of diabetes.[39] What the measurement of HbA_{1c} concentration does not do is to provide any additional information at a practical level on how to improve diabetes control in an individual patient. This is particularly true if one considers that the measurement of HbA_{1c} levels has only been compared to parameters that are normally used to monitor the therapy and progress of diabetes, namely, patient history, urinary glucose excretion, and FBG measurements.

CONCLUSIONS

Current methods of delivering insulin therapy, as well as methods of monitoring it, are crude. Attempts to achieve optimal glycemic control are probably worthwhile but at the present time these attempts must be tempered by recognition of the inaccuracies of methods for evaluating glucose control. Insulin therapy should be undertaken with the following liberal recommendations.

1. Avoid the symptoms of hyperglycemia or hypoglycemia.

2. Attempt to match the amount and type of injected insulin to the food and exercise habits of each patient with diabetes by examining the pattern and amount of glucosuria measured by the patient.

3. If FBG is measured during clinic visits recognize its limited value as a guide to making changes in insulin therapy.

4. Measurement of HbA_{1c} levels will be useful as a research tool to help relate long-term blood glucose levels to the development of diabetic sequelae, but the HbA_{1c} concentration offers no practical advantage over the conventional evaluation of patients with diabetes.

REFERENCES

1. Boyden, T.W., and Bressler, R. Asymptomatic hyperglycemia: to treat or not to treat. Edited by K.L. Melmon. In *Drug Therapeutics: Concepts for Physicians.* New York: Elsevier, 1979.

2. Siperstein, M.D. The glucose tolerance test: a pitfall in the diagnosis of diabetes mellitus. *Adv Intern Med.* 20:297–323, 1975.

3. Kobberling, J., and Creutzfeldt, W. Comparison of different methods for the evaluation of the oral glucose tolerance test. *Diabetes* 19:870–877, 1970.

4. Klint, C.R., Prout, T.E., Bradley, R.F. et al. Standardization of the oral glucose tolerance test (report of the Committee on Statistics of the American Diabetes Association, June 14, 1968). *Diabetes* 18:299–307, 1969.

5. McDonald, W.G., Fisher, F.G., and Burnham, C. Reproducibility of the oral glucose tolerance test. *Diabetes* 14:473–480, 1965.

6. Unger, R.H., Madison, K.L., and Adair, R.M. The significance of "normal" and "abnormal" oral glucose tolerance curves as determined by 5 to 10 year follow-up in 200 subjects. *Proceedings of the 19th American Diabetes Association Meeting,* 1959, p. 41.

7. O'Sullivan, J.B., and Mahan, C.M. Prospective study of 352 young patients with chemical diabetes. *N Engl J Med.* 278:1038–1041, 1968.

8. Kobberling, J., Kattermann, R., and Arnold, A. Follow-up of "nondiabetic" relatives of diabetics by retesting oral glucose tolerance after 5 years. *Diabetologia* 11:451–456, 1975.

9. Genuth, S.M., Houser, H.B., Carter, J.R. et al. Observations on the value of mass indiscriminate screening for diabetes mellitus based on a five-year follow up. *Diabetes* 27:377–383, 1978.

10. Houser, H.B., Mackay, W., Verma, N. et al. A three-year controlled follow up study of persons identified in a mass screening program for diabetes. *Diabetes* 26:619–627, 1977.

11. Seltzer, H.S., Fajans, S.S., and Conn, J.W. Spontaneous hypoglycemia as an early manifestation of diabetes mellitus. *Diabetes* 5:437–441, 1956.

12. Park, B.N., Kahn, C.B., Gleason, R.E. et al. Insulin-glucose dynamics in nondiabetic reactive hypoglycemia and asymptomatic biochemical hypoglycemia in normals, prediabetics, and chemical diabetes. *Diabetes* 21(suppl 1):373, 1972.

13. Burns, T.W., Bregnant, R., Van Peenan, H.J. et al. Observations on blood glucose concentration of human subjects during continuous sampling. *Diabetes* 14:186–191, 1965.

14. West, K.M. Substantial differences in the diagnostic criteria used by diabetes experts. *Diabetes* 24:641–644, 1975.

15. Sharp, C.L., Butterfield, W.J.H., and Keen, H. Diabetes survey in Bedford 1962. *Proc R Soc Med.* 57:193–202, 1964.

16. Hayner, N.S., Kjelsberg, M.D., Epstein, F.H. et al. Carbohydrate tolerance and diabetes in a total community, Tecumseh, Michigan. *Diabetes* 14:413–423, 1965.

17. O'Sullivan, J.B., and Mahan, C.M. Blood sugar levels, glycosuria, and body weight related to development of diabetes mellitus. The Oxford epidemiologic study 17 years later. *JAMA.* 194:587–592, 1965.

18. Jarrett, R.J., and Keen, H. Hyperglycaemia and diabetes mellitus. *Lancet* 2:1009–1012, 1976.

19. Jarrett, R.J., Keen, H., Fuller, J.H. et al. Worsening to diabetes in men with impaired glucose tolerance ("borderline diabetes"). *Diabetologia* 16:25–30, 1979.

20. Rushforth, N.B., Bennett, P.H., Steinberg, A.G. et al. Diabetes in the Pima Indians, evidence of bimodality in glucose tolerance distributions. *Diabetes* 20:756–765, 1971.

21. Zimmet, P., and Whitehouse, S. Bimodality of fasting and two-hour glucose tolerance distributions in a Micronesian population. *Diabetes* 27:793–800,1978.

22. Rushforth, N.B., Bennett, P.H., Steinberg, A.G. et al. Comparison of the value of the two- and one-hour glucose levels of the oral GTT in the diagnosis of diabetes in Pima Indians. *Diabetes* 24:538–546, 1975.

23. Bennett, P.H., Rushforth, N.B., Miller, M. et al. Epidemiologic studies of diabetes in the Pima Indians. *Recent Prog Horm Res.* 32:333–376, 1976.

24. Savage, P.J., Dippe, S.E., Bennett, P.H. et al. Hyperinsulinemia and hypoinsulinemia. Insulin responses to oral carbohydrate over a wide spectrum of glucose tolerance. *Diabetes* 24:362–368, 1975.

25. Dippe, S.E., Bennett, P.H., and Savage, P.J. How the fasting glucose relates to the two-hour post-load glucose level. *Diabetes* 23(suppl 1):350, 1974.

26. Kosaka, K., Hagura, R., and Kuzuya, T. Insulin responses in equivocal and definite diabetes, with special reference to subjects who had mild glucose intolerance but later developed definite diabetes. *Diabetes* 26:944–952, 1977.

27. National Diabetes Data Group. Classification and diagnosis of diabetes mellitus and other categories of glucose intolerance. *Diabetes* 28:1039–1057, 1979.

28. Service, F.J., Molnar, G.D., Rosevear, J.W. et al. Mean amplitude of glycemic excursions, a measure of diabetic instability. *Diabetes* 19:644–655, 1970.

29. Molnar, G.D., Taylor, W.E., and Langworth, A. On measuring the adequacy of diabetes regulation: comparison of continuously monitored blood glucose patterns with values at selected time points. *Diabetologia* 10:139–143, 1974.

30. Service, F.J., Molnar, G.D., and Taylor, W.F. Urine glucose analyses during continuous blood glucose monitoring. *JAMA.* 222:294–298, 1972.

31. Malone, J.J., Rosenbloom, A.L., Grgic, A. et al. The role of urine sugar in diabetic management. *Am J Dis Child.* 130:1324–1327, 1976.

32. Feldman, J.M., and Lebovitz, F.L. Tests for glycosuria. An analysis of factors that cause misleading results. *Diabetes* 22:115–121, 1973.

33. Bunn, H.F., Haney, D.N., Gabbay, K.H. et al. Further identification of the nature and linkage of the carbohydrate in hemoglobin A_{1c}. *Biochem Biophys Res Commun.* 67:103–109, 1975.

34. Peterson, C.M., Jones, R.L., Oenig, R.J. et al. Reversible hematologic sequelae of diabetes mellitus. *Ann Intern Med.* 86:425–429, 1977.

35. Trivelli, L.A., Ranney, H.M., and Lai, H.-T. Hemoglobin components in patients with diabetes mellitus. *N Engl J Med.* 284:353–357, 1971.

36. Koenig, R.J., Peterson, C.M., Jones, R.L. et al. Correlation of glucose regulation and hemoglobin A_{1c} in diabetes mellitus. *N Engl J Med.* 295:417–420, 1976.

37. Gonen, B., Rubenstein, A.H., Rochman, H. et al. An indicator of the metabolic control of diabetic patients. *Lancet* 2:734–736, 1977.

38. Tze, W.J., Thompson, K.H., and Leichter, J. HbA_{1c} — an indicator of diabetic control. *J Pediatr.* 93:13–16, 1978.

39. Gabbay, K.H., Hasty, K., Breslow, J.L. et al. Glycosylated hemoglobins and long-term blood glucose control in diabetes mellitus. *J Clin Endocrinol Metab.* 44:859–864, 1977.

3 Dietary Management of Patients with Diabetes Mellitus

Charles A. Nugent, MD

Unless a physician's practice is restricted to children, the great majority of his diabetic patients are non–insulin-dependent. Non–insulin-dependent patients are usually obese adults, often asymptomatic, and not prone to ketosis. Most of the discussion in this chapter will be directed toward their problems. Diabetic patients who are not prone to ketosis, but who are given insulin to correct hyperglycemia should not be classified as insulin-dependent.

The American Diabetes Association (ADA) has published two useful pamphlets[1,2] detailing the dietary management of insulin-dependent patients. The disease in these patients usually starts before age 30 and they are characteristically prone to ketosis and frequently not obese. For dietary management of these patients physicians need to use both of these ADA publications and patients need one of them.[1] Only the broad principles of dietary management of insulin-dependent patients will be discussed in this chapter.

NON-INSULIN-DEPENDENT PATIENTS

While heredity is a factor in the development of non-insulin-dependent diabetes in some patients, the disease would be uncommon in our society were it not for our physical inactivity and excessive consumption of calories leading to obesity.[3] The epidemiologic evidence relating obesity to diabetes is striking. West and Kalbfleisch[4] have shown that the correlation of the prevalence of diabetes with the prevalence of obesity is +0.89 in 12 age-matched populations in 11 countries. Racial differences in the prevalence of diabetes are small when racial groups are matched for obesity. There is a striking association of the prevalence of obesity with the percentage of the population engaged in sedentary occupations.[5,6] In the study by Keys,[5] the prevalence of both obesity and sedentary occupations was more than twice as frequent in the United States population examined than in any of the other 6 countries. It is estimated that in the United States 3% of middle-aged subjects and 5% of elderly subjects are known to have diabetes mellitus.[3] Because of the importance of obesity in the etiology and management of non-insulin-dependent diabetes, this problem will be discussed first.

Obesity

Obesity is frequently judged by comparing a patient's weight and height with the data presented in a table of Desirable Weights prepared by the Metropolitan Life Insurance Company.[7] Individuals judged to have desirable weights for their height and sex can have surprisingly large proportions of body fat. For example, Olefsky and his collegues[8] found that normal subjects (defined using the Desirable Weight table) had mean estimated body fats of 27% for men and 31% for women. In contrast, world class and nationally ranked male runners and wrestlers usually have body fats in the range of 5% to 12%.[9] Body fat in similarly trained women runners and gymnasts is usually higher than in the male athletes (10% to 20%).[9] In the absence of good information, firm advice cannot be given on the ideal percentage of body fat for optimal health. However, in managing diabetic patients, unless they have unusually well-developed muscles, it probably would be better to regard the Desirable Weight tables as providing overestimates of weight for height.

A number of methods have been used to estimate percentage of body fat. One of the most accurate techniques, determination of specific gravity, is time-consuming and requires special equipment.[10] If skin-fold calipers are available together with tables relating skin-fold thickness to percent body fat in men and women of different ages, estimates of percent body fat can be made.[11] For example, if the sum of skin-fold thickness in six areas (abdomen, thigh, chest, triceps, subscapular, and suprailium areas) is 60 mm in a 40- to 50-year-old individual, the estimated percent of body fat would be 12% to 13% in a man and 16% to 17% in a woman.[11]

Impaired glucose tolerance in the usual non–insulin-dependent diabetic patient is attributable to increased insulin resistance and often some degree of impairment of insulin secretion.[12] While obese non-insulin-dependent diabetics usually have higher plasma insulin levels than normal subjects these levels usually do not attain the elevated values seen in similarly obese subjects who are not diabetic.[12] Some obese patients with non–insulin-dependent diabetes eventually develop such marked impairment of insulin secretion that they make less insulin than non-obese subjects and may become insulin-dependent.[12]

Weight reduction of obese patients is effective in restoring insulin sensitivity to normal as well as increasing insulin secretion.[8,12,13] Even modestly obese patients can achieve dramatic improvements in glucose tolerance through weight loss.[8] Furthermore, obese diabetic patients need not reduce body weight to normal in order to improve glucose tolerance.[8] The first day of caloric restriction often results in a substantial reduction of blood sugar.

Current Management Practices

Treatment of non–insulin-dependent diabetics with drugs including insulin can lower blood sugar and free the patients from acute symptoms attributable to hyperglycemia. However, there is no convincing evidence that treating these patients with insulin, in contrast to placebo, lowers their mortality rate or their rate of development of complications attributable to diabetes.[14-17] Goldberg et al[18] in a survey at a diabetic clinic, concluded that management of patients frequently substituted treatment by drugs that were potentially harmful (oral hypoglycemic agents) for treatment that was physiologic (correcting obesity). Furthermore, treatment in their clinic ignored the correction of factors, such as hypertension and hyperlipidemia, that are as important or more important than hyperglycemia in the development of complications including death. This critical analysis of the deficiencies of their management of diabetic patients could probably be applied to many clinics and practices in this country.

Effective and Ineffective Techniques for Dietary Management

West[19] has published a thorough analysis of the usual failure of dietary management in controlling hyperglycemia in patients with diabetes mellitus. Most physicians are not skillful in the dietary management of these patients.[19]

However, there are physicians who know how to use diet control to manage diabetes in non–insulin-dependent diabetics and have published their results.[20-23] For example, Hadden and his colleagues[20] enrolled 98 adult-onset diabetics in a program of dietary management using traditional advice on restricting calories. At the time they prepared their report 85 were still attending their clinic and 57 had completed six months. At that time 36 of the 57 patients had restored their glucose tolerance to normal. This was achieved with an overall mean weight loss of only 8.2 kg.

Advice on restricting calories and increasing exercise, together with frequent follow-up visits has been an effective method, in many cases, for managing obese patients with non–insulin-dependent diabetes mellitus. However, because of compliance problems and poor long-term results,[19] other physicians have selected less traditional techniques.

Kempner and his associates[21] reported on their experience with 106 obese patients, some of whom were diabetic, and all of whom had lost at least 45 kg of body weight. The study subjects were outpatients managed on a rice diet, greatly restricted in calories, and followed a supervised daily exercise program. Their average weight loss was 63.9 kg. Forty-three of the patients achieved normal weights. No information was provided on the proportion of patients who did not succeed with the rice diet.

Another effective management method has been developed by Davidson, at Emory University.[22] His treatment begins with starving obese patients for a week. Subsequently the patient is managed with advice on caloric restriction and frequent outpatient visits. Davidson relies heavily on non-physician personnel (nurses and dieticians) for patient management. He reports success in dietary management of diabetes without the use of drugs in more than 80% of his patients. This success rate is particularly impressive in view of the fact that he is working with a predominantly inner city, black, impoverished population. His article should be consulted for details.[22]

We have found the Davidson approach to be far more satisfactory than just instructing the patients in dietary restriction of calories and arranging for frequent outpatient visits.

We have modified Davidson's approach somewhat. At our hospitals obese diabetics with no history of prior episodes of ketoacidosis and who do not have moderate or large amounts of ketones in their urine when glycosuric are candidates for this treatment. The patient is admitted to the hospital for a five-day period. If the patient is taking oral hypoglycemic agents or insulin, the drugs are stopped on the day of admission. For the first three days the patient is starved. He is allowed to drink water and to have up to three cups of coffee or tea and one carbonated, calorie-free beverage per day. Urine tests for sugars and ketones are done by the patient on double-voided urines obtained three times a day before meals and at bedtime. Ninety-five percent of our patients become aglycosuric within two or three days after admission. If the patient is not getting food, ketonuria usually develops by the second or third day and is a useful measure of compliance.

If moderate or large amounts of ketone appear in the urine while the fasting patient is still glycosuric, he needs prompt treatment with insulin and starvation should be halted. Glycosuric, ketonuric, fasting diabetic patients secrete so little insulin that they need insulin injections while following a calorie-restricted diet and further starvation would be hazardous.

After three days of starvation, rather then following Davidson's approach of prescribing a diet just restricted in calories, an attempt is made to change radically the type of food eaten by the obese non–insulin-dependent patient. On the fourth hospital day the patient is put on a calorically restricted vegan diet (no meat, milk, eggs, or their products, and no bread, potatoes, rice, nuts, seeds, pasta, or baked goods) and no more than one cup of cooked beans per day (mean intake less than 1000 cal/day). Following discharge the patient is urged to stay on this nutritionally inadequate diet for a two-month period before gradual introduction of nuts, seeds, potatoes, rice, and wheat and later minimal amounts of meat, milk, eggs, and their products (see *The Alternative Diet Book*[24] for details). The diet for long-term maintenance should be nutritionally adequate in all respects except for deficient calories until the patient's diabetes is cured, or he attains a normal weight.

Long-term follow-up of older programs that have been successful in inducing weight loss indicate that eventually a high proportion of patients regain their weight.[25,26] Permanent loss of weight demands major changes in lifestyle. To some extent one can modify the environment to which the patient is exposed by continuing close follow-up and ensuring that discussions of diet and exercise are major elements of each visit.

Alternatives

If it is not possible to eliminate diabetes mellitus in the obese non–insulin-dependent patient, it may be possible to minimize it or decrease the incidence of diabetic complications by dietary means. Continued caloric restriction with weight loss usually is helpful in ameliorating the disease in the obese patient.[12] However, even without changing the caloric intake of obese and non-obese non–insulin-dependent patients, it may be helpful to change the diet by 1) increasing the proportion of carbohydrates, 2) increasing the fiber content, 3) decreasing saturated fat and cholesterol, and 4) decreasing sodium. The first two of these measures have been shown in short-term studies to improve glucose tolerance in non–insulin-dependent diabetics but their long-term effectiveness and complications have not been studied. They cannot be regarded as widely accepted practices but they seem reasonable as supplementary forms of management if the patient cannot be managed with caloric restriction and is taking less than 30 units of insulin a day.[27] The last two measures, decreasing dietary saturated fat and cholesterol and decreasing salt intake, would not be expected to alter glucose tolerance but would be expected to decrease the risks of cardiovascular diseases. Epidemiologic studies have shown positive associations in diabetics between dietary intake of saturated fat and coronary artery disease and between sodium intake and strokes.[3] In patients with established atherosclerosis, regression or cessation of progression has been shown to follow lowering of serum cholesterol in a substantial proportion of patients.[28,29] These four noncaloric measures will now be discussed.

Increase the proportion of carbohydrates in the diet   Wood and Bierman[30] have published an excellent analysis of the historical basis for the past advocacy of carbohydrate restriction in the management of diabetes mellitus. Their review should be examined for details but their conclusions can be summarized.

"There no longer appears to be any need to restrict disproportionately the intake of carbohydrates in the diet of most diabetic patients."[30] Patient preference, cost, and other considerations (lowering the amount of saturated fat in the diet to decrease hypercholesterolemia) are now seen to be important considerations in determining the proportion of calories derived from carbohydrates.[30] Countries whose populations consume a high proportion of carbohydrates often have low rates of diabetes mellitus.[3] Furthermore, markedly increasing the proportion of calories derived from carbohydrate, without changing the calories consumed, tends to lower plasma glucose and improve oral and intravenous glucose tolerance tests in non–insulin-dependent diabetics.[30]

High-carbohydrate, high-fiber diets   Dietary fiber is the residue from plant foods resistant to hydrolysis by human alimentary enzymes.[31] Since dietary fiber is not digested by humans it does not provide calories. Dietary fiber includes complex carbohydrates associated with plant-cell contents (gums, mucilages, pectins, hemicelluloses) and substances associated with plant-cell-wall structures (cellulose, lignin).[32] Unfortunately food tables usually present information on the crude fiber content of foods (the material remaining after acid and alkaline hydrolysis of food), an unphysiologic measure that gives values in vegetables that range from 20% to 60% of those for dietary fiber while in fruits and grains the crude fiber content may be less than 10% of the dietary fiber content.[33]

There have been numerous reports on the improved control of hyperglycemia and decreased requirements for insulin and oral hypoglycemic agents in diabetic subjects given increased amounts of fiber.[34-38] For example, in one report examining the effects of increased fiber in addition to increased carbohydrate in the diet,[27] ten patients treated with less than 30 units of insulin per day or with oral hypoglycemic agents originally were given weight-maintaining diets with carbohydrates providing 43% of the total calories and 4.7 gm/day of crude fiber (ie, an ordinary American diet). When the diet was changed by increasing carbohydrate content to 75% of the calories and increasing crude fiber to 14.2 gm/day without changing caloric intake, all five patients on oral agents and four of the five patients on insulin were able to discontinue their medications. The single patient who continued to take insulin decreased the dose from 28 to 15 units/day. However, even with this marked decrease in drug therapy, fasting blood sugar levels decreased in all patients. Mean blood sugars were 170 mg/dl on the control diet and 119 mg/dl on the high-carbohydrate diet. The mean duration of the experimental diet was two weeks.[27] The effectiveness of high-fiber, high-carbohydrate diets on a short-term basis seems convincing. Controlled experience with these diets over long periods in the management of diabetes mellitus is not available.

Some of the specific components in fiber that are responsible for decreasing hyperglycemia have been identified. Pectin (in natural diets often derived from apples and oranges), guar gum and guar flour (guar is a galactomanan from the cluster bean), and cellulose are known to be effective. High-fiber diets have been effective in decreasing hyperglycemia in diabetics both when used as additives to the diet and when foods high in fiber were selected.

One practical way of advising patients on methods to increase the fiber content of their diet is to urge them to follow the advice of *The Alternative Diet Book*[24] of the Clinical Research Center of the University of Iowa.* American patients changing from a traditional diet to that advocated by this book will approximately triple their intake of crude

---

*Available for $3.95 from University of Iowa Publications Order Department, 17 West College Street, Iowa City, Iowa 52242.

fiber. Additional suggestions are contained in the original reports referred to above in the discussion of high-carbohydrate, high-fiber diets.

There may be some advantage to increasing the proportion of raw foods in the diet in order to decrease hyperglycemia.[39] Cell walls of plants are composed of cellulose and are impermeable to the digestive enzymes of humans. These cell walls are only slightly disrupted by chewing. Cooking causes starch in cells to swell rupturing cell walls and making the intracellular nutrients available for digestion.[39] An individual eating a constant amount of vegetables will derive fewer calories from the vegetables if they are uncooked. For health reasons, raw food in the diet should be restricted to fruits and vegetables and not include raw meat or fish, uncooked egg white or unpasteurized milk.[40]

Decrease the intake of saturated fat and cholesterol Coronary heart disease is the most common cause of death in patients with diabetes in Western societies.[41] The mortality rate from coronary heart disease is twice as high in men with diabetes and three times as high in women with diabetes as in nondiabetics.[42] The serum cholesterol concentration is an important risk factor for coronary heart disease and it is responsive to dietary alterations.[43]

Jarrett and his co-workers[44] in summarizing their experience with a five-year trial of dietary advice (decrease carbohydrate intake to 120 gm/day, eliminate sucrose) and drug therapy (phenformin) of non–insulin-dependent diabetics found no alteration in cardiovascular morbidity and mortality as a result of treatment. However, they did observe that the predominant risk factor for cardiovascular morbidity and mortality was the height of the systolic blood pressure while baseline plasma cholesterol concentration was a significant predictor of the onset of claudication. They concluded that treatment of hypertension and hyperlipidemia may be more effective in altering the progression of arterial disease in patients with mild to moderate glucose intolerance than conventional antidiabetic treatment.

Stone and Connor[45] reported in 1963 on the effectiveness of a high-fiber, high-carbohydrate, low-cholesterol diet in lowering serum cholesterol in diabetics. The mean serum cholesterol of the patients treated with the experimental diet was 49 mg/dl lower than that of the patients on the control regimen. Similar observations have been made by other investigators.[46,47] These isocaloric high-carbohydrate diets did not result in rises in serum triglycerides but instead serum triglyceride concentrations decreased.[30,46,47]

Connor and his associates, in *The Alternative Diet Book,*[24] outline a practical approach to decreasing serum cholesterol concentration and decreasing the risk of developing a number of diseases that frequently occur in our society. Overconsumption of rich foods is a major cause of coronary heart disease, cerebrovascular accidents, hypertension, obesity, and diabetes mellitus.[24] As factors in our diet partially responsible for these disorders these authors identify the following elements: high consumption of saturated fat, cholesterol, calories, sugar, and sodium together with inadequate intake of fiber and complex carbohydrates. The book details a staged progression of dietary alterations away from our traditional diet (Table 3-1). In the third (final) phase of the diet cereals, legumes, vegetables and fruit become the major sources of food while meat, fish, and chicken are used as condiments. In Phase III, 65% of the calories are derived from carbohydrates (mainly polysaccharides), 20% from fat (4% saturated) and 15% from protein while crude fiber amounts to 12 gm/day and cholesterol is only 100 mg/day.

Table 3-1
Changing to the Alternative Diet

Phase	Diet
I	Omit egg yolk, butter, cream, lard, organ meat, skin from poultry and fish, and visible fat in meat. Decrease use of salt. Alternative foods suggested.
II	In addition to above changes, decrease meat consumption to 6 to 8 oz per day. Also decrease fat, cheese, and salt consumption.
III	In addition to above changes, limit the total amount of meat, fish, and chicken to 3 to 4 oz per day. In baked products use only half the usual amount of salt but add none to other foods. Eat mainly cereals, legumes, vegetables, and fruit.

Decrease the intake of sodium Hypertension, a major risk factor for coronary heart disease,[31] is common in patients with diabetes mellitus. In the University Group Diabetes Program study 31% of the patients had hypertension at the beginning of the study.[14] The role of excessive sodium intake in the production of hypertension has been reviewed elsewhere.[48-50] The high prevalence of obesity and, usually after many years, some degree of renal impairment may be two factors that increase the tendency for diabetic patients to develop hypertension. It may seem overbearing to urge diabetics to add sodium restriction to the other limitations placed on their daily activities. Such advice might be given only after the physician has reviewed the evidence and discussed it with the patient. On epidemiologic grounds it would be expected that partial compliance with sodium restriction would decrease the likelihood of developing hypertension.[31,48,49] In patients with hypertension, restriction of the daily intake of sodium chloride to less than 5 gm[51] or 6 gm[52] has been shown to be therapeutically effective. Furthermore, the select Committee on Nutrition and Human Needs of the United States Senate has proposed as a dietary goal for all citizens that we decrease our intake of sodium chloride to approximately 3 gm per day.[53]

The first rule for decreasing sodium intake is to stop adding salt, both in the preparation of food and at the table. This is a difficult step. It may be reassuring for patients to realize that within a few weeks after they take this step they will begin detecting flavors in foods that they had not realized were there. It has been estimated that Americans eat 6 to 18 gm of sodium a day.[53] For most Americans, this salt is mainly derived from processed foods rather than being added to food in its preparation or at the table. If patients want to decrease salt intake but need some salt for particular dishes, it may be helpful to know that one-quarter teaspoon of salt contains only about 1.25 gm of sodium chloride.

The second rule for decreasing sodium intake is to eat no processed foods. These include bread, breakfast cereals, butter, cheese, frozen or canned foods, ice cream, ketchup, luncheon meats, margarine, pickles, spices with salt, TV dinners, and any other manufactured food. This makes one realize how difficult it is to restrict sodium intake in modern life. It is nearly impossible to eat no processed foods. If a choice can be made between eating a processed or a fresh food, however, the fresh item should be chosen, as its salt content is likely to be lower than that of the processed food. Specifically, fruits and vegetables, meat, fish, and poultry contain little sodium while canned or frozen vegetables, luncheon meats, ham, smoked fish, and sausage usually contain far more.

Some seasonings contain little sodium: basil, bay leaves, chili powder, cinnamon, curry, dry mustard, garlic, ginger, mint, onion powder, pepper, paprika, oregano, sage, salt substitute, and vinegar. Coffee and tea are low-sodium beverages. Certain processed foods are very low in sodium: macaroni, puffed rice, shredded wheat, salt-free bread, spaghetti, and unsalted margarine. Pamphlets providing details on dietary sodium restriction are available at local and national offices of the American Heart Association.

INSULIN-DEPENDENT PATIENTS

The objectives for the dietary management of insulin-dependent diabetics are: 1) provide for normal growth and development, 2) normalize and maintain body weight, 3) normalize glucose metabolism, 4) normalize lipid metabolism and decrease macrovascular complications, and 5) minimize microvascular complications. These objectives have been used to organize the presentation that follows.

Objectives of Dietary Management

The nutritional requirements for normal growth and development of patients with diabetes are the same as for all individuals, ie, an adequate quality and quantity of proteins, vitamins, minerals, and essential fatty acids and calories.[3] Our affluent status in the United States allows us to select a nutritionally adequate intake by eating a mixed diet composed of four traditional food categories, namely milk, meat, vegetables and fruits, and cereals and bread. Connor and his associates in *The Alternative Diet Book*[24] use different and possibly more appropriate food groupings, namely, legumes, nuts, and seeds; vegetables; whole grains; vegetable oils, margarines, and shortening; fruits; and low-fat animal products as condiments. These new food groupings of Connor et al have been devised to encourage selection of a diet likely not only to provide adequate nutrition but also likely to normalize serum lipid levels.

To normalize and maintain body weight, calories need to be adjusted. If insulin-dependent, ketosis-prone diabetics lose weight, their insulin requirements are likely to decrease. However, their ability to produce insulin is usually so deficient that their insulin requirement does not disappear. The dietary manipulations to decrease caloric intake or availability and increase satiety presented in the section on non–insulin-dependent patients is also applicable for insulin-dependent patients, with the exception of starvation. It is hazardous to starve insulin-dependent patients.

Daily subcutaneous administration of one or more doses of intermediate or short-acting insulin to insulin-dependent diabetics, even under the best of circumstances, only restores glucose metabolism to a condition approximating normality.[55] However, even this approximation cannot be obtained unless there is consistency in the amount and distribution of calories taken in day-by-day, a consistent balance of nutrients for each meal, ie, carbohydrates, fats and proteins, and consistent timing of meals[54] (see next section on Techniques for Prescribing Dietary Management).

To normalize lipid metabolism by dietary means one practical current method is to follow the advice given in *The Alternative Diet Book*.[24] The high-carbohydrate, high-fiber diet low in saturated fat and cholesterol, described in that book, corresponds to the diet eaten by populations in countries with far lower serum cholesterol concentrations than those in our country. On epidemiologic, experimental, and pharmacologic grounds there are excellent reasons for believing that measures that lower serum cholesterol are associated with decreases in the likelihood of development of coronary artery disease and atherosclerosis[28,29,41,56]; however, agreement among authorities is not universal.[57]

The experimental evidence in animals that hyperglycemia is responsible for many of the microvascular complications of diabetes mellitus is increasingly convincing.[55] Unfortunately, our ability to control hyperglycemia in insulin-dependent diabetics is very limited. The clinical evidence that control of hyperglycemia helps is, to date, suggestive.[55] Most of the remaining information in this chapter is directed to methods for improving the control of glucose metabolism.

Technique for Prescribing Dietary Management

In order to provide these patients with the information they need to select foods and to distribute them throughout the day in a consistent manner two publications are needed. One is the *Exchange Lists for Meal Planning.*[1]* This booklet provides information on the protein, carbohydrate, and fat content of foods assigned to six exchange groups that patients can use to help keep their diets stable and nutritionally adequate. It also has information on foods to avoid and foods that can be used in unlimited amounts.

It is very convenient if patients can be referred to dieticians for instructions in exchange meal planning. But even if a dietician is available, the physician needs to be involved in the selection of the content of calories, protein, carbohydrate, and fat in the diet and the distribution of calories in meals and snacks. Advice on the caloric content of the diet can be formulated by interview or by calculation. If the patient's weight approximates normal, the appropriate caloric content of the diet can be selected by determining the patient's current food intake and keeping the calories constant. The caloric content of a diet can be estimated by separating the components of the diet into the number and type of food exchanges consumed each day and using the *Exchange Lists for Meal Planning* for information on the caloric content of each exchange. A quicker way to do it is to make the estimates shown in Table 3-2. After the patient has been on the diet for several months, weight gains and losses can be handled by adjusting the diet in 500-calorie decrements and increments, respectively.

The American Diabetes Association[2] recommends that adults receive a minimum of 0.5 gm of protein per pound of desirable body weight. Growing children need 20% of their caloric intake as protein.

---

*Available from a local American Diabetes Association office, or it can be purchased for $0.50 per copy from the American Diabetes Association, 600 5th Avenue, New York, New York 10020.

Table 3-2
Estimating Caloric Needs

Activity	Calories
Basal	Body weight in lbs × 10
Sedentary	Basal + 30% of basal
Moderate	Basal + 50% of basal
Strenuous	Basal + 100% of basal

Carbohydrates and fats should be 50% to 70% and 30% to 50%, respectively, of nonprotein calories.

The *Alternative Diet Book*[24] advises that a higher proportion of calories be derived from carbohydrates. The difference between the maximum recommendation of the ADA with respect to the carbohydrate content of the diet and that of *The Alternative Diet Book* is not large. The maximum caloric intake of carbohydrate of a moderately active patient whose ideal and actual weight is 150 lbs would be 61% of total calories following the ADA recommendations and 65% following the advice in *The Alternative Diet Book*.

Initially the distribution of food in meals and snacks should follow the patient's usual pattern with 20% to 30% of the calories assigned to each meal and about 10% to each snack. The pattern of distribution of food during the day can be adjusted to improve control of blood sugar levels. Most patients using intermediate or long-acting insulins should have a snack before retiring and many need midafternoon or midmorning snacks to avoid hypoglycemic episodes. Extra food needs to be taken in association with unusual exercise. Insulin-dependent diabetics need to carry sugar cubes or hard candy at all times in case hypoglycemia occurs. If a meal is unavoidably delayed, patients should be advised to take a few crackers or a glass of fruit juice or sweet (not calorie-free) carbonated beverage.[3]

If the physician or the physician's aides have to instruct diabetic patients, in addition to the *Exchange Lists for Meal Planning*, a second pamphlet is needed. This is *A Guide for Professionals: The Effective Application of Exchange Lists for Meal Planning.*[2]* This publication contains helpful discussions on the importance of diet therapy for diabetics, the exchange list and its recent revision, individualization of meal planning, special dietary needs, and the details of preparing the diet prescription.

In the new edition (1976) of the *Exchange Lists for Meal Planning*[1] foods relatively low in saturated fat are printed in bold face type on the

---

*Published by the ADA and available for $1.50 per copy.

exchange lists. To decrease serum cholesterol and the risk of coronary artery disease patients should be encouraged to restrict their choices exclusively to foods low in saturated fats. After patients acquire some proficiency in using the exchange lists those patients who can be convinced to do more for themselves would be well-advised to modify the nature of the foods selected to conform with the recommendations in *The Alternative Diet Book.*[24]

Sugar

The ADA continues to recommend restriction of oligosaccharides.[1] Patients with diabetes mellitus are less able than normal individuals to handle a large load of easily assimilable carbohydrates. In the United States about 20% of the total caloric intake and about half of the carbohydrates we consume are in the form of oligosaccharides.[58] Our major dietary oligosaccharide is sucrose (table sugar) with smaller amounts of lactose (in milk and its products) while glucose, fructose and maltose (mainly in fruits) each account for about 1% of caloric intake.[58] The high content of oligosaccharides in many processed foods is often not apparent. For example, carbohydrates, mainly oligosaccharides, form one quarter of the weight of ketchup.[59] While overindulgence is not sensible, it is also not reasonable to regard sucrose and other oligosaccharides as poison for the diabetic. The combined weight of glucose and sucrose in a single apple is equal to the weight of one to two teaspoons of sucrose. A banana contains 3 to 4 teaspoons of sucrose and about one teaspoon of glucose.[60]

When glucose, sucrose, or starch are given as meals, the increase in blood sugar concentration is less than when they are given as liquids, suggesting that drinks sweetened with large amounts of sugar should be avoided.[61] A very interesting observation on the advantages of eating natural in contrast to processed foods has been made in regard to apples. Satiety is considerably greater when apples are eaten instead of isocaloric amounts of apple juice.[62] The chemical difference between the edible portion of an apple and its juice is the 3.1% of the weight of the apple that is fiber and unavailable for digestion.[62] As Mendeloff points out, the idea that something should be eaten (fiber) in addition to essential nutrients to assure optimal health is new.[32]

A number of studies have failed to reveal a substantial difference in blood sugar curves when equal amounts of carbohydrate are given as glucose (a monosaccharide), maltose (a disaccharide composed of glucose) or starch (a polysaccharide composed of glucose).[58,63,64] However, other observers have found increased blood sugar levels with ingestion of oligosaccharides in contrast to polysaccharides.[58,61] Furthermore, there are good arguments for reducing a high intake of sucrose, our major dietary oligosaccharide, without claiming that it has any marked direct adverse effect on diabetes. Sucrose contributes to the development of dental caries, and contains no vitamins, minerals, essential fatty or amino acids, or indigestible residue. Sucrose provides only taste and calories, supplements which overnourished Americans do not need. In addition, sucrose displaces from the diet potentially valuable nutrients and indigestible residues.[31]

Dietetic Foods

Patients should be cautioned about foods labeled "diet," "dietetic," and "diabetic." At the time this chapter was prepared these terms have no agreed-upon meaning. Patients tend to consume such foods without regard to their caloric content which is usually substantial and hardly different from the food product lacking the special label.[65] With the exception of canned fruit without added sugar, these "dietetic" products have little value for diabetics.

Excellent reviews have been published on the use of selected monosaccharides and disaccharides and their alcohols as sweeteners for patients with impaired glucose tolerance.[58,65] In brief, special diabetic foods and special sweeteners are not necessary to achieve recognized dietary objectives that could be more conveniently and less expensively met by informed selection of commonly available food items.[65] One well-designed study failed to show that the use of sweeteners increased success in adhering to a diabetic diet.[66]

Eating on Sick Days

On days that patients are ill, insulin requirements are likely to rise. This is attributable both to physical inactivity and the stress of the illness. If insulin-dependent patients do not eat their meals, outpatient management can become difficult. If the patient will not eat ordinary foods, sweet carbonated drinks (emphasize, not calorie-free) may be acceptable. If this is all the patient can consume, an attempt should be made to drink about 50 gm of carbohydrate for each meal as a substitute. The average sweet carbonated beverage contains about 100 calories or 25 gm of carbohydrate per 8 oz.[59] Clear soups can be used to replenish sodium and potassium losses. If the patient with insulin-dependent diabetes is vomiting and cannot keep down carbonated beverages, the patient should be admitted to the hospital. In the hospital the patient can be given intravenous electrolytes and glucose, 50 to 75 gm (500 to 750 ml of 10% dextrose in water) three times a day in a pattern spread out over the waking hours to make up for uneaten carbohydrate.

Alcohol

In small amounts alcohol is not hazardous for the insulin-dependent diabetic. Alcohol does contain 7 cal per gram and in food exchanges is best included with fats. One and a half oz of 100 proof whiskey contains 120 cal (one fat exchange contains 45 calories), 3½ oz of dry wine contains about 85 cal and 12 oz of beer contains about 150 cal.[54] Some patients taking oral hypoglycemic agents, especially chlorpropamide, may have reactions similar to those seen in patients taking disulfiram after ingesting small amounts of alcohol.[67]

Alcohol should never be consumed in excess. In large amounts it is a particular hazard to the diabetic. It provides the diabetic with calories that are usually not needed and may displace foods with greater nutritive value from the diet. It may depress cerebral function to the point where the diabetic is unable to take care of himself and observers will have difficulty distinguishing between alcohol intoxication and symptoms attributable to hypoglycemia or hyperglycemia. In large amounts alcohol impairs gluconeogenesis, may cause hypoglycemic reactions, and increases serum triglycerides. Finally, when consumed in large amounts over prolonged periods of time, it may add more chronic diseases to the burden of the diabetic.

Pregnancy

Good control of diabetes in pregnant mothers has an important influence on the health of the mother and the newborn. Management of this problem should probably be handled by a specialist. Excellent reviews are available detailing proper management techniques.[68]

Recent Advances

Since preparation of this chapter, there have been major advances in our knowledge of diabetes mellitus management. There is increasingly convincing evidence that many of the complications of diabetes mellitus in humans are attributable to hyperglycemia[69]. Furthermore, it is now possible in insulin-dependent patients to achieve near-euglycemia with a stable pattern of food and exercise and the use of either multiple daily injections of insulin or an insulin pump.[70]. The possibility of preventing and reversing[71] some of the complications of diabetes mellitus in insulin-dependent patients should revive the interest of professional personnel and patients in dietary management.

REFERENCES

1. *Exchange Lists for Meal Planning.* New York: American Diabetes Association, 1976.

2. *A Guide for Professionals: The Effective Application of "Exchange Lists for Meal Planning."* New York: American Diabetes Association, 1977.

3. West, K.M. Diabetes mellitus. Edited by H.A. Schneider, C.E. Anderson, and D.B. Coursin. In *Nutritional Support of Medical Practice.* New York: Harper & Row, 1977.

4. West, K.M., and Kalbfleisch, J.M. Influence of nutritional factors on prevalence of diabetes. *Diabetes* 20:99–108, 1971.

5. Keys, A. Coronary heart disease in seven countries. *Circulation* 41(suppl 1):1–212, 1970.

6. Bray, G.A. *The Obese Patient.* Philadelphia: W.B. Saunders, 1976.

7. New weight standards for men and women. *Stat Bull Metropol Life Ins Co.* 40:1–4, 1959.

8. Olefsky, J., Reaven, G.M., and Farquhar, J.W. Effects of weight reduction on obesity. *J Clin Invest.* 53:64–76, 1974.

9. Wilmore, J.H., Brown, C.H., and Davis, J.A. Body physique and composition of the female distance runner. *Ann NY Acad Sci.* 301:764–776, 1977.

10. Behnke, A.R., and Wilmore, J.H. *Evaluation and Regulation of Body Build and Composition.* Englewood Cliffs: Prentice-Hall, 1974.

11. Jackson, A.S., and Pollock, M.L. Generalized equations for predicting body density of men. *Br J Nutr.* 40:497–504, 1978.

12. Berger, M., Muller, W.A., and Renold, A.E. Relationship of obesity to diabetes: some facts, many questions. Edited by H.M. Katzen and R.J. Mahler. In *Diabetes, Obesity and Vascular Disease,* Part 1. New York: John Wiley & Sons, 1978.

13. Stanik, S., and Marcus, R. Insulin deficiency in obese patients with severe diabetes improves after weight loss. *Clin Res.* 27:51A, 1979.

14. University Group Diabetes Program. A study of the effects of hypoglycemic agents on vascular complications in patients with adult onset diabetes. *Diabetes* 19:747–830, 1970.

15. Audit confirms conclusions of UGDP study on oral diabetic drugs. *FDA Bull.* 8:34–36, 1978–79.

16. Effects of hypoglycemic agents on vascular complications in patients with adult onset diabetes. VII. Mortality and selected nonfatal events with insulin treatment. *JAMA.* 240:37–42, 1977.

17. University Group Diabetes Program. A study of the effects of hypoglycemic agents on vascular complications in patients with adult onset diabetes. VI. Supplementary report on nonfatal events in patients treated with tolbutamide. *Diabetes* 25:1129–1153, 1976.

18. Goldberg, R.B., Bersohn, I., Joffe, B.I. et al. Hyperlipidemia, obesity and drug misuse in a diabetic clinic. *S Afr Med J.* 48:277–280, 1974.

19. West, K.M. Diet therapy of diabetes: an analysis of failure. *Ann Intern Med.* 79:425–434, 1973.

20. Hadden, D.R., Montgomery, D.A.D., Shelly, R.J. et al. Maturity onset diabetes mellitus: response to intensive dietary management. *Br Med J.* 3:276–278, 1975.

21. Kempner, W., Newberg, B.C., Peschel, R.L. et al. Treatment of massive obesity with rice/reduction diet program. *Arch Intern Med.* 135:1575–1584, 1975.

22. Davidson, J.K. Controlling diabetes mellitus with diet therapy. *Postgrad Med.* 59:114–122, 1976.

23. Doar, J.W.H., Thompson, M.E., Wilde, C.E. et al. Influence of treatment with diet on oral glucose-tolerance test and plasma sugar and insulin levels in patients with maturity-onset diabetes mellitus. *Lancet* 1:1263–1266, 1975.

24. Connor, W.E., Connor, S.L., Fry, M.M. et al. *The Alternative Diet Book.* Iowa City: University of Iowa Press, 1978.

25. Sohar, E., and Sneh, E.D. Follow up of obese patients: 14 years after a successful reducing diet. *Am J Clin Nutr.* 26:845–848, 1973.

26. Johnson, D., and Drenick, E.J. Therapeutic fasting in morbid obesity. *Arch Intern Med.* 137:1381–1382, 1977.

27. Kiehm, T.G., Anderson, J.W., and Ward, K. Beneficial effects of a high carbohydrate, high fiber diet on hyperglycemic diabetic men. *Am J Clin Nutr.* 29:895–899, 1976.

28. Barndt, R., Blankenhorn, D.H., Crawford, D.W. et al. Regression and progression of early femoral atherosclerosis in treated hyperlipoproteinemic patients. *Ann Internal Med.* 86:139–146, 1977.

29. Kuo, P.T., Hayase, K., Kostis, J.B. et al. Use of combined diet and colestipol in long-term (7–7½ years) treatment of patients with Type II hyperlipoproteinemia. *Circulation* 59:199–211, 1979.

30. Wood, F.C., Jr., and Bierman, E.L. New concepts in diabetic dietetics. *Nutr Today* 7:4–11, 1972.

31. Nugent, C.A., and Van Haldren, L.L. Diet and coronary heart disease. *Family and Community Medicine* 1:53–68, 1979.

32. Mendeloff, A. Dietary fiber and human health. *N Engl J Med.* 297:811–814, 1977.

33. Anderson, J.W., Wen-Ju, L., and Ward, K. Composition of foods commonly used in diets for persons with diabetes. *Diabetes Care* 1:293–302, 1978.

34. Jenkins, D.J.A., Goff, D.V., Leeds, A.R. et al. Unabsorbable carbohydrates and diabetes: decreased postprandial hyperglycemia. *Lancet* 2:172–174, 1976.

35. Jenkins, D.J.A., Wolever, T.M.S., Hockday, T.D.R. et al. Treatment of diabetes with guar gum. *Lancet* 2:779–780, 1977.

36. Jenkins, D.J.A., Leeds, A.R., Gassul, H.A. et al. Decrease in postprandial insulin and glucose concentrations by guar and pectin. *Ann Intern Med.* 86:20–23, 1977.

37. Miranda, P.M., and Horwitz, D.L. The effects of dietary fiber content on plasma glucose levels in diabetics. *Diabetes* 26(suppl 1):356, 1977.

38. Mounier, L., Pham, T.C., Aguirre, L. et al. Influence of indigestible fibers on glucose tolerance. *Diabetes Care* 1:83–88, 1978.

39. Horwitz, D.L., and Slowie, L. Raw diet in diabetes mellitus. *Ann Intern Med.* 82:853–854, 1975.

40. Douglass, J.M. Raw diet and insulin requirements. *Ann Intern Med.* 82:61–62, 1975.

41. Hockaday, T.D.R., Hockaday, J.M., Mann, J.I. et al. Prospective comparison of modified-fat-high-carbohydrate with standard low-carbohydrate advice in the treatment of diabetes: one year follow-up study. *Br J Nutr.* 39:357–362, 1978.

42. Kannel, W.B., and McGee, D.L. Diabetes and cardiovascular risk factors: the Framingham Study. *Circulation* 59:8–13, 1979.

43. Turpeinen, O. Effect of cholesterol-lowering diet on mortality from coronary heart disease and other causes. *Circulation* 59:1–7, 1979.

44. Jarrett, R.J., Keen, H., Fuller, J.H. et al. Treatment of borderline diabetes: controlled trial using carbohydrate restriction and phenformin. *Br Med J.* 2:861–865, 1977.

45. Stone, D.B., and Connor, W.E. The prolonged effects of a low cholesterol, high carbohydrate diet upon the serum lipids in diabetic patients. *Diabetes* 12:127–132, 1963.

46. Albrink, M.J., Davidson, P.C., and Newman, T. Lipid-lowering effect of a very high carbohydrate high fiber diet. *Diabetes* 25:324, 1976.

47. Anderson, J.W., and Ward, K. Long-term effects of high carbohydrate, high fiber diets on glucose and lipid metabolism: a preliminary report on patients with diabetes. *Diabetes Care* 1:77–82, 1978.

48. Dahl, L.K. Salt and hypertension. *Am J Clin Nutr.* 25:231–244, 1972.

49. Freis, E.D. Salt, volume and the prevention of hypertension. *Circulation* 53:589–595, 1976.

50. Nugent, C.A. Salt and essential hypertension. *Ariz Med.* 34:29–32, 1977.

51. Hunt, J.C. Management and treatment of essential hypertension. Edited by J. Genest, E. Koiw, and O. Kuchel. In *Hypertension.* New York: McGraw-Hill, 1977.

52. Parys, J., Joossens, J.V., Van der Linden, L. et al. Moderate sodium restriction and diuretics in the treatment of hypertension. *Am Heart J.* 85:22–34, 1973.

53. Select Committee on Nutrition and Human Needs, United States Senate. *Dietary Goals for the United States.* Stock #052-070-03913-2, Washington, DC: US Government Printing Office, 1977.

54. Skylar, J.S. Nutritional management of diabetes mellitus. Edited by H.M. Katzen, and R.J. Mahler. In *Diabetes, Obesity and Vascular Disease,* Part 2. New York: John Wiley & Sons, 1978.

55. Raskin, P. Diabetic microangiopathy revisited. Medical Grand Rounds, Parkland Memorial Hospital. 20 Jan 1977.

56. Blackburn, H. Progress in the epidemiology and prevention of coronary heart disease. *Prog Cardiol.* 3:1–36, 1974.

57. Ahrens, E., Jr. The management of hyperlipidemia: whether, rather than how. *Ann Intern Med.* 85:87–93, 1976.

58. Brunzell, J.D. Use of fructose, xylitol, or sorbitol as a sweetner in diabetes mellitus. *Diabetes Care* 1:223–230, 1978.

59. Adams, C.F. *Nutritive value of American food in common units.* Agriculture Handbook 456. Washington, DC, US Government Printing Office, 1975.

60. Hardinger, M.G., Swarner, J.B., and Crooks, H. Carbohydrates in foods. *J Am Diet Assoc.* 46:197–204, 1965.

61. Crapo, P.A., Reaven, G., and Olefsky, J. Plasma glucose and insulin responses to orally administrated simple and complex carbohydrates. *Diabetes* 25:741–747, 1976.

62. Haber, G., Heaton, K.W., Murphy, D. et al. Depletion and disruption of

dietary fiber: effects on satiety, plasma glucose and serum insulin. *Lancet* 2:679–682, 1977.

63. Lenner, R.A. Studies of glycemia and glycosuria in diabetics after breakfast meals of different compositions. *Am J Clin Nutr.* 29:716–725, 1976.

64. Lutjins, A., Verleur, H., and Plooij, M. Glucose and insulin levels on loading with different carbohydrates. *Clin Chim Acta.* 62:239–243, 1975.

65. Talbot, J.M., and Fisher, K.D. The need for special foods and sugar substitutes by individuals with diabetes mellitus. *Diabetes Care* 1:231–240, 1978.

66. Farkas, C.A., and Forbes, C.E. Do non-caloric sweeteners aid patients with diabetes to adhere to their diets? *J Am Diet Assoc.* 46:482–484, 1965.

67. Leslie, R.D.G., and Pyke, D.A. Chlorpropamide-alcohol flushing: a dominantly inherited trait associated with diabetes. *Br Med J.* 2:1519–1521, 1978.

68. Franz, M. Nutritional management of diabetes and pregnancy. *Diabetes Care* 1:264–270, 1978.

69. Unger, R.H. The management of Type 1 diabetes mellitus in the 1980's. Medical Grand Rounds, Parkland Memorial Hospital. 24 July, 1980.

70. Rizza, R.A., Gerich, J.E., Haymond, M.W. et al. Control of blood sugar in insulin-dependent diabetes: comparison of an artificial endocrine pancreas, continuous subcutaneous insulin infusion, and intensified conventional insulin therapy. *N Eng J Med.* 303:1313–1318, 1980.

71. Pietri, A., Ehle, A.L., and Raskin, P. Changes in nerve conduction velocity after six weeks off glucoregulation with portable insulin pumps. *Diabetes* 29:668–671, 1980.

4 Insulin Therapy

Rubin Bressler, MD

It has not yet been proved definitively that more precise control of the blood glucose in diabetics (closer simulation of physiologic control) affords protection against the complications of diabetes mellitus. However, recent evidence of its benefits have caused many investigators and practitioners to advocate a regimen that affords as much physiologic control of the blood glucose as is possible without producing wide glycemic fluctuations with periodic hypoglycemic and hyperglycemic episodes.[1-4] The value of control of blood glucose in preventing the development and slowing the progression of the complications of diabetes is covered in Chapter 7.

In response to an oral challenge of carbohydrate or a mixed meal, the normal person secretes sufficient insulin to promote utilization of the ingested glucose and/or amino acids for energy and anabolic requirements. Pancreatic insulin secretion is regulated partially by the quantitative nature of the challenge (levels of circulating glucose or amino acids) and is responsive in both time and quantity to the stimulus (Figure 4-1).[5,6]

The diabetic patient matches his food to his insulin intake, in contrast to the normal person who matches his insulin to his food intake. The patient with insulin-dependent diabetes mellitus receives a predetermined dose of insulin and must match his food intake to the resultant peaks of the injected insulin's activity. The diabetic's food intake (diet) must be matched in both time and amount to the insulin dosage and type. Currently available patterns of diet, activity, and exercise have resulted in an imperfect balance of food and insulin.[7-10]

Insulin is an anabolic-anticatabolic hormone. These dual effects of building body tissues and preventing their breakdown depend on the circulating levels of insulin.[5,6,11] During challenges of glucose and amino acids (meals) plasma levels of insulin are in the 30 to 150 μU/ml range. These higher levels promote the use of ingested nutrients for energy and for storage as glycogen, protein, and lipids. Anabolic levels of insulin stimulate glycolysis in a number of tissues and augment the uptake of glucose and amino acids by adipose tissue and muscle, where they are converted to glycogen, protein, and lipids. In the fasting state (between meals) insulin levels are in the 1 to 10 μU/ml range, which is sufficient to control catabolism. This insulin concentration decreases the rates of glycogenolysis, proteolysis, lipolysis, and gluconeogenesis.[5,6,11,12] Thus, basal concentrations of insulin control the rate of break down to tissue stores for energy needs in the fasting state. Lack of the anticatabolic actions of low levels of insulin results in a rapid breakdown of muscle and adipose tissue with severe weight loss and eventual development of diabetic ketoacidosis.

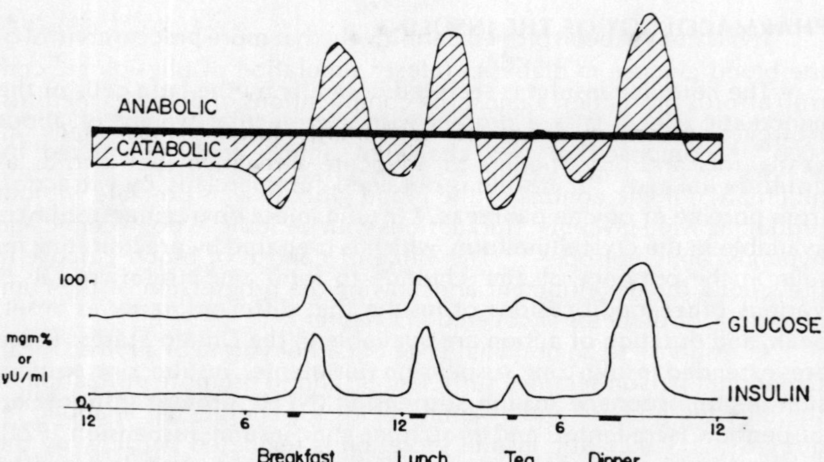

Figure 4-1 Blood glucose and insulin levels of a normal subject in response to meals. In a normal individual, each time a meal is eaten, the brisk rise in insulin facilitates peripheral storage of all three circulating fuels: glucose, amino acids, and fatty acids.

GOALS OF INSULIN THERAPY

The viewpoint of this chapter is that the aim of insulin therapy for patients with insulin-dependent diabetes mellitus is normoglycemia with minimal pathophysiologic abnormalities.[7,9,10,13] The following considerations must be held in mind:

1. The patient should be able to carry out normal activities, including gainful employment and/or routine household duties and family activities.

2. The patient should be free of episodes of diabetic ketoacidosis or hypoglycemic reactions.

3. Body weight should be maintained at a low-normal level for sex, age, height, and body build.

4. The patient should have little or no glucosuria and should have blood glucose levels, fasting, and postprandial, as near the normal range as feasible.

5. He should maintain a healthy mental attitude, neither totally dependent upon the care of others, nor denying the illness or using it as a defense against problems.

The attainment of optimum blood glucose control requires a thorough understanding by the physician of the use of diet, the properties of the various insulin preparations, and patient factors that influence the interaction of the first two factors. In addition, the complications of insulin therapy must be recognized and anticipated.

In this chapter, the clinical pharmacology of insulin and the strategy of insulin use will be discussed.[7,9,10,14]

PHARMACOLOGY OF THE INSULINS

The hormone insulin is secreted normally by the beta cells of the pancreatic islet.[11] It is a protein with a molecular weight of about 6000[15,16] composed of two chains of amino acids connected by disulfide linkages.[15-18] Insulin is obtained commercially by extraction from porcine or bovine pancreas.[19] Insulin injection (regular insulin) is available in the crystalline form, which is prepared by precipitating insulin in the presence of zinc chloride to form zinc-insulin crystals.[20] Various other modifications of insulin that differ primarily in onset, peak, and duration of action are available in the United States. These are: extended insulin zinc suspension (ultralente), insulin zinc suspension (lente), isophane insulin suspension (NPH), prompt insulin zinc suspension (semilente), and protamine zinc-insulin suspension (PZI). Sulfated insulin, which is composed of zinc-insulin crystals modified with concentrated sulfuric acid, is an investigational insulin modification in the United States, but is commercially available in Canada.[21]

54

Recent advances in chromatographic techniques have resulted in an improved manufacturing process and insulin preparations of increased purity.[19,22,23] All commercially available insulin preparations are now of "single-peak" purity and contain 99% insulin and insulin-like materials (eg, desamido insulin, arginine insulin, esterified insulin) and 1% or less pro–insulin-like materials, insulin aggregates, and non-insulin.[22-24] A purer form, "single component" or "monocomponent" insulin, which contains more than 99% pure insulin,[22-24] is now also available.

Uniformity of insulin potency was achieved with the availability of crystalline insulin. The earlier standards were based on the hypoglycemic effect of insulin on rabbits. Today the standard used is based on an absolute dry weight of highly purified crystalline zinc-insulin prepared from a composite sample. The present standard contains 24 units per milligram. The USP standard and the international standard are the same.

The basic bioassay for the assignment of potency to insulin products is the USP rabbit assay. This official test follows a "twin crossover" design; it has been the biologic test of choice and has received the greatest use in this country since its introduction in the early 1920s. It measures the decrease in blood glucose concentration produced by graded doses of insulin.[7,10]

During the production of bulk quantities of zinc-insulin crystals an immunoassay procedure is used to monitor the process. The assay is relatively simple, specific, rapid, and accurate.[25,26]

INSULIN PREPARATIONS

The most widely used available insulin preparations differ in their speed of onset of hypoglycemic action, their peak of hypoglycemic activity, and the duration of action following subcutaneous administration. These data are shown in Table 4-1.[7,9,10] These data were obtained in part from studies on stable, well-controlled diabetic patients with relatively low daily insulin requirements. After the patients were stabilized on a metabolic ward, insulin therapy was interrupted, and the blood sugar was permitted to become elevated. When the blood sugar value rose to more than 200 mg/100 ml, a single large dose (usually about 80 units) was given; the blood sugar curve was then followed every four hours—one-sixth of the total diet being given after each blood sample drawn. Such studies were usually pursued for more than 36 hours; therefore, the blood sugar levels on which they are based are not strictly analogous to those encountered in clinical practice in patients on long-term insulin therapy receiving three or four feedings

Table 4-1
Insulin Preparations Used in the United States

Type of Insulin	Appearance	Onset of Action (hr)	Action	Peak Activity (hr)	Duration (hr)	Zinc Content (mg/100 units)	pH Buffer	Protein Type	Protein mg/100 units
Regular crystalline	Clear	(½–1)	Rapid	2–4	5–7	0.01–0.04	None 7.2	None	—
NPH	Turbid	(1–2)	Intermediate	6–12	24–28	0.01–0.04	Phosphate 7.2	Protamine	0.4
Protamine zinc	Turbid	(4–8)	Prolonged	14–24	36+	0.15–0.25	Phosphate 7.2	Protamine	1–1.5
Semilente	Turbid	(½–1)	Rapid	2–4	12–16	0.14–0.25	Acetate 7.2	None	—
Lente	Turbid	(1–4)	Intermediate	6–12	24–28	0.14–0.25	Acetate 7.2	None	—
Ultralente	Turbid	(4–8)	Prolonged	18–24	36+	0.14–0.25	Acetate 7.2	None	—

daily. Nevertheless, these curves have provided a useful means of comparing the onset, peak, and duration of action of the various insulins available for clinical use.

Crystalline Zinc (Regular, CZI)

Insulin is an acidic protein with an isoelectric point (pH of minimal solubility) of 5.3. At physiologic pH of 7.4, it is highly soluble in body fluids and is rapidly absorbed from its injection site. Crystalline zinc-insulin (CZI) is a solution of insulin that contains zinc, required for the process of purification and crystallization. CZI, also called regular insulin, is ordinarily administered subcutaneously one-half to two hours before a meal so that its physiologic effects will parallel the absorption of glucose.[9,10,14]

Improved processing techniques have yielded a crystalline insulin of high purity that remains in solution at physiologic pH. This insulin is called neutral regular insulin. It has the same onset and duration of action as crystalline zinc-insulin but has a greater shelf-life.[27,28]

Protamine Zinc-Insulin (PZI)

The addition of a basic protein (protamine) to insulin results in the formation of large insoluble particles. Hagedorn and co-workers[29] produced a PZI that had poor solubility and was slowly absorbed. Subcutaneous injection of a suspension of the precipitate, whose pI (pH of least solubility) is around pH 7.3, makes available a deposit from which insulin is slowly dissolved by the body fluids. The use of zinc in the preparation of the precipitate yielded a more uniform suspension. PZI is prepared by mixing insulin, protamine, and zinc in a buffered solution.

In the 1930s, multiple doses of CZI were relied on for control of hyperglycemia in insulin-dependent diabetics. When doses of CZI at midnight or 2 AM were omitted in juvenile diabetics, nocturnal hyperglycemia was associated with diabetic dwarfism. The introduction of PZI in 1936–1937, with its prolonged action, permitted control of nocturnal hyperglycemia. In conjunction with multiple doses of CZI in juvenile diabetics, normal growth and development was achieved. When PZI was given to adult diabetics who required insulin, many did well on a single daily injection.[7,14,29]

Estimates of the duration of action of protamine insulin preparations have varied with the methods employed for its measurement. It has been demonstrated that, in a patient receiving food at two-hour intervals, the greatest effect of a large dose of PZI develops from 14 to 20 hours after its administration. There is also evidence of duration of action well beyond a 24-hour period. In fasting patients, a single injection of PZI has maintained hypoglycemic levels for as long as 48 to 72 hours. As with the administration of all types of insulin, the larger the dose given, the more prolonged will be the effect.

PZI consists of a two-to-one ratio of protamine to insulin. This excess of protamine is an important consideration when other insulins such as CZI are mixed in the same syringe with PZI. Insulin mixtures will be discussed later in this chapter.

Neutral Protamine Hagedorn (NPH) Insulin

NPH insulin was developed as a consequence of clinical investigations of a large series of intermediate-acting insulin modifications and of mixtures of CZI and PZI given as a single daily dose. In the majority of cases, it was found that such mixtures (usually in the ratio of two of CZI to one part of PZI), administered once in the morning, would have the pharmacologic effect of doses of PZI supplemented by separate injections of CZI. This was true even when CZI alone was required once or twice a day for overall control of glycosuria and hyperglycemia.

Because of the possibility of errors in dosage and the relative inconvenience of extemporaneous mixtures, a preparation was sought that would be as stable as PZI yet incorporate the desirable time activity of a mixture. At the Hagedorn Laboratories in Copenhagen, it was discovered that careful control of the ratio of protamine and insulin made it possible to produce a crystalline entity that contained both insulin and the modifier. Isophane, the generic name applied to this insulin, was coined by Hagedorn and was based on the Greek words *iso* meaning equal and *phane* meaning appearance. The isophane point describes these conditions in which the amounts of protamine and insulin are in near stoichiometric proportions, so that the crystals being formed leave behind no excess of protamine or insulin. This is in contrast to PZI, which consists of about a two-to-one stoichiometric excess of protamine. The resulting product became known as NPH insulin. (NPH was a code designation used during the clinical trial; the "N" indicated a neutral pH, the "P" denoted the presence of protamine, and the "H" referred to Hagedorn, its discoverer.)[29]

NPH insulin was found to duplicate very closely the clinical effects and timing that seem most suitable for the greatest number of cases. Because of its more rapid onset of action after injection plus its moderate overlapping effect, NPH insulin incorporates some of the advantages of CZI and eliminates some of the disadvantages of PZI. The duration of effect of NPH insulin, although not as great as that of PZI, is sufficiently long to protect the patient from one day to the next (see Table 4-1).

Lente Insulins

In 1951 Hallas-Møller and co-workers[31] reported on the development of a retarded action insulin that did not depend on the presence of a modifying basic protein for its relative insolubility at physiologic pH. These investigators ascertained that when the zinc concentration of the buffer solutions was increased and the buffer changed from phosphate to acetate, the higher concentration of zinc would combine with insulin to yield a zinc-insulin complex that was insoluble at pH 7.4.

Two physical forms of the high-zinc insulin compound can be produced by adjustment of the pH, one crystalline and one either amorphous or microcrystalline. The crystalline form is more insoluble and, therefore, long-acting. The microcrystalline form presents more surface area to the body fluids per amount of insulin used and is more quickly absorbed. The two physical preparations used are ultralente (large insulin crystals) and semilente (small insulin crystals). Their rapidity of onset of action is inversely proportional to their crystal size, whereas their durations of action are directly proportional to crystal size.[31,32] With the basic term lente to indicate slow action, the two preparations were designated ultralente for the very long-acting crystalline form, and semilente for the shorter-acting amorphous form (see Table 4-1).

Clinical evaluation disclosed that perhaps the most practical timing could be achieved by using a portion of each physical form in a mixture combining approximately 70% of the ultralente and 30% of the semilente form. This mixture, designated as lente insulin, has almost precisely the same characteristics as NPH insulin or the 2:1 mixture of CZI and PZI. These preparations are similar in clinical effectiveness, but lente insulin is free of any modifying protein. By the addition of ultralente or semilente, mixtures can be tailor-made to suit patients who may not be adequately controlled by lente alone.

Ultralente insulin has been found to be satisfactory when given in a single daily dose and its time course is similar to PZI. Semilente insulin is particularly useful in accelerating the action of lente insulin.[31,33]

SUMMARY OF INSULIN ACTION[7,9,10,14]

The proper use of insulin requires an awareness of the pharmaceutical composition and clinical properties (advantages and limitations) of the several insulin preparations shown in Table 4-1. Although certain patients derive benefit from fast-acting or long-acting insulin alone, the intermediate-acting insulins (NPH or lente) either alone or in combination with fast-acting insulin (CZI or semilente) constitute the treatment for the majority of diabetic patients. NPH and lente have similar pharmacologic effects but are based on different physical-chemical principles.

Unmodified insulin is an acidic protein with an isoelectric point of 5.3. At physiologic body pH of 7.4, it is very soluble in body fluids and is therefore rapidly absorbed from subcutaneous injection sites. Unmodified insulin has a rapid onset of action and short duration of activity.

The combination of the acidic protein, insulin, and a basic protein, protamine, results in an insulin-protamine complex with an isoelectric point of 7.2. Insulin is thus released from a depot that is very insoluble at body pH of 7.4. The complex slowly dissolves accounting for the extended action of protamine-insulin complexes (NPH, PZI).

In NPH insulin, the amounts of protamine and insulin are in near (1:1) stoichiometric proportion so that there is no excess of uncomplexed insulin or protamine. This is in contrast to PZI, which consists of a two-to-one ratio of protamine to insulin.

There are three preparations of lente insulin:

Ultralente	—	crystalline; slowly absorbed; long-acting. Equivalent to PZI.
Semilente	—	amorphous or microcrystalline; rapidly absorbed; short-acting. Equivalent to CZI (regular insulin).
Lente	—	70% ultralente plus 30% semilente. Equivalent to NPH.

INSULIN COMBINATIONS

In order to gain a more uniform insulin coverage in response to the periodic and episodic challenges of daily food intake, physicians have increasingly resorted to the use of insulin combinations. These mixtures of insulin have afforded more flexibility per injection, because long-acting, intermediate-acting, and short-acting insulins may be adjusted to the patient's diet and activity schedule. Some important constraints regarding insulin mixtures must be considered before undertaking this type of therapy.

Neutral and acidified regular insulin may be added to NPH insulin in any ratio desired, but the mixing should be done immediately prior to use in order to prevent physical changes that may lead to unpredictable time activities of the combination.[9,27,28,34,35]

Acidified regular insulin may be mixed with zinc-insulin suspensions (lente triad, semilente, lente, ultralente) but, in order to preserve the duration of action of each, the ratio cannot exceed 1:1.[9,34,35] Neutral regular insulin may be mixed with insulin-zinc suspension (lente triad) in any proportion.[27,28,34]

Both neutral regular and acidified regular insulins may be mixed with PZI, but the ratio must not be less than 1:1, or the added insulin will be bound by the excess protamine present in the PZI. This will result in a mixture with the same duration of action as PZI alone.[9,35] Mixtures of regular insulin and PZI may be prepared at any time.

A mixture of two parts of regular insulin and one part of PZI has a duration of action similar to that of NPH alone.[7,9,35] A mixture of regular insulin and PZI in proportions greater than 2:1 approximates the duration of a mixture of regular insulin and NPH.[14,35]

Mixtures of acidified regular insulin with NPH, the lente triad, or PZI must be used immediately after mixing.[35,36] Mixtures of neutral regular insulin with NPH or the lente triad are stable for two to three months.[36]

Semilente, ultralente, and lente may be combined in any ratio desired, and their combination differs from the regular-lente or regular-NPH mixture in that it can be made at any time. Therefore, the physician may prepare the mixtures during patient visits for those who require a combination of the lente triad but who are incapable of preparing it themselves.[9]

INSULIN BIOAVAILABILITY AND PHARMACOKINETICS

Because antibodies to exogenous insulin complicate its measurement in the serum, and because of the wide spontaneous fluctuations of the blood glucose in diabetics, several investigators have evaluated the pharmacokinetics of insulin in normal humans. These studies have yielded information that has relevance to diabetic patients being treated with insulin.[28,37-41]

The fraction of insulin dose absorbed by normal subjects is shown in Table 4-2. The bioavailability of insulin is estimated by dividing the area under the serum concentration curve over time following the subcutaneous administration by that following the intravenous administration of the same dose for the same time period.[42] Thus, for subcutaneous doses of insulin in normal fasting subjects, only on the order of 50% of the exogenously administered hormone is available. This fractional absorption of insulin from injection sites could be less in

Table 4-2
Effect of Route of Administration on the Bioavailability of Regular Insulin*

Subject	Intravenous Area	Subcutaneous (26 gauge ½″ needle)		Intramuscular (22 gauge 1″ needle)		Intramuscular (21 gauge 1½″ needle)	
		Area	% Bioavailable	Area	% Bioavailable	Area	% Bioavailable
GUI.	395	201	51	201	51	193	51
BRO.	172	197	51	116	85	204	55
Katz.	418	197	63	188	45	228	55
Mow.	459	212	46	233	51	224	55
Mean	411	218	53	235	58	220	54

*Studies were performed in normal, fasting subjects who received 0.15 units/kg by the means indicated. All area measurements are the 0 to 10 hour area under the insulin curve determined by trapezoidal rule. "Single component" pork regular insulin was used in all studies.[38]

diabetic patients with insulin antibodies. However, other pharmacokinetic factors such as local destruction of insulin at the injection site could be responsible for the 50% insulin bioavailability.[9,10,38]

It has also been found that the fractional absorption of insulins of intermediate-duration administered subcutaneously is even less than 50%. Table 4-2 also shows the bioavailability of NPH to be 27% and lente 38%.[38] Table 4-3 shows that the bioavailability of mixtures of short-acting and intermediate-acting insulins is midway between the two types of insulin.[38]

Table 4-3
Insulin Bioavailability in Eight Subjects

Treatment (Type SC Insulin)	Fractional Absorption
Neutral Regular (NR)	0.483
NR + Lente 3:1	0.438
NR + Lente 2:1	0.452
NR + Lente 1:1	0.442
NR + Lente 1:2	0.547
NR + Lente 1:3	0.347
Lente	0.381
NR + NPH 3:1	0.408
NR + NPH 2:1	0.303
NR + NPH 1:1	0.423
NR + NPH 1:2	0.274
NR + NPH 1:3	0.184
NPH	0.271

Source: Galloway, J.A., Unpublished data.

The low, apparent bioavailability of subcutaneously administered insulin may be related to enzymatic destruction at the injection site, or may be artifactual and related to non-linearity in either the absorption, distribution, or elimination kinetics of insulin.[9,38]

Absorption rates of subcutaneously administered insulin vary with the size of injection and the volume and concentration of the insulin.[9,28,39,43,44] Absorption from the arm is more rapid than absorption from the thigh.[9,39] With regular insulin larger injection volumes result in more rapid absorption rates whereas with NPH the reverse occurs.[7,9] Absorption may be decreased or delayed by the presence of insulin-binding antibodies that develop in all patients after two to three months of insulin treatment.[40,45]

Insulin is rapidly distributed throughout extracellular fluids.[46] The hormone has a plasma half-life of approximately 6.5 to 15 minutes in normal subjects; however, the half-life may be prolonged for up to 13 hours in diabetic patients.[46-48]

Insulin is rapidly metabolized primarily in the liver by the enzyme, glutathione insulin transhydrogenase, and to a lesser extent in the kidneys and muscle tissue.[49-51] Insulin is filtered at the glomerulus and almost completely (98%) reabsorbed in the proximal renal tubules.[51-54] About 40% of this reabsorbed insulin is returned to venous blood and 60% is metabolized in the cells lining the proximal convoluted tubules.[51] In normal patients, only a small quantity (less than 2%) of an insulin dose is excreted in the urine.[51,52,54]

Exercise in the insulin-dependent diabetic patient has long been known to augment the hypoglycemic effect of subcutaneous insulin.[55] Recent studies have shown that exercise increases the affinity of insulin for its tissue receptor sites.[56] This observation is consonant with the potentiating effect of exercise on insulin action.[57,58] However, a body of information also supports the effect of exercise in increasing the mobilization of subcutaneously administered insulin from injection sites.[59] The effects of leg exercise on the absorption of ^{125}I-labeled insulin showed that a 135% increase of insulin mobilization occurred in the first 10 minutes of exercise, but remained 50% above resting absorption levels after 60 minutes.[59] This effect of exercise has obvious clinical implications. However, since most athletic activity and work efforts use a variety of muscles (leg, arm, abdominal), injecting insulin in nonexercised areas is difficult. It is more reasonable to either increase the patient's carbohydrate intake or decrease his dose of insulin when exercise is planned.

Differences in bioavailability of subcutaneously administered insulin are usually of no concern where control of blood glucose is a goal of therapy because insulin dose in a patient is a composite of variables (weight, diet, activity) and is dealt with individually. However, there are some patients requiring larger doses of insulin, whose insulin dose appears to be a function of poor bioavailability. Six insulin-dependent diabetic patients were studied who were maintained in states of poor blood glucose control on large doses (120 to 3000 units/day) of subcutaneous insulin.[60] The subjects did not have sufficient antibody titers to account for the large insulin requirement. The patients were brought into states of adequate glucose homeostasis with much smaller doses of intravenous insulin (50 to 60 units/day). It is probable that these patients represent extremes of poor subcutaneous bioavailability of insulin. The larger insulin doses were not a function of the usual causes of insulin resistance such as antibodies, obesity, or infection.

CLINICAL PHARMACOLOGY OF THE INSULINS

A patient's response to insulin administration is subject to a variety of physiologic (eg, counter-insulin hormones, insulin antibodies, insulin-receptor status, infections), pharmacologic (absorption, distribution, metabolism), and emotional inputs.

Time of Onset and Duration of CZI and Semilente Insulins[7,9,14]

CZI is generally thought of as a short-acting insulin with peak effect in two to four hours and virtual disappearance of effect within six to eight hours after a single subcutaneous injection. In normal man and in rabbits, these time activity values are valid. However, as a result of the formation of antibodies to insulin and other factors present in diabetics, the onset of action is slower and the duration longer than in normal subjects (Figure 4-2). This retarded and prolonged effect of CZI is a fairly frequent response to CZI in patients with insulin-dependent diabetes mellitus of two years' or more duration. The duration of action of CZI also correlates with the magnitude of the dose, with larger doses having a more prolonged hypoglycemic effect. For the same reasons, although semilente insulin has been thought to act only slightly longer than CZI, some diabetic patients being treated with this short-acting insulin occasionally have hypoglycemic episodes much longer after the last insulin injection than one would expect.

Although an explanation for these observations could only be speculative at present, the clinical implications should enter into the

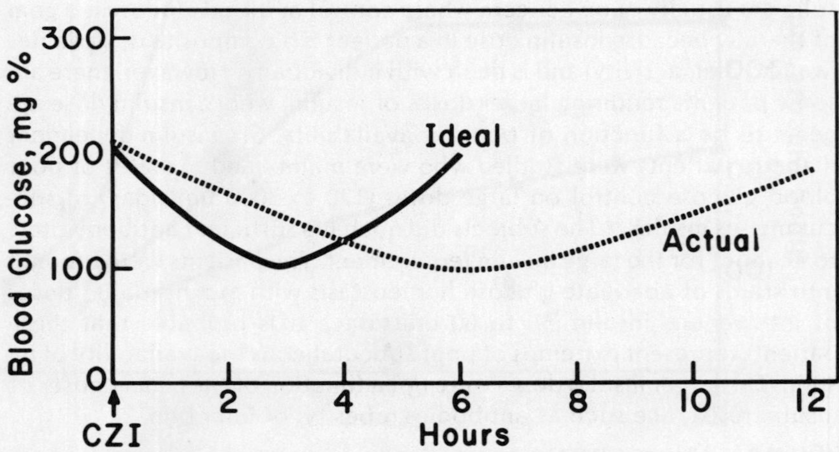

Figure 4-2   Duration of action of regular insulin (CZI).

use of CZI (or semilente) in day-to-day diabetic management.

1. The so-called "sliding scale" insulin management of the diabetic state is not a rational therapy. Because the maximum hypoglycemic effects of CZI may not be seen until from four to ten hours after a subcutaneous injection, it is not reasonable to give a second dose of CZI based on a urine (or blood) sugar assessment at a time prior to four hours after the last dose of CZI. An effective and safer approach is the use of CZI every six hours.

2. By using CZI as a major part of the morning dose of insulin, one can take advantage of its prolonged effect. In such a regimen, at least two daily doses of insulin are usually needed.

3. CZI should be given at least one to one and one-half hours before a meal, in order to allow adequate plasma concentrations of insulin to correspond to peak carbohydrate absorption.

The delayed onset of action of CZI is shown by the data of Figure 4-3. The figure shows the blood glucose response of three individual diabetic patients who received doses of regular insulin (CZI) at 8 AM. These patients had been on regular insulin on order for three days prior to the study. On the fourth day a single subcutaneous dose of regular insulin was administered. Breakfast was given, but lunch was withheld. The blood glucose was followed at hourly intervals following insulin administration (zero hour).

Patient 1 was given 40 units. His blood sugar level was unchanged

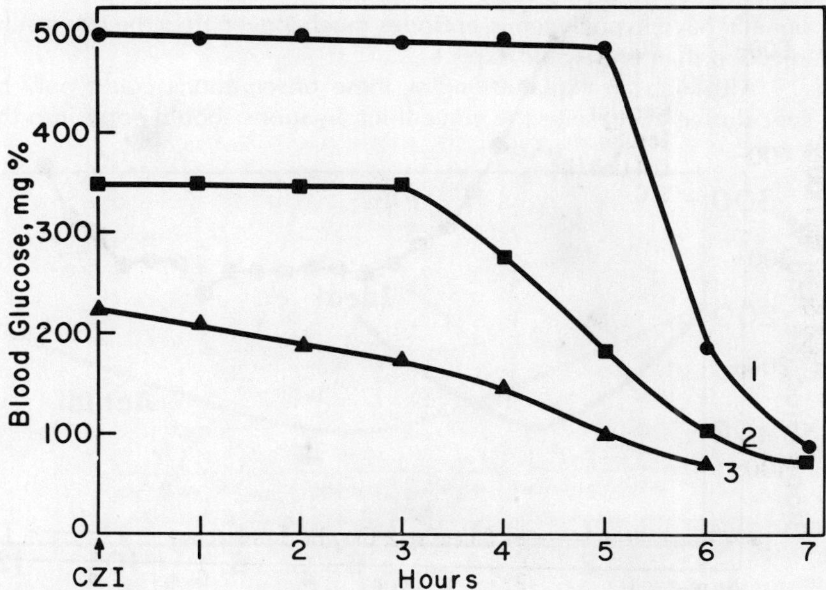

Figure 4-3 Delayed onset of action of CZI.

for the first five hours, after which time it fell, reaching its lowest value at seven hours.

Patient 2 received 28 units. His blood sugar began to fall at three hours, but did not reach its nadir until seven hours.

Patient 3 received 24 units. His blood sugar began a gradual decline almost immediately, but it did not reach its lowest value for six hours.[61,62]

More quantitative information about the duration of action of CZI in an insulin-dependent patient is illustrated in Figure 4-4. Glucose was infused intravenously at a constant rate, into patients who had received no insulin for at least 12 hours, and no long-acting insulin for two days or more. After a stable, high level of blood glucose was present, a single dose of regular insulin was given subcutaneously. The glucose infusion was continued. A typical response is shown in Figure 4-4.

The maximum lowering of blood sugar was not reached until about five hours after the insulin was given (in other patients this varied from 3½ to 9 hours). The blood sugar in this patient remained low for up to nine to ten hours. This prolonged effect of regular insulin was a fairly frequent response to regular insulin in patients with insulin-dependent diabetes mellitus of two years' or more duration. As men-

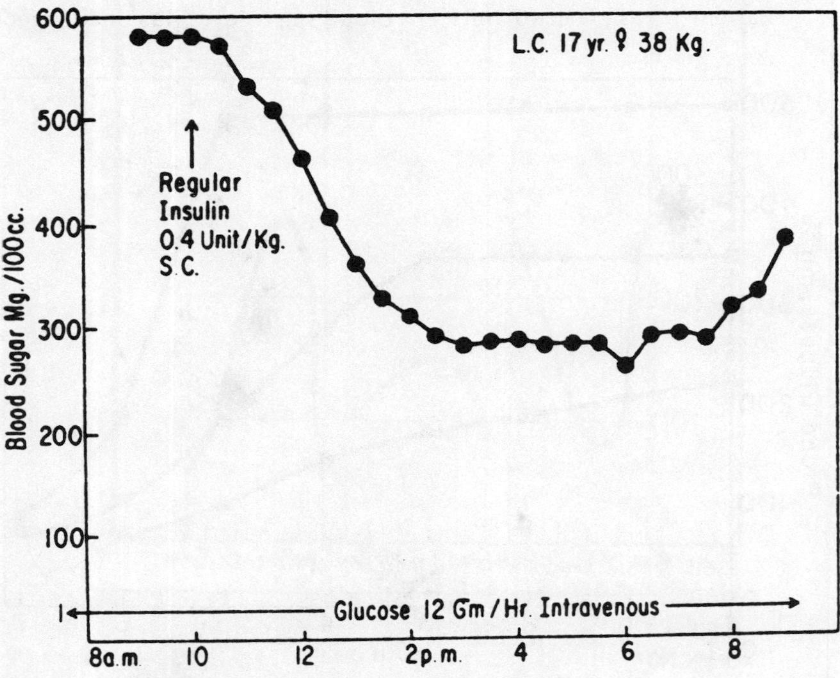

Figure 4-4 Prolonged duration of action of regular insulin.

tioned earlier, the duration of action of regular insulin also correlates with the magnitude of the dose, with larger doses having more prolonged hypoglycemic effects.[61]

Responses to NPH and Lente Insulins[7,9,14,31,32,62]

Whereas many insulin-dependent patients with diabetes mellitus can be well-controlled by means of a single daily dose of NPH or lente insulin, others cannot be so regulated and frequently present as problems of control. (Excellent control is defined here as normoglycemia: blood sugar level two hours after meals of 140 mg/100 ml, and the absence of glycosuria or hypoglycemia.)

In order to understand the pathogenesis of such problems, it is important to recognize that diabetic patients may differ in response to a single daily dose of intermediate-acting insulin (NPH or lente). These responses to a single daily injection of HPH (or lente) insulin have been characterized and are shown in Figure 4-5.

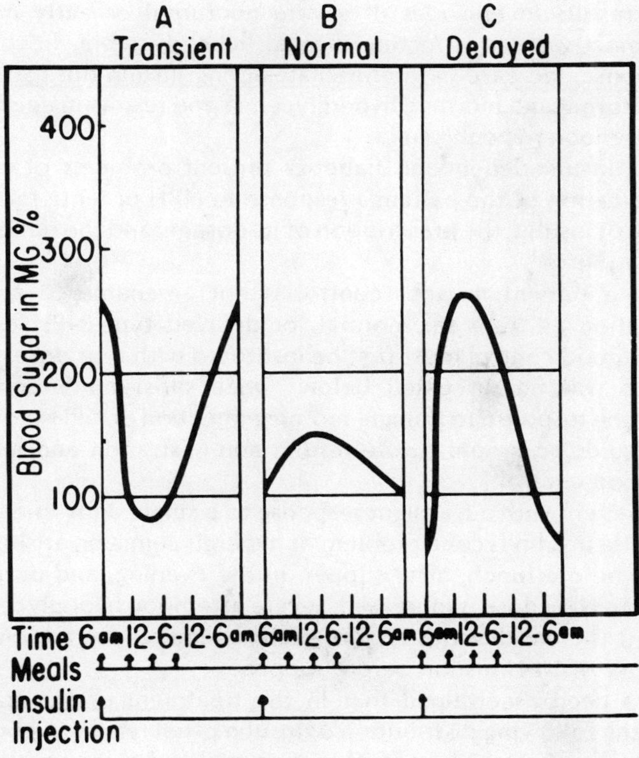

Figure 4-5 Responses to a single daily dose of NPH insulin.

The response of a patient who remains normoglycemic throughout the 24-hour period on diet and a single daily dose of NPH is designated as a B, or normal response. He develops a tendency toward hyperglycemia only in relation to food ingestion.

The response of a patient who is hyperglycemic during the day and normoglycemic to hypoglycemic at night is designated as a C, or delayed response. These patients have a delayed onset of action of the NPH dose and may be characterized by hypoglycemic reactions at night or in the early morning hours.

The response of a patient with fasting hyperglycemia, hyperglycemia during the morning and during the evening is designated as an A or transient response. These patients have periods of normoglycemia restricted to the afternoon, and, when their insulin doses are excessive, they experience hypoglycemic reactions at that period of the day.

Problems of control often arise when a patient who has been well-controlled by means of a single daily dose of intermediate-acting insulin at the onset of diabetes gradually loses the normal response and develops either a transient or a delayed response. Increase in intermediate-acting insulin dosage in the patient with a delayed response results in episodes of severe nocturnal or early morning hypoglycemia without affecting diurnal hyperglycemia. In the transient response, increase in intermediate-acting insulin dosage fails to affect nocturnal and morning hyperglycemia and results in episodes of severe afternoon hypoglycemia.

When insulin-dependent diabetics present problems of control, the classification of the patient's response to NPH or lente facilitates the choice of insulin, the prescription of its dosage, and the timing of its administration.

Since a patient in poor control is not amenable to accurate categorization as transient, normal, or delayed type NPH or lente responses, good control must first be instituted with four doses of CZI daily. This will be discussed below. Once satisfactory control is achieved, the response to a single morning injection of NPH serves as a valuable guide to proper future insulin administration and maintenance of good control.

The patient with a transient response to a single daily injection of NPH or lente insulin faces a problem of hyperglycemia on arising, after breakfast, before lunch, after supper, in the evening, and during the night. As the NPH dose is increased, severe afternoon hypoglycemia intervenes. It is clear that this type of patient requires the addition of a second dose of NPH insulin before supper.

It has been ascertained that in the treatment of the transient response the following distribution of insulin often results in good control: before breakfast, 2 parts CZI to 1 part NPH; before lunch, no insulin; and before supper, 1 part CZI to 1 part NPH. The quantitative distribution varies so that the combined morning insulin contributes about two thirds of the total daily dosage, and more CZI than NPH is used.

There also exists a group of patients who demonstrate a transient response to a single daily dose of NPH insulin (A response) but who are well-controlled without the use of CZI. These patients achieve excellent control on injections of NPH insulin before breakfast and before supper. This group may represent an early transition from the normal or B response.

Patients with a transient response to NPH or lente insulin may also be treated with mixtures of lente and ultralente in one daily injection. In this regimen, the prolonged action of ultralente serves to afford sufficient retarded insulin release to obviate the need for a second dose of lente or NPH before supper in spite of the transient nature of the response to the lente or NPH.

The patient with a long delay in response to NPH insulin faces a problem of nocturnal or early morning hypoglycemia and daytime hyperglycemia (C response). By increasing the morning dose of NPH insulin, these patients may experience severe nocturnal hypoglycemia.[7,9,13,14,62]

The addition of CZI before breakfast and before supper, if necessary, permits reduction of the NPH dose and abolishes nocturnal hypoglycemia and diurnal hyperglycemia. This use of NPH and CZI is perhaps one of the most effective procedures in insulin therapy and properly utilized obviates the need for other insulins. The use of two daily doses of intermediate- and short-acting insulins to offset the basal hyperglycemia of diabetes with its food-related spikes is depicted in Figure 4-3. In treatment of the delayed response, we have found that a 2:1 mixture of NPH to CZI given before breakfast often results in excellent control. Here, the total daily dose of NPH usually exceeds that of CZI, although it is sometimes necessary to use an additional dose of CZI before supper.

Patients with a delayed response to NPH or lente insulin may also be treated with mixtures of lente and semilente insulin in one daily injection. In this regimen, the more rapid onset of action of semilente affords an earlier insulin effect, which may be prolonged enough to cover the patient until the delayed onset of action of lente becomes manifest.

The described responses to a single dose of NPH or lente insulin have been found to be clearly separable. The patient's response has often been ascertained merely by noting the time of hypoglycemia as the morning NPH dose was raised in an attempt to achieve better control. The transient responder experiences hypoglycemia in the afternoon and the delayed responder at night. Many of our young patients have been transient or delayed responders.

The response to a single daily dose of NPH may change with time. Most newly discovered, insulin-dependent diabetics start off in good control with a single daily dose of NPH insulin. However, with time, the response to a single daily dose of NPH may become insufficient and the insulin dose is usually increased.[7,9,62]

INSULIN THERAPY FOLLOWING THE TREATMENT OF KETOACIDOSIS

The use of insulin in ketoacidosis is understood by most physicians. However, management immediately after the acute episode frequently leads to problems. One approach is to place these patients on CZI every six hours for two to four days after the ketoacidosis has been successfully treated. The CZI dosage distribution based on the work of Haunz[63] and Wildberger and Ricketts[64] is roughly: one-third total daily dosage, one and one-half hours after breakfast; one-sixth, one hour before lunch; one-third, one and one-half hours before supper, and one-sixth at midnight. These times permit the period of maximum hypoglycemic effect to coincide more closely with food intake. Owing to the danger of nocturnal hypoglycemia with CZI, the midnight dose has been limited to five units of CZI or replaced entirely with a full sixth of the daily dose as NPH.[63,64] The total insulin dose to be administered is calculated on a weight basis: 0.75 to 1.0 units per pound. The well-controlled patient requires 0.25 to 0.5 units per pound. Consideration is given to the range of dose that previously afforded good control in the patient.[7,9,62]

Recent studies on the regulation (normalization) of plasma glucose in diabetic patients were carried out by the subcutaneous administration of insulin by means of an infusion pump. Insulin was delivered at a basal rate with pulse-dose increments before meals.[65] In regard to the preprandial insulin doses required to achieve normoglycemia in these studies, it is noteworthy that elimination of postprandial morning hyperglycemia required a 40% to 55% larger insulin dose before breakfast than was necessary before lunch or dinner. This was true despite a 50% larger caloric intake at those meals. These findings are in keeping with observations in normal subjects that the endogenous insulin response to the breakfast meal exceeds that observed after lunch or dinner.[66,67] In a like manner, a higher insulin dose before breakfast has been employed in preprogrammed intravenous insulin delivery systems,[68] and is consonant with the four CZI doses recommended above for patient management following ketoacidosis.

INSULIN THERAPEUTICS

Effect of the Natural History of Diabetes Mellitus on Insulin Requirements

Insulin-dependent diabetes is usually characterized as a state of insulin deficiency.[69] Shortly after onset of the disease and after appropriate treatment, a substantial number of patients recover from the absolute exogenous insulin dependence and a partial or complete remission of the disease can occur.[70-74] The duration of this remission period of juvenile diabetes may last from a few weeks to several months or even years during which time the patient can be effectively treated with diet alone or with diet and small amounts of insulin.[75,76]

The natural history of insulin-dependent diabetes mellitus is summarized in Figure 4-6. The patient's carbohydrate tolerance is normal at birth. Onset of diabetes most frequently occurs between 3 and 12 years of age. The disease progresses slowly at onset, but once the cardinal signs and symptoms are manifest, the severity of the untreated disease progresses rapidly. The patient passes from the initial stage to one of little or no carbohydrate tolerance in only a few weeks or months. Following regulation with insulin, there is a remarkable tendency for most patients to regain tolerance. The typical patient soon passes to a phase of steadily ameliorating diabetes, so that his insulin can be cut

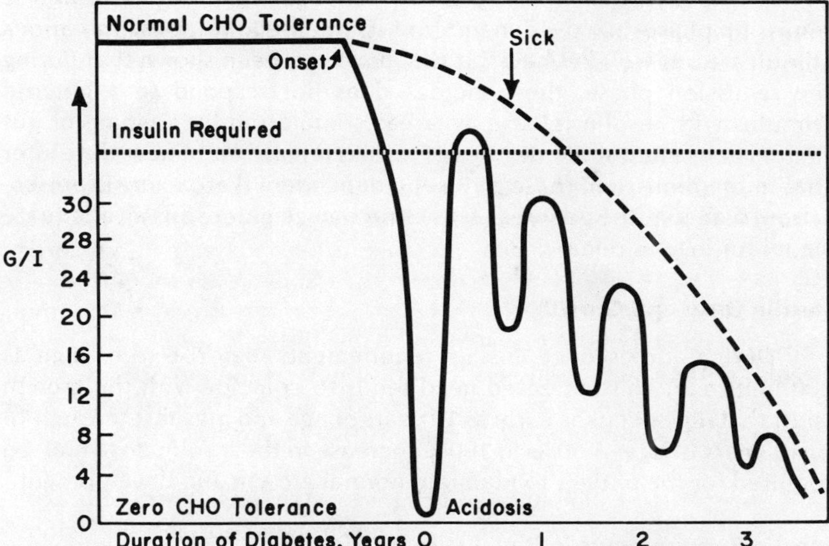

Figure 4-6   The course of insulin-dependent diabetes. G/I = Total available carbohydrate in diet (gm) minus Glucose loss in urine (gms)/Insulin dose (units).

repeatedly, and eventually in about 10% of patients admitted with an initial episode of diabetic ketoacidosis, no insulin at all is needed. This occurs without relation to the type or even adequacy of therapy. Patients lose their tolerance again, however, and in the course of several months to two or three years they become permanent insulin-dependent diabetics. A succession of rapid and perhaps severe losses of carbohydrate tolerance is followed by a slower partial recovery, as shown in Figure 4-6.

There are several characteristic events that usually precede these episodes of loss of tolerance (sickness). The child may have been constantly hyperglycemic and glucosuric due to insufficient insulin, infections, insufficient exercise, or severe emotional upsets. Sometimes these dips in tolerance appear to be the result of insulin overdosage.

It is the policy of many physicians to initiate lifelong insulin therapy in all juvenile patients, regardless of the degree of remission occurring after treatment of the initial breakdown of glucose tolerance. This serves to underscore the fact that diabetes is forever and avoids the psychologic impact of a later need for insulin therapy, which is often interpreted by the patient as a worsening of his state of health. The early use of insulin (at times in doses as little as two to four units) commits the patient to a lifelong schedule of insulin, food intake, and physical activity that optimizes his potential for a normal life. Moreover, by continuing the use of insulin, the likelihood of developing insulin allergy is reduced.[10]

It is known that the diabetic has endogenous insulin during the remission phase, but the dynamics of its release in response to various stimuli are not well-defined.[77] It has, however, been shown that during the remission phase, the pancreas does not respond to a glucose stimulus with insulin release, whereas stimulation by arginine or gut factors does elicit some degrees of insulin release.[77,78] These data infer that in the remission phase of insulin-dependent (ketoacidosis presentation) diabetes, the pancreas fails to recognize glucose as an adequate signal for insulin release.[77]

Insulin Dose and Growth

During adolescence, insulin requirements may rise to as high as 200 units/day. This increased need tends to coincide with the growth spurt that may occur as early as 10 years of age and may last through 18 or 19 years of age. A 50% to 100% increase in the insulin dose may be required for the patient to maintain normal growth and development.[7]

Insulin Requirements in Renal Disease

The insulin requirement of diabetics with impaired renal function relates in part to the stage of the renal disease.[79,80] Impaired glucose tolerance, or azotemic pseudodiabetes, is found in nondiabetic patients with substantial uremia.[81] The patient with diabetes and primary renal disease becomes insensitive to both endogenous and exogenous insulin,[79-81] a state that requires increased insulin. The basis of the insulin resistance is not known, but it is not likely to be immunogenic.[10,79]

With progression of the renal disease in the diabetic, a decrease in insulin requirement is seen.[79,80,82] This heightened sensitivity to insulin has been attributed to decreased nutritional intake; and diminished catabolism of insulin by the kidney, resulting in a longer insulin half-life in plasma; and perhaps to substances in uremic plasma that potentiate glucose uptake.

Because of these changes in insulin sensitivity, insulin requirements must be carefully followed in diabetics with renal disease. Reduction of insulin doses of 50% or more may be necessary.[80,82]

Etiology of Unstable ("Brittle") Insulin-Dependent Diabetes Mellitus

Unstable, or brittle, diabetes mellitus is a syndrome found in nonobese insulin-dependent patients of any age.[83] It has been estimated to be found in the 2% to 10% range of insulin-dependent patients.[83] The syndrome is characterized by rapid, wide fluctuations in blood glucose control in spite of careful and appropriate regulation of insulin, diet, and exercise. The wide glycemic swings range from hypoglycemia to hyperglycemia and ketosis and ketoacidosis. The patients experience unexplainable short- and long-term periods of erratic blood glucose control.[84,85]

Investigations of the hormonal status of these patients have suggested several etiologies for their unstable blood glucose control.[86-92] The unstable patients exhibit low to absent residual endogenous insulin and absence of an adequate glucagon response to hypoglycemia.[88]

In normal subjects rapid fluctuations of plasma insulin modulate moment-to-moment changes in blood glucose and keep it in a narrow range. The absence of sufficient endogenous (residual) insulin results in an inability to modulate the changes in blood glucose engendered by diet, emotions, hormones, and drugs.

The counterregulatory response to a decrease in blood glucose in nondiabetics includes a prompt release of glucagon.[93] Glucagon's stimulatory effect on glycogenolysis and gluconeogenesis elevates the depressed blood glucose levels.[11,12] Impairment of the glucagon response to hypoglycemia has been found in diabetics. The decreased glucagon responses were most pronounced in the insulin-dependent diabetic patients.[87] The lack of glucagon response during hypoglycemic episodes in diabetic patients would accentuate the hypoglycemic state by failing to elicit release of an important counterinsulin hormone.[11,12,88]

It is likely that the two abnormalities, absent insulin reserve and failure of glucagon to respond to blood glucose depressions, play important roles in the pathogenesis of unstable diabetes mellitus.

STRATEGY OF INSULIN USE IN INSULIN-DEPENDENT DIABETES MELLITUS

CZI and Semilente Insulins

These insulins have rapid onsets of action (around one hour), peak activities at two to four hours and durations of action of six to twelve hours (see Table 4-1). They provide high anabolic levels of plasma insulin when administered one to three hours before a meal, and establish glucose tolerance across the meal. They also provide some degree of glucose tolerance across the following meal, which is usually taken five to six hours later. The duration of action of these insulins, which ranges six to twelve hours permits this coverage.

Attempts to treat diabetics with three to four injections of either CZI or semilente have resulted in lower mean diurnal glycemic levels, but have also produced significant hypoglycemic reactions and little in the way of improvement of the wide glycemic swings of the unstable diabetic patient.[83-85]

NPH and Lente Insulins

These insulins are the most widely used in the therapy of insulin-dependent diabetes mellitus. They are both mixtures rather than pure types of insulin. Both insulin mixtures consist of two parts of long-acting and one part of short-acting insulin. In the case of NPH, there is one part of unbound insulin (CZI) for every two parts bound to protamine. Lente consists of three parts of semilente (small crystals, fast onset of action, shorter duration of action) and seven parts of ultralente (large crystals, slower onset of action, long duration of action). The pharmacology of these insulin preparations has been discussed previously (see Table 4-1).

A dose of 0.25 units/kg of lente or NPH produces a serum concentration after ten hours of approximately 10 μg/ml.[9,10] Since serum concentration is considered to be a linear function of dose, it would be expected that 0.5 units/kg (35 units in a 70 kg person) would produce a serum concentration of approximately 20 μU/ml. If, as demonstrated in Figure 4-7, the normal subject in response to the evening meal achieves a serum concentration of 80 μU/ml, it is somewhat surprising that a diabetic patient can be controlled on a single daily dose of intermediate-acting insulin (NPH or lente). The diabetic patient on a single daily dose of NPH or lente taken before breakfast would theoretically require a morning dose of around 140 units in order to achieve a serum concentration of 80 μU/ml ten hours later. Other factors must be considered in these estimations. These include the

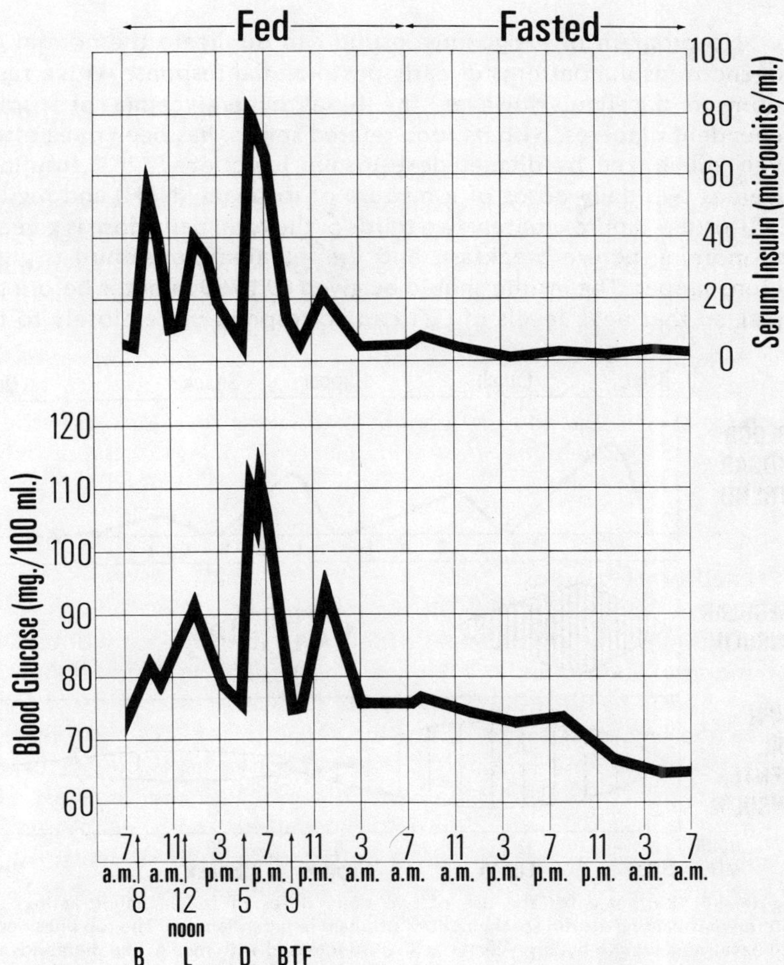

Figure 4-7 Blood glucose and serum insulin changes with meals. B = breakfast; L = lunch; D = dinner; BTF = bedtime food.

possibility that many diabetic patients on insulin therapy possess residual capacity to secrete some endogenous insulin. Moreover, in many instances serum antibodies bind the exogenous insulin as it is being absorbed from the injection site and delay its release to the tissues, a phenomenon described by Kurtz et al.[94] On the other hand, there are unquestionably a number of patients who in fact need two doses daily of insulin in order to achieve serum concentrations that are adequate to meet the metabolic demands of meals.

Insulin Mixtures

No program of exogenous insulin can duplicate the normal endogenous insulin patterns of early postprandial response with a rapid return to baseline. However, the basal hyperglycemia of insulin-dependent diabetes, with its food-related spikes, has been most effectively minimized by divided-dose insulin injections.[7,9,10,13] Insulin is given as two daily doses of a mixture of isophane (NPH) and regular (CZI) insulin. Approximately two thirds of the total daily dose is given in the morning before breakfast, and the remaining one third is given before supper. The insulin should be given 60 to 90 minutes before the meal, so that peak levels of CZI can correspond more closely to the

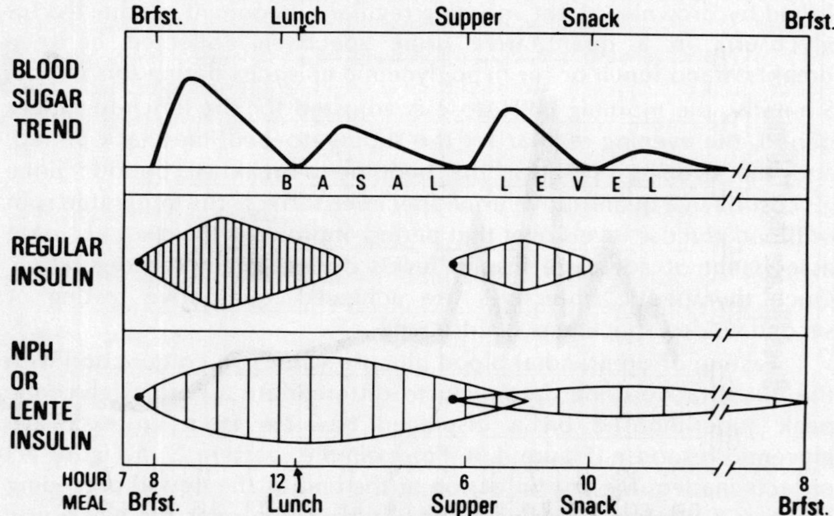

Figure 4-8 Rationale for the use of two daily doses of regular (short-acting) and intermediate-acting insulin for the control of juvenile-type diabetes. The top lines depict the basal tendency to hyperglycemia, which is increased with meals. The diamonds and ellipses represent the duration of action of the insulin dose indicated, and the density of the vertical lines is intended to demonstrate the intensity of action (dose) of insulin usually needed.[7]

time of maximum carbohydrate absorption.[7,13] This schedule of insulin administration is shown in Figure 4-8.

This schedule frequently obviates the need to choose between postprandial glycosuria and frequent hypoglycemia at the peak of CZI action. The ratio of NPH to regular insulin in the morning mixture is 2:1, and the evening dose is either 2:1 or 1:1. It is also essential to the success of this regimen to distribute the daily caloric intake over three meals and three between-meal snacks to minimize postprandial hyperglycemia and fasting hypoglycemia.[7,9,13,14]

The pattern of insulin levels achieved with this program coincides most closely with the caloric loads provided by meals (see Figure 4-7). The evening NPH component provides important basal levels of insulin to control excessive nocturnal lipolysis and gluconeogenesis. The duration of the insulin effect correlates in part with the magnitude of the dose. In addition, insulin absorption varies from patient to patient. Consideration of these features will facilitate the prescription of insulin dosage and the timing of its administration in relation to the meal times of individual patients.

Although there is actually some overlap of effect between insulins in an individual dose and between morning and evening insulin doses, dosage adjustments can be made by considering the four insulin components—morning regular, morning NPH, evening regular, and evening NPH—separately in relation to four daily periods by a method published by Brownlee.[13] The morning regular component is adjusted for glycosuria in a quantitative urine specimen collected between breakfast and lunch or for hypoglycemic episodes during this period. Similarly, the morning NPH dose is adjusted for the lunch-to-supper period, the evening regular for the supper–to–bedtime-snack period, and the evening NPH for the bedtime-to-breakfast period. Since glycosuria in a quantitative urine specimen reflects the integrated sum of blood glucose levels over that period, it provides the most accurate assessment of adequate insulin levels during attempted regulation. Once therapeutic objectives are achieved, qualitative testing of second-voided specimens is sufficient.

Fasting or preprandial blood glucose values, in conjunction with the quantitative urine data, help to differentiate a normal glycemic peak superimposed on a displaced baseline from an excessive glycemic response (Figure 4-9). For example, pattern B in Figure 4-9 reflects inadequate insulin action at the end of the period preceding glycosuria. Pattern C indicates too little insulin over the glycosuric period. A common error is to increase the insulin during the glycosuric period for pattern B. This adjustment leads to hypoglycemia at the peak of insulin action in the subsequent period, with a resultant compensatory reduction of insulin during that period. This reduction results in insufficient insulin effect at the end of that period, which then necessitates another cycle of dosage adjustments.

Correct interpretation of the glycosuric pattern will help avoid inappropriate, destabilizing insulin adjustments. Occasionally, an excessive glycemic response is exacerbated by increasing the appropriate insulin component (posthypoglycemic hyperglycemia).[85,95-97] In such instances, a gradual decrease of the insulin dose is indicated. Insulin adjustments should be made on the basis of trends and patterns, not individual values. Perseverance and patience are required, since it may take many weeks of attentive effort to achieve the desired therapeutic goals.

SENSITIVITY TO INSULIN AND INSULIN-RECEPTOR STATUS

The physiologic responses to injected insulin involve a number of separate and distinct phenomena. These include:

1. Absorption of insulin from subcutaneous injection sites into the plasma. One uncommon mechanism of insulin insensitivity is due to circulating antibodies to insulin.[10,98,99] These antibodies are produced in response to insulin use and delay and impair the delivery of the hormone to tissues.[10,99,100]

2. Binding of insulin to specific receptors in tissues and subse-

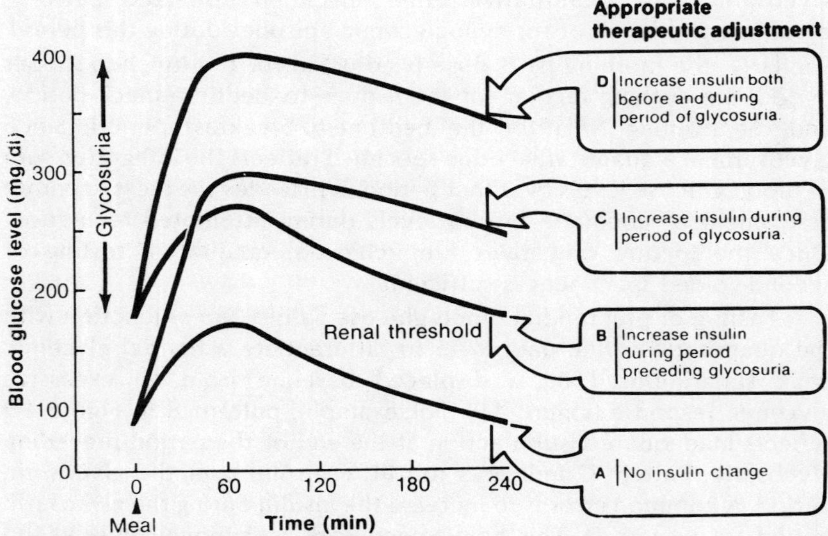

Figure 4-9 Glycemic patterns resulting in glycosuria. Brownlee, M. Normoglycemia as a therapeutic goal in insulin-dependent diabetes. *Drug Therapy* 3:13–20, 1978. Reprinted with permission.

quent activation of the several biochemical (anabolic-anticatabolic) effect of insulin in these tissues. The binding of insulin to cell receptors has recently been characterized,[56,101,102] and receptor status in a number of pathophysiologic states of altered sensitivity to the usual biologic effects of insulin has been studied.[56,101] It has been found that these states of altered insulin sensitivity differ in either the concentration of insulin receptors or in the affinity of the receptor for insulin.[56,101] These data are shown in Table 4-4.[56]

Table 4-4
Insulin-Receptor Status in States of Altered Insulin Sensitivity

Pathophysiologic State	Receptor Concentration	Receptor Affinity for Hormone
Insulin Insensitivity		
Obesity	Low	Normal
Hyperinsulinemic diabetes	Low	Normal
Glucocorticoid excess	Normal	Low
Growth hormone excess	Low	High
Uremia	Low	Normal
Insulin Sensitivity		
Glucocorticoid deficiency	Normal	High
Growth hormone deficiency	High	High
Exercise	Normal	High

The characterization as insulin-insensitive does not imply anything about the glucose tolerance. The insulin-insensitive state (obesity, corticosteroid use) means that a normal amount of insulin produces a less-than-usual effect. However, augmented levels of insulin can produce a usual biologic effect (normal glucose tolerance). This is the situation usually seen in obesity and corticosteroid use. Subjects with insulin resistance range from normal glucose tolerance to severe diabetes. The two factors that, together, determine the state of glucose tolerance in any insulin-insensitive patient are the severity of the insensitivity and the capacity of the beta-cells to compensate through increased insulin secretion.

Obesity is the most frequent and most studied state of insulin insensitivity. It has been found that insulin-receptor concentrations are reduced in liver, muscle, and fat, in animals and man. This reversible defect seems to result from the hyperinsulinemia induced by overeating.[56,101-104] Receptor impairment appears to be the predominant cause of insulin resistance. Glucocorticoid excess, whether of endogenous or exogenous origin, is another well-known cause of insulin insensitivity. In a carefully studied animal model reduced affinity of insulin receptors seemed to be the major cause of the insulin insensitivity.[56]

The alterations in insulin sensitivity explain many of the clinical impressions of the past 55 years. The insulin sensitivity that accompanies exercise and the insulin insensitivity of the posthypoglycemic state can now be understood in terms of receptor concentrations and affinity.[56]

Several syndromes of extreme resistance to insulin have been described. One of these states is thought to be attributable to antibodies to the insulin receptor.

These altered states of insulin sensitivity and insensitivity are reversible and thus are amenable to therapeutic intervention.[56,103] Insulin per se appears to be the impetus for the down regulation of insulin-receptor concentration in human subjects.[105] This might in part account for the difficulty in regulating the blood glucose of patients who have experienced hypoglycemic reactions. The excess insulin by down-regulating insulin receptors would make the patient less sensitive to insulin. Such posthypoglycemic hyperglycemia has been well characterized.[89,95-97]

DRUG-INSULIN INTERACTIONS

Because insulin-dependent diabetic patients have nearly normal lifespans, there is ample opportunity to experience other diseases that need to be treated with drugs. The use of other drugs in addition to insulin raises the possibility for drug-insulin interactions. A number of these have been reported and will be discussed briefly. There are three clinically significant types of drug-insulin interactions and several of lesser clinical importance. The classification of interactions can be made functionally:

1. Drugs that potentiate insulin action by increasing the amount of insulin (residual) secreted, augmenting the usual effects of insulin, or overcoming the effects of counterinsulin hormones.
2. Drugs that decrease insulin sensitivity.
3. Drugs that decrease or abolish residual insulin secretion.
4. Other drugs interacting with insulin.

Potentiators of Insulin Action

Salicylates in large doses (4 to 6 gm/day) are known to potentiate the hypoglycemic action of insulin.[106-109] Two mechanisms have been proposed. Salicylates increase (residual) plasma insulin[109] and also have intrinsic hypoglycemic activity, the mechanism of which is not known.[108]

Anabolic steroids appear to sensitize the diabetic patient to the effects of insulin.[110,111] The increased sensitivity to exogenous insulin has been most studied in the case of methandienone.[110] The mechanism is not known.

Ethanol ingestion in large amounts can markedly potentiate the hypoglycemic action of insulin.[112] This severe hypoglycemia is usually seen in alcoholic patients who have been eating poorly, and have depleted glycogen stores.[113] Ethanol diminishes hepatic gluconeogenesis. Since glycogen is depleted, these patients have no mobilizable carbohydrate with which to combat the hypoglycemic action of insulin.[114]

Monoamine oxidase inhibitors (MAOI) such as tranylcypromine and pargyline[115-117] have been reported to potentiate the hypoglycemic action of insulin. An interference of the MAOIs with compensatory adrenergic hyperglycemic responses (glycogenolysis and gluconeogenesis) to decreases in blood glucose have been suggested as the mechanism of action.[118]

Propranolol, a β-adrenergic blocking drug has also been found to potentiate insulin hypoglycemia.[119-122] It has been postulated that this is due to interference of propranolol with catecholamine-induced glycogenolysis and perhaps gluconeogenesis.[120,121] This potentiation is especially dangerous because the β-adrenergic blockade also blocks the tachycardic response to hypoglycemia, creating a more insidious clinical picture.

Guanethidine is an antihypertensive drug that is a ganglionic blocking agent. It has been thought to potentiate insulin action because withdrawal of the drug in insulin-dependent diabetic patients results in a worsening of the blood glucose status and an increased insulin requirement.[123-125] Moreover, control of the blood glucose in non–insulin-dependent diabetic subjects was improved by the use of guanethidine.[124-126]

Oxytetracycline (OTC) has been found to potentiate the hypoglycemic action of insulin in human subjects.[127,128] The antibiotic has been found to facilitate insulin secretion in mice.[129] Animal studies also suggest that OTC intensifies and prolongs the action of insulin.[130]

Drugs that Decrease Insulin Sensitivity

These drugs include corticosteroids and steroidal oral contraceptives. Corticosteroids oppose the hypoglycemic action of insulin in several ways. They decrease the affinity of insulin for its tissue receptors thus creating a peripheral insulin insensitivity.[56] They also act as counterinsulin hormones in stimulating gluconeogenesis, which raises the blood glucose.[12,131-133] Steroidal oral contraceptives can also produce a state of peripheral insulin insensitivity.[134-136]

Drugs that Diminish Insulin Output from the Pancreas

Many insulin-requiring diabetic patients have some capacity to secrete insulin. Although their insulin secretion is small and limited, it may be sufficient to maintain a stable blood glucose control in association with exogenous insulin. Unstable ("brittle") diabetics have been found generally to be devoid of residual insulin.[88] Both thiazide-type (sulfonamide) diuretics[137-140] and phenytoin[141-144] have been found to decrease insulin secretion in animals and humans. These effects of the thiazides are more pronounced at higher drug concentrations and may be due partially to drug effects on pancreatic islet cell ions (Na^+, K^+).[145-147]

Other Drugs that Oppose Insulin's Hypoglycemic Action

Epinephrine stimulates glycogenolysis and inhibits insulin secretion.[148]

Nicotinic acid worsens blood glucose control by worsening glucose tolerance by unknown mechanisms.[149]

The deleterious effects of drug-insulin interactions on control of the blood glucose are reversible and can be remedied either by withdrawal of the interacting drug or appropriate adjustment of the insulin dose. Raising the dose of insulin will compensate for either drug-induced insulinopenia or drug-induced insensitivity to insulin. Caution must be exercised in withdrawal of the interacting drug because a rapid return of endogenous insulin secretion or insulin sensitivity may occur, resulting in hypoglycemia on the same dose of exogenous insulin.

REFERENCES

1. Bressler, R. The controversy over blood glucose control. *Drug Therapy* 8:24–41, 1978.

2. Bressler, R. Control of the blood glucose in diabetes mellitus: Is it valuable? Is it feasible? *Drugs* 17:461–470, 1979.

3. Raskin, P. Diabetic regulation and its relationship to microangiopathy. *Metabolism* 27:235–252, 1978.

4. Cahill, G.F., Etzwiler, D.D., and Freinkel, N. Blood glucose control in diabetes. *Diabetes* 25:237–239, 1976.

5. Cahill, G.F. Physiology of insulin in man. *Diabetes* 20:785–799, 1971.

6. Felig, P. Pathophysiology of diabetes. Edited by R. Sussman, and R. Metz. In *Diabetes Mellitus,* 4th Edition. New York: American Diabetes Association, 1975, pp 1–9.

7. Bressler, R., and Galloway, J.A. Insulin treatment of diabetes mellitus. *Med Clin North Am.* 55:861–876, 1971.

8. Molnar, G., Taylor, W., and Langworthy, A. Plasma immunoreactive insulin pattern in insulin-treated diabetes. *Mayo Clin Proc.* 47:709–719, 1972.

9. Bressler, R., and Galloway, J.A. The insulins: pharmacology and uses. *Drug Therapy* 8:43–61, 1978.

10. Galloway, J.A., and Bressler, R. Insulin treatment in diabetes. *Med Clin North Am.* 62:663–679, 1978.

11. Williams, R.H., and Porte, D., Jr. The pancreas. Edited by R.H. Williams, In *Textbook of Endocrinology.* Philadelphia: W.B. Saunders, 1974, pp 502–626.

12. Schade, D.S., and Eaton, R.P. The controversy concerning counterregulatory hormone secretion. *Diabetes* 26:596–599, 1977.

13. Brownlee, M. Normoglycemia as a therapeutic goal in insulindependent diabetes. *Drug Therapy* (Hospital Edition) 3:13–20, 1978.

14. Bressler, R., and Galloway, J.A. The insulins. *Ration Drug Ther.* 5:1–6, 1971.

15. Holcomb, G.N. Current concepts in antidiabetics. *Am J Pharm.* 34:648–661, 1970.

16. Sanger, F. Chemistry of insulin: determination of the structure of insulin opens the way to greater understanding of life processes. *Science* 129:1340–1344, 1959.

17. Chance, R.E. Amino acid sequences of proinsulins and intermediates. *Diabetes* 21(suppl 2): 461–467, 1972.

18. Sanger, F. Chemistry of insulin. *Br Med Bull.* 16:183–188, 1960.

19. Rosenbloom, A.L. Advances in commercial insulin preparations. *Am J Dis Child.* 128:631–633, 1974.

20. Goodman, L.S., and Gilman, S.G. (Eds.). *The Pharmacological Basis of Therapeutics,* 5th Edition. New York: Macmillan, 1975, pp 1507–1533.

21. Little, J.A., and Arnott, J.H. Sulfated insulin in mild, moderate and severe insulin resistant diabetes mellitus. *Diabetes* 15:457–465, 1966.

22. Galloway, J.A., and Root, M.A. New forms of insulin. *Diabetes* 21(suppl 2): 637–648, 1972.

23. Galloway, J.A., Root, M.A., Chance, R.E. et al. New forms of insulin. Edited by P.J. Kryston and R.A. Shaw. In *Endocrinology and Diabetes.* New York: Grune & Stratton, 1975, pp 329–343.

24. Root, M.A., Chance, R.E., and Galloway, J.A. Immunogenicity of insulin. *Diabetes* 21(suppl):657–660, 1972.

25. Yalow, R.S., and Berson, S.A. Plasma insulin in man. *Am J Med.* 29:1–8, 1960.

26. Arquilla, E.R., and Stavitsky, A.B. The production and identification of antibodies to insulin and their use in assaying insulin. *J Clin Invest.* 35:458–466, 1956.

27. Jackson, R.L., Storvick, W.O., Hollinden, C.S. et al. Neutral regular insulin. *Diabetes* 21:235–245, 1972.

28. Galloway, J.A., Root, M.A., Rathmacher, R.P. et al. A comparison of acid regular and neutral regular insulin. *Diabetes* 22:471–479, 1973.

29. Hagedorn, H.C., Jensen, B.N., Karup, N.B. et al. Protamine insulinate. *JAMA.* 106:177–180, 1936.

30. Peck, F.P. Actions of insulin. *Proc Am Diabetes Assoc.* 2:69–83, 1942.

31. Hallas-Møller, K., Peterson, K., and Schlichtkrull, J. Crystalline and amorphous insulin-zinc compounds with prolonged action. *Science* 116:394–398, 1952.

32. Hallas-Møller, K. The lente insulins. *Diabetes* 5:7–14, 1956.

33. Whitehouse, F., Lowrie, W.L., Redfern, E. et al. The lente insulin triad. *Ann Intern Med.* 55:894–902, 1961.

34. Rosenbloom, A.L. Advances in commercial insulin preparations. *Am J Dis Child.* 128:631–633, 1974.

35. Rosenberg, J.M., Simon, W.A., Sangkachand, P. et al. Mixing insulin preparations. *Hosp Pharm.* 11:186–191, 1976.

36. Young, L.Y., and Kimble, M.A. (Eds.). *Applied Therapeutics for Clinical Pharmacists.* San Francisco: Applied Therapeutics, Inc., 1975, pp 225–260.

37. Yue, D.K., and Turtle, J.R. New forms of insulin and their use in the treatment of diabetes. *Diabetes* 26:341–345, 1977.

38. Nelson, R.L., Galloway, J.A., Wentworth, S.M. et al. The bioavailability, pharmacokinetics and time action of regular and modified insulins in normal subjects. *Diabetes* 25:325, 1976.

39. Bender, C. Mechanism of insulin absorption. *Acta Pharmacol Toxicol.* 27(suppl 2):23–49, 1969.

40. Ginsberg, I., Block, M.B., Mako, M.E. et al. Serum insulin levels following administration of exogenous insulin. *J Clin Endocrinol Metab.* 36:1175–1179, 1973.

41. Guerra, S.M.O., and Kitabchi, A.E. Comparison of the effectiveness of various routes of insulin injection: insulin levels and glucose response in normal subjects. *J Clin Endocrinol Metab.* 42:869–874, 1976.

42. Greenblatt, D.J., and Koch-Weser, J. Clinical pharmacokinetics. *N Engl J Med.* 293:964–970, 1973.

43. Nora, J.J., Smith, D.W., and Cameron, J.R. The route of insulin administration in the management of diabetes mellitus. *J Pediatr.* 64:547–551, 1964.

44. Binder, C., Nielson, A., and Jorgensen, K. The absorption of an acid and a neutral solution after subcutaneous injection into different regions in diabetic patients. *Scand J Clin Lab Invest.* 19:156–163, 1967.

45. Yalow, R.S., and Berson, S.A. Immunologic aspects of insulin. *Am J Med.* 31:882–891, 1961.

46. Tomasi, T., Sledz, D., Wales, J.K. et al. Insulin half-life in normal and diabetic subjects. *Proc Soc Exp Biol Med.* 126:315–317, 1967.

47. Orskov, H., and Christensen, N.J. Plasma disappearance rate of injected human insulin in juvenile diabetic, maturity-onset diabetic and non-diabetic subjects. *Diabetes* 18:653–659, 1969.

48. Levine, R. Concerning the mechanism of insulin action. *Diabetes* 10:421–431, 1961.

49. Tomizawa, H.H. Mode of action of an insulin-degrading enzyme from beef liver. *J Biol Chem.* 237:428–431, 1962.

50. Van Rooyen, R.J., De Bruin, E.J.P., Bieler, E.U. et al. The half-life of ^{131}I-insulin in different groups of patients compared with normal subjects. *S Afr Med J.* 46:1927–1931, 1972.

51. Rubenstein, A.H., and Spitz, I. Role of the kidney in insulin metabolism and excretion. *Diabetes* 17:161–169, 1968.

52. Chamberlain, M.J., and Stimmler, L. The renal handling of insulin. *J Clin Invest.* 46:911–919, 1967.

53. Rabkin, R., Simon, N.M., Steiner, S. et al. Effect of renal disease on renal uptake and excretion of insulin in man. *N Engl J Med.* 282:182–187, 1970.

54. Malone, J.J., and Root, A.W. Renal wastage of insulin in children with diabetes mellitus. *Diabetes* 25:989–993, 1976.

55. Lawrence, R.D. The effect of exercise on insulin action in diabetes. *Br Med J.* 1:648–650, 1926.

56. Flier, J.S., Kahn, R., and Roth, J. Receptors, antireceptor antibodies and mechanisms of insulin resistance. *N Engl J Med.* 300:413–419, 1979.

57. Murray, F.T., Zinman, B., McClean, P. et al. The metabolic response to moderate exercise in diabetic men receiving intravenous and subcutaneous insulin. *J CLin Endocrinol Metab.* 44:708–720, 1977.

58. Berger, M., Halban, P., Müller, W.A. et al. Mobilization and distribution of subcutaneously injected ^{3}H-insulin: effects of exercise. *Diabetes* 26:357, 1977.

59. Koivisto, V.A., and Felig, P. Effects of leg exercise on insulin absorption in diabetic patients. *N Engl J Med.* 298:79–83, 1978.

60. Dandona, P., Healey, F., Foster, M. et al. Low-dose insulin infusions in diabetic patients with high insulin requirements. *Lancet* 2:283–285, 1978.

61. Gibson, R.C., Stretcher, G.S., and Williams, T.F. Duration and magnitude of insulin effect in juvenile-onset diabetics. *Clin Res.* 14:63, 1966.

62. Marler, E., Bressler, R., and Styron, C. The use of insulin in unstable diabetes mellitus. *South Med J.* 57:1447–1451, 1964.

63. Haunz, E.A. An approach to the problem of the "brittle" diabetic patient. *JAMA.* 142:168–173, 1950.

64. Wildberger, H.L., and Ricketts, H.T. Multiple injections of crystalline insulin in treatment of labile diabetes. *JAMA.* 172:655–658, 1960.

65. Tamborlane, W.V., Sherwin, R.S., Genel, M. et al. Reduction to normal of plasma in juvenile diabetes by subcutaneous administration of insulin with a portable insulin pump. *N Engl J Med.* 300:573–578, 1979.

66. Hansen, A.P., and Johansen, K. Diurnal patterns of blood glucose, serum free fatty acids, insulin, glucagon and growth hormone in normals and juvenile diabetics. *Diabetologia* 6:27–33, 1970.

67. Genuth, S.M. Plasma insulin and glucose profiles in normal, obese, and diabetic persons. *Ann Intern Med.* 79:812–822, 1973.

68. Genuth, S.M., and Martin, P. Control of hyperglycemia in adults by pulsed insulin delivery. *Diabetes* 26:571–581, 1977.

69. Parker, R.L., Pildes, R.S., Chao, K.I. et al. Juvenile diabetes mellitus, a deficiency in insulin. *Diabetes* 17:27–32, 1968.

70. Hernandez, A., Zorrilla, E., and Gersberg, H. Serum-insulin in remission of juvenile diabetes. *Lancet* 2:223, 1968.

71. Park, B.N., Soeldner, J.S., and Gleason, R.E. Diabetes in remission. Insulin secretory dynamics. *Diabetes* 23:616–623, 1974.

72. Weber, B. Glucose-stimulated insulin secretion during "remission" of juvenile diabetes. *Diabetologia* 8:189–195, 1972.

73. Baker, L., Kaye, R., and Root, A.W. The early partial remission of juvenile diabetes mellitus. *J Pediatr.* 71:825–831, 1967.

74. Genuth, S.M. Clinical remission in diabetes mellitus. Studies in insulin secretion. *Diabetes* 19:116–121, 1970.

75. Jackson, R.I., Onofrio, J., Waiches, H. et al. "The honeymoon period." Partial remission of juvenile diabetes mellitus. *Diabetes* 20(suppl 1):361, 1971.

76. Carlström, S., and Ingemanson, C.A. Juvenile diabetes with long-standing remission. *Diabetologia* 3:465–467, 1967.

77. Heinze, E., Beischer, W., Keller, L. et al. C-peptide secretion during the remission phase of juvenile diabetes. *Diabetes* 27:670–676, 1978.

78. Block, M.B., Mako, M.E., Steiner, D.F. et al. Diabetic ketoacidosis. Evidence for C-peptide and proinsulin following recovery. *J Clin Endocrinol Metab.* 35:402–406, 1972.

79. Westervelt, F.B., Jr. Clinical aspects of uremia and dialysis. Edited by S.G. Massry and A.L. Sellers. In *Carbohydrate Metabolism.* Springfield, Ill.: Charles C. Thomas 1976, pp 212–230.

80. De Fronzo, R.A., Andres, R., Edgar, P. et al. Carbohydrate metabolism in uremia. *Medicine* 52:469–481, 1973.

81. Horton, E.S., Johnson, C., and Lebovitz, H.E. Carbohydrate metabolism in uremia. *Ann Intern Med.* 68:63–74, 1968.

82. Zubrod, C.G., Wilson, J.E., Root, H.F., et al. Amelioration of diabetes and striking rarity of acidosis in patients with Kimmelstiel-Wilson lesions. *N Engl J Med.* 245:513–517, 1951.

83. Molnar, G.D. Observations on the etiology and therapy of "brittle" diabetes. *Can Med Assoc J.* 90:953–959, 1964.

84. Service, F.J., Molnar, G.D., Rosevear, J.W. et al. Mean amplitude of glycemic excursions, a measure of diabetic instability. *Diabetes* 19:644–655, 1970.

85. Molnar, G.D., Taylor, W.E., and Ho, M.M. Day-to-day variation of continuously monitored glycemia: a further measure of diabetic instability. *Diabetologia* 8:342–348, 1972.

86. Maher, T.D., Tanenberg, R.J., Greenberg, B.Z. et al. Lack of glucagon response to hypoglycemia in diabetic autonomic neuropathy. *Diabetes* 26:196–200, 1977.

87. Gerich, J.E., Langlois, M., Noacco, C. et al. Lack of glucagon response to hypoglycemia in diabetes: evidence for an intrinsic pancreatic alpha cell defect. *Science* 182:171–173, 1973.

88. Shima, K., Tanaka, R., Morishita, S. et al. Studies on the etiology of "brittle diabetes." *Diabetes* 26:717–725, 1977.

89. Bloom, M.E., Mintz, D.H., and Field, J.B. Insulin-induced posthypoglycemic hyperglycemia as a cause of "brittle" diabetes. Clinical clues and therapeutic implications. *Am J Med.* 47:891–903, 1969.

90. Cremer, G.M., Molnar, G.D., Taylor, W.F. et al. Studies of diabetic instability. II. Tests of insulinogenic reserve with infusions of arginine, glucagon, epinephrine, and saline. *Metabolism* 20:1083–1098, 1971.

91. Dixon, K., Exon, P.D., and Hughes, H.R. Insulin antibodies in aetiology of labile diabetes. *Lancet* 1:343–347, 1972.

92. Johansen, K., and Hansen, A.P. Diurnal serum growth hormone levels in poorly and well-controlled juvenile diabetics. *Diabetes* 20:239–245, 1971.

93. Gerich, J.E., Schneider, V., Dippe, S.E. et al. Characterization of the glucagon response to hypoglycemia in man. *J Clin Endocrinol Metab.* 38:77–82, 1974.

94. Kurtz, A.B., Mustaffa, B.E., Daggett, P.R. et al. Effect of insulin antibodies on free and total plasma insulin. *Lancet* 1:56–58, 1977.

95. Bruck, E., and MacGillivray, M.H. Posthypoglycemic hyperglycemia in diabetic children. *J Pediatr.* 84:672–680, 1974.

96. Somogyi, M. Exacerbation of diabetes by excess insulin action. *Am J Med.* 26:169–191, 1959.

97. Somogyi, M. Diabetogenic effect of hyperinsulinism. *Am J Med.* 26: 192–198, 1959.

98. Boshell, B.R., Barrett, J.C., Wilensky, A.S. et al. Insulin resistance:

response to insulin from various animal sources including human. *Diabetes* 13:144–152, 1964.

99. Shipp, J.C., Cunningham, R.W., Russell, R.O. et al. Insulin resistance: clinical features, natural course and effects of adrenal steroid treatment. *Medicine* 44:165–186, 1965.

100. Berson, S.A., Yalow, R.S., Bauman, A. et al. Insulin I-131 metabolism in human subjects: demonstration of insulin binding globulin in circulation of insulin treated subjects. *J Clin Invest.* 35:170–190, 1956.

101. Bar, R.S., and Roth, J. Insulin receptor status in disease states of man. *Arch Intern Med.* 137:474–481, 1977.

102. Olefsky, J.M. The insulin receptor: its role in insulin resistance of obesity and diabetes. *Diabetes* 25:1154–1162, 1976.

103. Archer, J.A., Gorden, P., and Roth, J. Defect in insulin binding to receptors in obese man: amelioriation with caloric restriction. *J Clin Invest.* 55:166–174, 1975.

104. Soll, A.H., Kahn, C.R., Neville, D.M. et al. Insulin receptor deficiency in genetic and acquired obesity. *J Clin Invest.* 56:769–780, 1975.

105. Wigand, J.P., and Blackard, W.G. Down-regulation of insulin receptors in obese man. *Diabetes* 28:287–291, 1979.

106. Seltzer, H.O. Drug induced hypoglycemia: a review based on 473 cases. *Diabetes* 21:955–966, 1972.

107. Fang, V. Hypoglycemic activity and chemical structure of the salicylates. *J Pharm Sci.* 57:2111–2116, 1968.

108. Field, J., Boyld, C., and Remer, A. Effect of salicylate infusion on plasma insulin and glucose tolerance in healthy persons and mild diabetics. *Lancet* 1:1191–1194, 1967.

109. Chen, M., and Robertson, R.P. Restoration of the acute insulin response by sodium salicylate: a glucose dose-related phenomenon. *Diabetes* 27:750–756, 1978.

110. Landon, J., Wynn, V., Cooke, J. et al. Effects of anabolic steroid methandienone on carbohydrate metabolism in man. *Metabolism* 11:501–512, 1962.

111. Landon, J., Wynn, V., and Samols, E. The effect of anabolic steroids on blood sugar and plasma insulin levels in man. *Metabolism* 12:924–935, 1963.

112. Arky, R., Veverbrants, E., and Abramson, E. Irreversible hypoglycemia: a complication of alcohol and insulin. *JAMA.* 206:575–578, 1968.

113. Field, J., Williams, H., and Mortimore, G. Studies on the mechanism of ethanol-induced hypoglycemia. *J Clin Invest.* 42:497–506, 1963.

114. DeMoura, M., Correia, J., and Madeira, F. Clinical alcohol hypoglycemia. *Ann Intern Med.* 66:893–905, 1967.

115. Adnitt, P.I. Hypoglycemic action of monoamine oxidase inhibitors (MAOI's). *Diabetes* 17:628–633, 1968.

116. VanPraag, H.M., and Leijnse, B. The influence of some antidepressives of the hydrazine type on the glucose metabolism in depressed patients. *Clin Chim Acta.* 8:466–475, 1963.

117. Cooper, A., and Ashcroft, G. Potentiation of insulin hypoglycemia by MAOI antidepressant drugs. *Lancet* 1:407–409, 1966.

118. Wickstrom, L., and Pettersson, K. Treatment of diabetics with monoamine oxidase inhibitors. *Lancet* 2:995–997, 1964.

119. Kotler, M.N., Berman, L., and Rubenstein, A.H. Hypoglycemia precipitated by propranolol. *Lancet* 2:1389–1390, 1966.

120. McBride, J.T., McBride, M.C., and Viles, P.H. Hypoglycemia associated with propranolol. *Pediatrics* 51:1085–1087, 1973.

121. Byers, S., and Friedman, M. Insulin hypoglycemia enhanced by β-adrenergic blockade. *Proc Soc Exp Biol Med.* 122:114–115, 1966.

122. Sussman, K., and Vaughn, G. Propranolol and hypoglycemia. *Lancet* 1:626, 1967.

123. Davidoff, F. Guanidine derivatives in medicine. *N Engl J Med.* 289: 141–146, 1973.

124. Kansal, P.C., Buse, J., Durling, F.C. et al. Effect of guanethidine and reserpine on glucose tolerance. *Curr Ther Res.* 13:517–522, 1971.

125. Gupta, K., and Lillicrap, C. Guanethidine and diabetes. *Br Med J.* 2: 697–698, 1968.

126. Gupta, K. The antidiabetic action of guanethidine. *Postgrad Med.* 45:455–456, 1969.

127. Miller, J. Hypoglycemic effect of oxytetracycline. *Br Med J.* 2:1007, 1966.

128. Sen, S., and Mukerjee, A. Hypoglycemic action of oxytetracycline. *J Indian Med Assoc.* 52:366–369, 1969.

129. Begin-Heick, N., Heick, H.M.C., and Norman, M.G. Regranulation of islets of Langerhans and normalization of *in vivo* insulin secretion in ob/ob mice treated with oxytetracycline. *Diabetes* 28:65–70, 1979.

130. Hiatt, N., and Bonorris, G. Insulin response in pancreatectomized dogs treated with oxytetracycline. *Diabetes* 19:307–310, 1970.

131. Thorn, G. Clinical considerations in the use of corticosteroids. *N Engl J Med.* 274:775–781, 1966.

132. Wagle, S. Studies on the mechanism of glucose synthesis in diabetic and normal rat liver. *Diabetes* 12:19–23, 1966.

133. Owen, E., Patel, M.S., Block, B.S. et al. Gluconeogenesis in normal, cirrhotic and diabetic humans. Edited by R.W. Hanson and M.A. Mehlman. In *Gluconeogenesis: Its Regulation in Mammalian Species.* New York: John Wiley & Sons, 1976, pp 533–558.

134. Beck, P. Effects of gonadal hormones and contraceptive steroids on glucose and insulin metabolism. Edited by H. Salhanick, D. Kipnis, and R. Weile. In *Hormones and Contraceptives.* New York: Plenum Press, 1969, pp 97–125.

135. Gershberg, H., Javier, Z., and Hulse, M. Glucose tolerance in women receiving an ovulatory suppressant. *Diabetes* 13:378–382, 1964.

136. Durand, J., and Bressler, R. Clinical pharmacology of the steroidal oral contraceptives. *Adv Intern Med.* 24:97–119, 1979.

137. Remenchik, A., Hoover, C., and Talso, P. Insulin secretion by hypertensive patients receiving hydrochlorthiazide. *JAMA.* 212:869, 1970.

138. Runyan, J.W. Influence of thiazide diuretics on carbohydrate metabolism in patients with mild diabetes. *N Engl J Med.* 267:541–543, 1962.

139. Chazan, J.A., and Boshell, B.R. Etiological factors in thiazide-induced or aggravated diabetes mellitus. *Diabetes* 14:132–136, 1965.

140. Goldner, M.G., Zarowitz, H., and Akgun, S. Hyperglycemia and glycosuria due to thiazide derivatives administered in diabetes mellitus. *N Engl J Med.* 262:403–405, 1960.

141. Kizer, J.S., Vargas-Cordon, M., Brendel, K. et al. The *in vitro* inhibition of insulin secretion by diphenylhydantoin. *J Clin Invest.* 49:1942–1948, 1970.

142. Fariss, B.L., and Lutcher, C.L. Diphenylhydantoin-induced hyperglycemia and impaired insulin release. *Diabetes* 20:177–181, 1971.

143. Levin, S.R., Reed, J.W., King-Nien, C. et al. Diphenylhydantoin: its use in detecting early insulin secretory defects in patients with mild glucose intolerance. *Diabetes* 22:194–201, 1973.

144. Stambaugh, J.E., and Tucker, D.C. Effect of diphenylhydantoin on

glucose tolerance in patients with hypoglycemia. *Diabetes* 23:679–683, 1974.

145. Rappaport, M., and Hurd, H. Thiazide-induced glucose intolerance treated with potassium. *Arch Intern Med.* 113:405–408, 1964.

146. Maronde, R., Milgrom, M., and Dickey, J. Potassium loss with thiazide therapy. *Am Heart J.* 78:16–21, 1969.

147. Kizer, J.S., and Bressler, R. Drugs and mechanism of insulin secretion. *Adv Pharmacol Chemother.* 7:91–115, 1969.

148. Robertson, R.P., and Porte, D., Jr. Adrenergic modulation of basal insulin secretion in man. *Diabetes* 22:1–8, 1973.

149. Molnar, G., Berge, K., Rosevear, J. et al. The effect of nicotinic acid in diabetes mellitus. *Metabolism* 13:181–189, 1964.

5 **The Complications of Insulin Therapy**

John A. Galloway, MD

The complications of insulin therapy include allergy (both local and systemic), the lipodystrophies (atrophic or lipoatrophy, and hypertrophic or hypertrophy), and antibody formation including immunologic resistance. In addition, hypoglycemia and insulin edema will be discussed. Moreover, since conventional insulin treatment only occasionally normalizes the blood glucose, and since chronic hyperglycemia is increasingly being cited as the principal cause of the complications of diabetes,[1,2] it is reasonable to categorize the complications of diabetes as complications of insulin therapy. This theory is covered in Chapter 4. Additional information on the complications of insulin therapy is contained in other articles by Bressler and Galloway[3,4] and by Kahn and Rosenthal.[5]

Since the terms "single peak" and "single component" are unofficial, a word of explanation or review is in order. On gel chromatography single peak insulin yields a profile consisting chiefly of a single peak (Figure 5-1).[6-8] The primary improvement seen in this insulin compared to those insulins commonly available in the early 1970s is a reduction of the amount of large molecular substances that elute as the A and B peaks. The disc-gel electrophoresis profile of single peak insulin is shown in "D" on the upper left-hand panel, and demonstrates the presence of insulin, the major band, and smaller amounts of desamido insulin and arginine insulins, which have been shown to be intermediates in the conversion of proinsulin to insulin.

Single component insulin is single peak insulin that has been further purified by DEAE cellulose chromatography.[6] The chief difference between these two insulins is that single component is 99% insulin and has only miniscule amounts of large-molecular-weight material.

The species from which the insulin is derived has a bearing on the treatment of the complications of insulin therapy. Therefore, it is helpful to know that over 95% of insulin sold in the United States is mixed beef-pork. The remainder is monospecies pork and monospecies beef material.

In addition to chromatography, new technology has made it possible to measure in minute quantities other substances, such as proinsulin, somatostatin, vasoactive intestinal peptide (VIP), pancreatic polypeptide (PPP), and glucagon, in commercial insulin. While there are little data on the clinical significance of most of these substances,[9-11] it is becoming increasingly evident that proinsulin is a

G-50(F) SEPHADEX CHROMATOGRAPHY OF PORCINE INSULIN

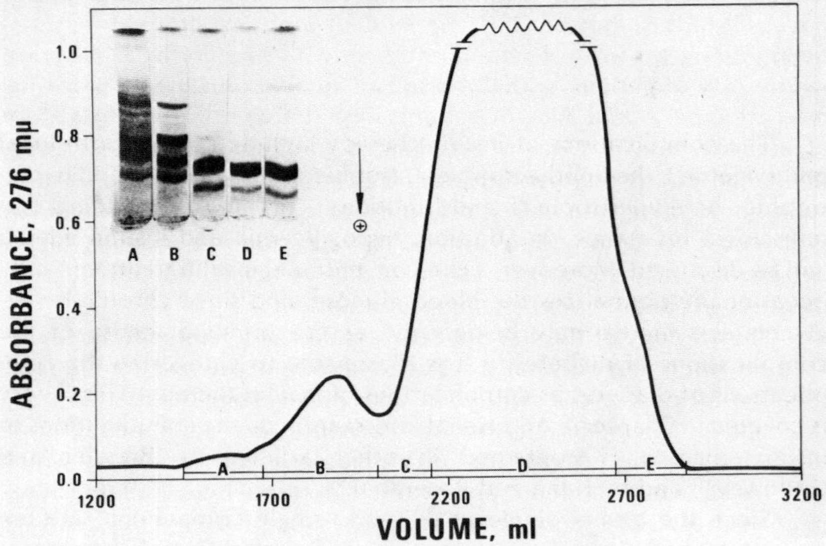

Figure 5-1 Polyacrylamide disc gel electrophoresis of pork insulin. Peak A contains proteins with a molecular weight of 10,000 and greater; peak B, proinsulin and structurally similar material plus a "dimer" of insulin; and peak D "single peak" insulin. Identical chromatograms are obtained with beef insulin.

useful absolute index of insulin purity and complements chromatographic analyses.[9,11] The proinsulin contents of insulins available in the United States are listed in Table 5-1.

Table 5-1
Proinsulin Content (parts per million, PPM)

Conventional USP	>10,000
Single peak*	<3,000
Improved single peak†	<50
Purified pork‡	<10

*All Lilly insulin manufactured from 1972–1979.
†All Lilly mixed beef-pork insulins marketed in April 1980.
‡Lilly Iletin II, Pork, and Lilly Iletin II, Beef; Novo Purified and Insulins in the U.S. (marketed as "Monocomponent" outside of the U.S.); and Nordisk Purified Insulins in the U.S. (marketed as "Rarely Immunogenic" out side of U.S.).

INSULIN-INDUCED LIPOATROPHY

Insulin lipoatrophy (ILA) is a complication of diabetes occurring in approximately 10% of patients receiving unchromatographed insulin.[12] ILA occurs most frequently in young children and young women. However, older women and men are now being recognized as having ILA. ILA does not become evident until insulin treatment has been in progress from several months to two years. In the Lilly series[9] nearly 25% of patients with ILA also had local insulin allergy of the immediate type. About 30% of patients with ILA demonstrate loss of fat at sites where insulin was never injected.[9] Twenty-four percent of patients had co-existing hypertrophy. It is important not to confuse insulin lipoatrophy with classical lipoatrophic diabetes.[13] Although ILA is a benign condition, the cosmetic disfiguration is frequently highly detrimental to the patient's self-image. As a result, successful treatment results in an exceedingly grateful patient.

The etiology of ILA has not been established. However, the available evidence suggests that it is due to both lipolytic and immune factors. The efficacy of the purified insulins clearly suggests that lipolytic substances have been removed. The contribution of immune factors is suggested by the efficacy of unchromatographed insulin to which steroids have been added,[14] and by the high frequency of allergy in patients with ILA. The sequence of pathophysiologic events that leads to ILA might include sensitization of the subject to the lipolytic substances in impure insulin with development of homocytotropic antibody (IgE) with deposition not only where insulin has been given but at distant sites. When impure insulin is used repeatedly the lipolytic

94

substances combine with the antibody, in some way triggering local factors to produce lipolysis.

The treatment of ILA consists of switching the patient to a more pure form of insulin. If ILA developed while the patient was taking unchromatographed mixed beef-pork insulin, then a switch to single peak mixed beef-pork insulin should be made with the expectation that in 90% of cases resolution can be expected.[9] (See Figure 5-2.) For the patient who does not improve or develops ILA while taking single peak mixed beef-pork insulin, then purified pork insulin (Lilly), or the purified porcine insulins prepared by the Novo or Nordisk Companies in Denmark should be used. If the purified insulins are injected into the affected areas, then improvement should become evident in two to four weeks with complete resolution in a few months. The filling in of the excavated areas is probably due to the lipogenic effect of insulin. Many patients report that the newly filled in areas have a "doughy" feel, which over four to eight weeks takes on the consistency of normal fat. Once an atrophic area fills in another site should be injected until it is filled in. The patient should then begin rotating injection sites; otherwise hypertrophy may occur. If local allergy co-exists, the allergy will improve, usually completely, with the use of the purified pork insulins. Once started on purified porcine insulins patients should remain on these for the rest of their lives, for use of less pure insulin may result in excavation of all the sites that had previously filled in. Reinstitution of treatment with the purified insulins usually produces unsatisfactory results.[4,9]

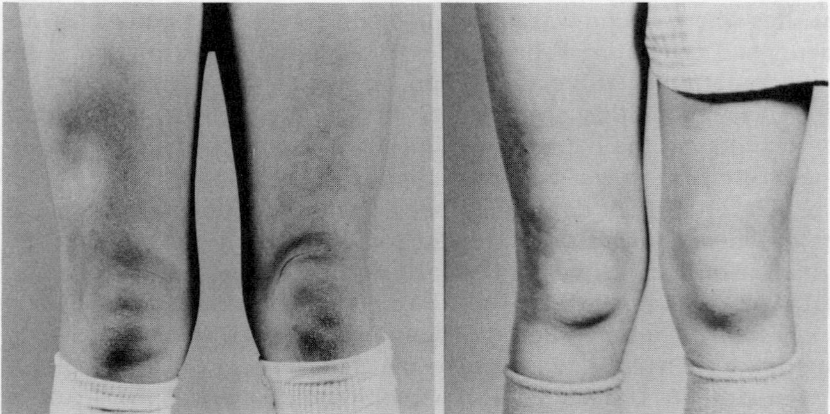

Figure 5-2   B.J., age 8, developed insulin-induced lipoatrophy on mixed beef-pork conventional insulin at the age of 3½ (left). "Single peak" beef-pork Lente and Regular insulins were injected into the site and improvement was noted within 30 days (right). Photographs courtesy of Dr. Gordon Gibbs, University of Nebraska, Omaha.

INSULIN HYPERTROPHY

This condition consists of areas of swelling where insulin has been administered, namely in the arms, anterior thighs, abdomen, and buttocks (Figure 5-3). These are usually soft in consistency and many occur adjacent to areas of atrophy, a finding that accentuates the appearance of both conditions. The cause is unknown but may, at least in part, be due to a local lipogenic effect of insulin. Treatment consists of avoiding the affected areas by rotation of the sites of insulin injection. Over 50% of patients with insulin hypertrophy will improve if treated with the purified pork insulins.[9]

INSULIN ALLERGY

Allergy to insulin occurs in two forms—local and generalized. Local allergy usually consists of itching at the injection site at the time of injection followed by the development over the next two to four hours of a hard, indurated area (immediate reaction). A few patients with local insulin allergy have no reaction for four or more hours after injection (delayed reaction). Occasionally, patients will present with both immediate and delayed reactions.[15]

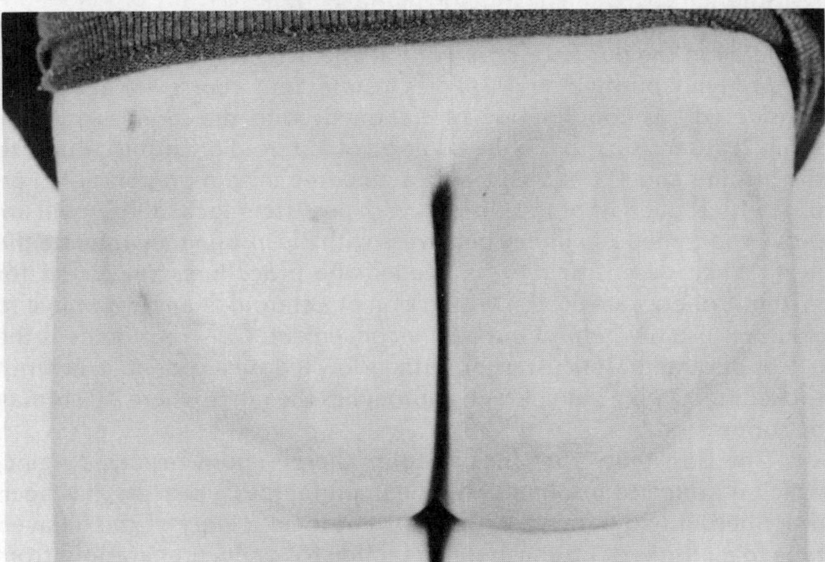

Figure 5-3 J.B.L. was nine years old when the above picture was taken in August, 1973. He had been diabetic since age one. He had been treated with unchromatographed NPH and Regular insulin and later "single peak" mixed beef-pork insulin, but with no improvement. He was lost to follow-up before highly purified pork insulin could be prescribed.

Systemic allergy consists of generalized symptoms and signs varying from itching and hives to angioedema, laryngospasm, hypotension, and, very rarely, anaphylaxis and death. Immediate local and systemic allergy are mediated by IgE antibody.[16,17] About 25% of patients with systemic allergy have a history of local allergy and/or have local reactions concurrent with the systemic manifestations.

In both forms of insulin allergy there is frequently a history of allergies to food and drugs, notably penicillin, or interrupted insulin treatment (which augments the immune response). Moreover, 30% of patients are 20% or more overweight. The frequency of local insulin allergy has been reduced by the availability of the purified insulins.[11] Local allergy may be due to impurities in the insulin,[7] the species source, protamine in the NPH,[18] or to zinc.[19]

Ordinarily, we do not treat local reactions unless they persist for over four to six weeks, sooner if they are a source of particular distress to the patient. Before initiating treatment it is important to rule out errors of injection technique and to be certain the patient is using a high quality alcohol designed specifically for injection site cleansing. Most local reactions will improve if the patient is switched from beef-containing insulins (mixed beef-pork or monospecies beef) to monospecies pork insulin. The purified pork insulins are beneficial in over three quarters of the cases. A small minority of patients, usually children and patients with Type I (juvenile-onset or ketosis-prone) diabetes,[10] improve when monospecies beef insulin is used. This, too, is available in the purified form. For patients who fail to respond to the use of highly purified monospecies insulin, four courses of action are considered[4]: 1) continuation of treatment with the monospecies insulin, 2) desensitization, 3) the addition of a steroid or antihistaminic to the insulin, and 4) treatment with a zinc-free insulin preparation. Fortunately, about half of the patients with persistent local allergy will improve spontaneously if they persevere with the insulin they tolerate the best. When desensitization is needed the procedures suggested for systemic allergy are used. The addition of a steroid or antihistaminic to insulin is usually helpful but also inconvenient. Our first choice is the use of dexamethasone, starting with as low a dose as possible, and not exceeding 0.75 mg daily, which approaches the range where ACTH may be suppressed.[4]

The possibility that local insulin allergy could be due to zinc, which is added to insulin during the manufacturing process, has been described in two patients with persistent local allergy of the delayed type to all forms of insulin, but no reaction to insulin preparations from which the zinc had been removed.[19] The patients had negative intradermal tests to the zinc-free insulins but positive tests to zinc insulin and zinc sulfate. Studies on the peripheral white cells of both patients were consistent with allergy to zinc. The zinc-free insulins are prepared by a chelation reaction which removes the zinc. The resulting material is called "Neutral Sodium Insulin" (NSI), which is soluble and behaves like neutral regular insulin. The time action of NSI may be extended by adding protamine. NSI containing protamine 0.3 mg/100 units has absorption characteristics and bioavailability similar to a 1:1 or 2:1 NPH:Regular mixture. These are investigational drugs and can be obtained only through the Lilly Research Laboratories.

Desensitization to Insulin

An occasional patient with systemic allergy to insulin may tolerate the purified insulins without desensitization. However, such patients can be identified only by trial and error, and the error could be a severe allergic reaction. Therefore,desensitization is recommended for all patients who have systemic and/or refractory local allergy and need insulin. We have used modifications of the methods of Corcoran[21] and Marble.[22] Eli Lilly and Company makes available insulin allergy desensitization kits with the dilutions of insulin in prepared form (Table 5-2). Human serum albumin is added to prevent binding of low concentrations of insulin to glassware. The kits are available as purified monospecies beef and purified monospecies pork.

In order to allow a washout of all insulin in the patient we recommend discontinuing insulin for two to four days before the desensitization procedure is initiated. Since discontinuing insulin in a Type I

Table 5-2
The Dilutions of Regular Insulin Found in the Insulin Allergy Desensitization Kits Prepared by Eli Lilly and Company*

Bottle Label Letter	Unit/0.1 ml	Dilution (in decimal)	Units/ml
A	1/1000	U-0.01	1/100
B	1/500	U-0.02	1/50
C	1/250	U-0.04	1/25
D	1/100	U-0.10	1/10
E	1/50	U-0.20	1/5
F	1/25	U-0.40	2/5
G	1/10	U-1	1
H	1/5	U-2	2
J	1/2	U-5	5
K	1	U-10	10

*Supplied on a complimentary basis on request of the physician.

diabetic is a hazardous procedure, the benefits of which must be carefully weighed, we recommend hospitalization. To shorten the time the patient is without insulin in cases of true insulin-dependency, we switch from intermediate to regular insulin for four days. The latter is given in divided doses every six hours. Desensitization may be initiated 24 hours after the last dose. In ketosis-prone patients, careful attention is given to fluid and electrolyte balance during the period of insulin withdrawal and desensitization by monitoring the serum electrolytes every four to six hours and maintaining a continuous infusion of isotonic saline. Potassium and sodium bicarbonate are used when needed. In one case (a middle-aged woman with labile Type I diabetes), somatostatin was used to delay the deterioration of the metabolic status (Dail, R.W., and Galloway, J.A., personal communication).

Before desensitization is started the patients should be advised of the possibility of severe allergic reactions during the procedure and the necessity of maintaining the desensitized state once it has been achieved (injection of insulin is required at least once—and in many cases, twice—a day). Also, prior to desensitization intradermal skin testing is usually performed using a saline control and 0.1-ml volumes from bottles A and B (1/1000 and 1/500 unit).* Unless the reaction to beef is clearly less than that to pork, desensitization is undertaken with pork insulin. The rationale for this is that over 40% of patients with systemic allergy to insulin have IgG serum antibody titers directed to beef insulin. This falls within the range compatible with a diagnosis of immunologic resistance to beef insulin, the treatment of which is usually pork insulin (see below). No drugs (eg, antihistamines or steroids) that might obscure an allergic reaction are used during the procedure. Desensitization is initiated using 0.1 ml of bottle A either intradermally or subcutaneously. Subsequent doses are given every 30 minutes subcutaneously. If a reaction occurs we drop back two dilutions. Patients with severe allergy may require beginning with 1:10,000 or even 100,000 of a unit, with interpolation of several doses between those supplied in the kit (Table 5-2). In these cases the doses are given every two hours and continued until the procedure is complete.

Over 90% of patients with systemic allergy can be desensitized using the methods described above. The remainder must endure the allergy to insulin, lose weight if they are overweight, tolerate hyperglycemia and its consequences, or be placed on chronic low-dose steroid treatment as suggested by Cockel and Mann.[23]

---

*Allergists prefer to use 0.025-ml volumes, which require special syringes. If this is done, then skin testing is started with bottles C and D (1/250 and 1/100 unit).

INSULIN ANTIBODIES

All patients receiving insulin for more than a few weeks develop antibodies to it of the IgG class.[24] The degree of antibody formation is a function of 1) the patient's inherent immune response, 2) the species source of the insulin—beef insulin, differing at positions 8 and 10 on the α-chain from pork and human, is more immunogenic than the latter two insulins, 3) pharmaceutical form—Lente is more immunogenic than regular,[25] and 4) purity—the purified pork insulins, are the least immunogenic of all insulin preparations. The significance of these antibodies is not known. Clearly they delay the onset and peak action of administered insulin.[26,27] However, Dixon et al[28] have suggested that the presence of some antibody is useful in labile diabetics, acting as a buffer to reduce the immediate effects of absorbed insulin.

Wehner et al[29] have demonstrated that rabbits immunized with A and B component (see Figure 5-1) from commercial insulin develop serum antibodies to insulin. Moreover, insulin:insulin antibody complexes in the kidneys of the animals were found using light and electron microscopy and the lesions were indistinguishable from those of nodular glomerulosclerosis seen in human diabetics. The animals treated with saline or purified pork insulin had neither these lesions nor insulin antibodies in their serum. The significance of these findings is reduced by the fact that patients who have never received insulin develop nodular glomerulosclerosis. Yue and Turtle[30] point out that it will require many years to ascertain whether insulin immunogenicity is causally related to the development of this diabetic complication.

Finally, the use of insulin of low immunogenicity has been related to preservation of endogenous beta-cell function. Thus, Ludvigsson and Heding[31] have demonstrated in Type I diabetes that increased serum antibody titers to insulin are associated with unmeasurable fasting serum C-peptide concentrations. If insulin antibodies have a deleterious effect on endogenous insulin secretion in diabetics, then it is attractive to consider the purified pork insulins for all newly discovered Type I diabetics.

INSULIN RESISTANCE

The presence of this condition is defined as "hyporesponsiveness to or a tolerance of 200 units of insulin daily over a period of time in the absence of infection or coma."[32] However, many patients requiring much lower doses have mechanisms operating in them that result in the need for higher than usual doses than others. The following points should be considered in treating patients with increased insulin requirements:

1. Obesity is the most common cause of increased insulin requirements. The degree of severity of the diabetes in many patients is a function of the extent to which excess weight is present. For a classical case study, the reader's attention is directed to an article by Genuth.[33]

2. Immunologic resistance is the result of high titers of IgG antibody in the serum directed to beef insulin, patients with insulin resistance having values of at least 30 to 50 mU/ml. In evaluating patients with suspected immunologic resistance it is important to know that some commercial laboratories report antibody titers to both beef and pork insulin and the latter may be elevated. Since this elevation is usually not associated with resistance to pork insulin, we ascribe it to cross-reaction in the assay between the anti-insulin antibody and pork insulin. The treatment for immunologic resistance is use of insulin with an amino acid sequence more like human than beef, namely pork insulin. Serum antibodies to beef insulin may cross-react with and bind pork insulin, thereby imparting to it a repository effect otherwise achieved by modifying the insulin with excess zinc (as in Lente) or protamine (as in NPH). Thus, two doses daily of pork regular insulin usually will result in adequate blood glucose control for a 24-hour period. If the diabetes is uncontrolled when pork insulin is about to be started, then the initial doses are the same as those the patient was taking when using mixed beef-pork or monospecies beef insulin. If, on the other hand, a response to mixed beef-pork or monospecies beef insulin has been observed, then the initial doses of pork insulin should be about two thirds of the previous dose of insulin. Although serum antibody titers change slowly, the response to pork insulin, if it is to be favorable, is usually immediate.[34] Consequently, patients should be under careful surveillance when species source is being changed. Once patients have been controlled with moderate doses of monospecies pork insulin, they may be switched to monospecies pork Lente or NPH insulin.

For patients who fail to respond to pork insulin, steroids are recommended. The usual course consists of 40 to 80 mg of prednisone daily for ten days.[35,36] The response to steroids may be striking with the patient demonstrating hypoglycemia after the fifth or sixth day and not requiring insulin treatment for several days thereafter.

For patients who cannot take steroids we recommend sulfated beef insulin, which is an investigational drug, as proposed by Davidson and DeBra.[37] Sulfated insulin is an investigational drug manufactured by the Connaught Laboratories, Toronto, Canada.

Physicians interested in insulin resistance should be aware of two recently characterized forms of insulin resistance. One is apparently due to destruction of the insulin at the injection site,[38,39] and the other to impairment of insulin interaction with its receptors.[5] Fortunately, these conditions are rare. Marked destruction of insulin at the injection site is suggested when patients are controlled on conventional doses of insulin intravenously, but require hundreds or thousands of units when given intramuscularly or subcutaneously. Patients with receptor interference fail to respond to large doses of insulin regardless of the route of administration. The elucidation of the nature of the impairment of the interaction of insulin with its receptors requires special analyses. These are available only at specialized centers such as the National Institutes of Health.[5] Patients with both forms of resistance are subject to spontaneous remission.

OTHER IMMUNOLOGIC PHENOMENA ASCRIBED TO INSULIN AND OTHER SUBSTANCES IN INSULIN

Antibodies to glucagon have been demonstrated in 12% of children from an outpatient department.[40] The antibodies were demonstrated to predispose the patients to nocturnal hypoglycemia, presumably by interfering with the action of endogenous glucagon.

In a study[10] of the concentration of hormonal contaminants in commercial and purified insulins significant quantities of pancreatic glucagon, pancreatic polypeptide (PPP), vasoactive intestinal peptide (VIP) and somatostatin were found in the commercial insulins but not in the highly purified insulins. (PPP is a recently discovered substance that has a molecular weight of 4200 daltons and has been found to be elevated in the plasma of normal subjects in response to meals. VIP, also recently discovered, has a molecular weight of 3300, is widely distributed in the body, and thought to be a neurotransmitter.) Determination of the frequency of increased antibody titers to the contaminants in the sera of 442 insulin-treated diabetic patients disclosed that over half of the diabetics had elevated serum titers to PPP and VIP. Immunocytochemical studies revealed that plasma from diabetics with positive titers to the various insulin contaminants reacted with their respective hormone-producing cells. While the clinical significance of these findings is not known, such reports will undoubtedly increase the use of purified insulins.

Finally, hemolytic anemia is a rare complication of insulin treatment as indicated by the report of a child, age nine, with insulin-resistant diabetes, lymphadenopathy, hepatosplenomegaly, and a Coomb's positive hemolytic anemia.[41] Investigations disclosed that the patient's plasma cells contained anti-insulin antibody (IgG) that was characterized as being identical to serum IgG insulin antibody. Since the child's serum was determined to contain more insulin anti-insulin soluble immune complexes than free anti-insulin antibodies, the authors postulated that these complexes coated the patient's erythrocytes making them Coomb's positive. The patient was treated with porcine insulin and 40 mg of prednisone every other day.

INSULIN EDEMA

Fluid accumulation with or without frank localized (pretibial, presacral, or periorbital) or generalized edema is the rule following institution of proper insulin therapy in poorly controlled diabetic subjects.[42] Insulin edema occurs in patients with normal renal function[42] as well as in patients with renal disease.[43] The diagnosis of insulin edema should be suspected in any patient whose diabetic control has been acutely improved and whose weight gain is disproportionate to the number of calories retained. The mechanisms responsible for insulin edema have not been precisely determined. Marked elevations in serum antidiuretic hormone (ADH) have been reported in uncontrolled diabetes.[44] These are ascribed to the hypovolemia secondary to the osmotic diuresis associated with glycosuria. The importance of ADH in insulin edema is reduced by the fact that marked sodium retention occurs even in the absence of hypovolemia when diabetic control is restored with the weight gain being commensurate with the amount of sodium retained.[42] Since reduction of the blood glucose in poorly controlled diabetics results in an improvement of carbohydrate utilization, the mechanism for the edema may be explained by the hormonal changes that accompany fasting and refeeding.[45] If so, then the fluid retention of insulin edema could be due to a cessation of the natriuretic effects of the hyperglucagonemia present during poor diabetic control (fasting) and the influx of gastrointestinal fluid into the extracellular and subsequently intracellular space during refeeding.[45] Since insulin edema is a self-limited condition, treatment is usually not necessary. On the other hand, if edema is pronounced, then treatment with a diuretic such as a thiazide or furosemide is suggested.

HYPOGLYCEMIA

The single greatest acute hazard for the insulin-dependent diabetic is that of hypoglycemia. The reality of this problem can be appreciated by comparing the insulin and food patterns of the normal person and the insulin-requiring diabetic. Whereas the normal subject matches his insulin to his food, the insulin-requiring diabetic matches his food to his insulin. Because of the inherent problems associated with variations in absorption and bioavailability of the modified insulins, alone or in combination with regular,[46,47] the attempt of the diabetic to synchronize his life-style with injected insulin and to control his blood glucose is fraught with hypoglycemic risks.

The availability of assays that can measure minute amounts of hormones in plasma has made it possible to assess the roles in response to hypoglycemia of various substances known to elevate the blood glucose; the importance of some has been discounted. For instance, in both normals and diabetics the hyperglycemic effects of growth hormone during hypoglycemia have been found to be minimal.[48,49] Also, cortisol appears not to be of consequence in the counterregulation of hypoglycemia.[49] While glucagon is known to protect against hypoglycemia during fasting,[50,51] the degree to which endogenous glucagon prevents or corrects insulin-induced hypoglycemia in diabetics is not clear. In a comparison of plasma glucagon concentrations in normal and insulin-dependent diabetics,[52] equivalent levels of hypoglycemia produced glucagon levels in diabetics that were only 15% of that observed in normals. Also, the blood glucose concentrations of the diabetics were slower to recover than normals. However, it was not possible to ascertain whether the slow response of the diabetics was due to hypoglucagonemia or to a continuing release of insulin from antibodies.

The roles of epinephrine (E) and norepinephrine (NE) have been reviewed by Christensen.[53] The fact is incontrovertible that plasma E rises when the blood glucose falls below normal.[54] Moreover, the two parameters are related roughly inversely, ie, the lower the blood glucose the higher the plasma E. Of interest is the fact that a falling plasma glucose evokes an increase in NE but E does not increase until the blood glucose falls to hypoglycemic levels.

The response of the sympathetic nervous system and change in plasma E and NE in the counterregulation of hypoglycemia has been studied by the use of 2-deoxy-D-glucose, which enters nervous tissue, including brain cells, and simulates intracellular glucopenia. In comparison with normals, in a person with a severed spinal cord there is no change in blood glucose, lactate, or free fatty acids. When 2-deoxy-D-glucose is given to adrenalectomized subjects, a rise in the blood glucose occurs, although it is less than normal. Since lactic acid and free fatty acids do not change, the hyperglycemic effects have been ascribed to NE. The importance of E in the counterregulation of hypoglycemia is reduced by the finding that adrenalectomized patients have normal blood glucose (and glucagon) responses to insulin hypoglycemia.[55] Thus, E and NE appear to be the chief hormones released in response to insulin-induced hypoglycemia. E is released from the adrenal medulla and NE from sympathetic nerve endings and to a lesser extent the adrenal medulla.

Finally, studies in normals[54] have disclosed that insulin-induced hypoglycemia is the result of both a decrease in insulin production and an increase in glucose utilization. The initial phase of the counter-regulatory response is due to hepatic glycogenolysis. Over time gluconeogenesis utilizing alanine is the dominant contributor. Of all the hormones studied, changes in the catecholamines correlated best with the responses observed.[53,54]

It is not clear whether the counterregulatory responses seen in "hypoglycemia" are a falling blood glucose or a low blood glucose or both. In normal subjects studied with a glucose clamp in which the arterial blood glucose was artificially raised to 200 mg/dl and then permitted to fall spontaneously,[56] and in which exogenous insulin was not used, no increase in growth hormone, cortisol, glucagon, or catecholamines was demonstrated when the blood glucose was above normal levels.[56] On the other hand, when an increase in sweating (as indicated by a decrease in skin resistance to galvanic current) was used as a marker for clinical hypoglycemia, insulin-dependent diabetics demonstrated hypoglycemic reactions occurring at a mean blood glucose concentration of 280 ± 192 mg/dl, 70 ± 30 minutes following the administration of regular insulin.[26] The symptoms and signs present during hyperglycemia were identical to those observed when the blood glucose was normal or low. Thus, it is possible that chronic hyperglycemia may result in a higher setting of the level at which the counter-regulatory mechanisms for hypoglycemia are initiated.

Several authors have investigated the prevalence and effects of hypoglycemia in insulin-dependent diabetics. In one study[57] marked "overcontrol" was found in 22 of 135 children being evaluated for diabetic instability. In another,[58] overtreatment with insulin was observed in 70% of 101 unselected juvenile diabetics whose diabetes was regarded as unstable. In a group of 39 unstable diabetics who were monitored overnight, hypoglycemia was documented in 22. In 17 the episode lasted three hours or more.[59] Finally, while electroencephalographic analyses of 40 patients with uncomplicated diabetes disclosed no increased incidence of cerebral dysrhythmia over normals, 51% of patients with a history of frequent insulin reactions had abnormal EEGs.[60]

The clinical picture of a hypoglycemic reaction varies. Not only do the symptoms and signs, listed in Table 5-3, differ from patient to patient, but they frequently vary in the same patient from episode to episode. A useful and often overlooked finding in hypoglycemia is change in body temperature. Slight reductions (0–2°C) occur in mild hypoglycemia.[61] These are ascribed to reduction in heat production and to secretion of sweat, as well as to peripheral vasodilatation and hyperventilation. On the other hand, when the hypoglycemia is severe, fever may occur.[62] In 16 bouts of hypoglycemia in 14 patients, the recorded temperature varied from 1° to 2.5°C. The mechanism was thought to be related to cerebral edema.[62]

Table 5-3
Findings Common in Insulin-Induced Hypoglycemia

Inward nervousness	
Fatigue	
Headache	
Hunger	
Sweating	
Nausea	
Dizziness	
Weakness	Night sweats
Diplopia	Convulsions
Blurred vision	"Night fits"
Lassitude, lethargy	Stertorous breathing
Paresthesia	Focal neurologic deficit
Depression	Stupor
Psychopathic behavior	Coma
Vivid or disturbing dreams	Fever

Clinical studies have made it possible to identify the various stages of a hypoglycemic reaction; a typical full-blown reaction is characterized by a response of the autonomic nervous system as well as by progressive changes of the central nervous system. Sussman et al[63] have pointed out the four stages of an insulin reaction in a diabetic: 1) parasympathetic, characterized by hunger, nausea, eructation, and occasionally bradycardia and mild hypotension; 2) diminished cerebral function, indicated by lethargy, lassitude, frequent yawning, diminished spontaneity of conversation, and inability to do simple calculations; 3) sympathetic, in which epinephrine signs dominate, such as an increase in the systolic and mean blood pressure, sweating, and tachycardia; and 4) hypoglycemic coma and occasionally convulsions. It is important to recognize that whereas some patients demonstrate and are aware of the autonomic nervous system response, others demonstrate and are not aware of it, and still others progress from consciousness to coma with no evidence of autonomic nervous system hyperactivity.[63]

The symptoms and signs of a reaction are especially variable in children. Autonomic symptoms frequently include voracious hunger and faintness. Therefore, a hungry diabetic youngster should be allowed to eat. Motor symptoms may include a feeling of heaviness in the extremities, unsteadiness of gait, a tremor of the hands, or simply easy fatigability. The early cortical signs may include confusion, somnolence, apathy, nervousness, and occasionally hallucinations and delusions.

Two frequent manifestations of hypoglycemia are rebound hyperglycemia with deteriorating blood glucose control, the Somogyi effect,[64,65] and weight gain. The former occurs in Type I diabetics and the latter in Type II (adult-onset, insulin-dependent, nonketotic) diabetics. While the classic Somogyi effect is usually recognized, weight gain as a sign of overtreatment with insulin is occasionally overlooked. Although human investigations of diabetics have apparently not quantitated the lipogenic effects of chronic insulin overdosage,[66] studies in normal rats have clearly shown that sustained hyperphagia results from repeated injections of protamine zinc insulin.[67] The treatment of the Somogyi effect is reduction of the insulin dose. In Type I diabetics the reduction may be in the range of 10% of the daily dose each day. In Type II diabetics the insulin reduction may be as much as 25% of the daily dose.

It should be pointed out that many conditions may mimic and/or occur in conjunction with insulin-induced hypoglycemia. Transient ischemic attacks[68] and hypertensive crises and acute myocardial infarction fall into this category. Hypoglycemia increases the frequency and/or severity of changes in the electrocardiogram, in enzyme concentration, and evidence of myocardial damage in dogs with artificial coronary occlusions over controls, eg, dogs with occluded coronaries but no hypoglycemia. However, human diabetics rarely develop acute myocardial infarction during hypoglycemia. Bradley[70] ascribes the low frequency of myocardial damage during hypoglycemia to the ability of the myocardium to utilize substrates other than glucose, eg, acetoacetate, free fatty acids, and lactic acid.

A final entity to be considered in the differential diagnosis of insulin hypoglycemia is that of postural hypotension, which may be an acute effect of insulin administration in patients with autonomic neuropathy.[71] In such patients systolic and diastolic hypotension follow the intravenous, subcutaneous, or intramuscular injection of insulin. This coincides with the fall in the blood glucose and may persist for several hours after the blood sugar has risen to hyperglycemic levels. Patients frequently cannot distinguish between hypoglycemia and postural hypotension.

Factors and conditions that have been clearly implicated in the development of insulin hypoglycemia are listed in Table 5-4. While most are self-explanatory, a few deserve special comment.

1. With the availability of the new, purified pork insulins, physicians need to be aware of the possibility of a dosage change when patients are switched from conventional mixed beef-pork or monospecies

Table 5-4
Factors and Conditions Resulting in
or Associated with Insulin-Induced Hypoglycemia

Injection technique
  Failure to agitate vial before use
  Improper measurement of insulin
  Injection of insulin into area of hypertrophic lipodystrophy
  Use of insulin in which precipitate has become clumped or granular

Reduction of insulin requirement as a result of natural course of disease
  Spontaneous remission as in Type I diabetes
  Response to diet and weight reduction as in Type II diabetes

Excessive insulin dose
  Exercise
  More rapid absorption as a result of injection into an exercising limb[72]
  Iatrogenic hyperinsulinism, including Somogyi effect
  Factitious hyperinsulinism
  In susceptible patients switching from mixed beef-pork or monospecies beef
    to monospecies pork insulins and rarely switching from a less pure to more
    pure insulin with or without a change in species source

Correction of conditions known to increase insulin requirements
  Infection
  "Hyperendocrinopathies"
  Removal of stress (emotional or surgical)
  Menstruation[79]

Termination of pregnancy

Onset of concurrent diseases resulting in lowering of the blood glucose, eg, islet
cell adenomas, "hypoendocrinopathies," and liver disease

Use of drugs that have hypoglycemic activity or block hyperglycemic counterregulatory mechanism, eg, alcohol and propranolol

---

beef to the pork insulins. Thus, Asplin et al[74] found an average overall
reduction in dosage to be 22%. Our experience in switching patients
from single peak insulins demonstrates very little change in dosage
(Clinical Research Files, Eli Lilly and Company, Indianapolis).
Nonetheless, the possibility of a marked reduction should be considered in all patients being switched from unchromatographed or
single peak insulins, regardless of species source, to the purified pork
insulin preparations. Unfortunately, it is not possible to identify such
patients a priori.

2. Arky et al [75] have pointed out the disastrous potential of the
hypoglycemic effect of insulin in diabetics who drink alcohol. The
mechanism is related to the shut-down of hepatic glucose output by
ethanol.

3. Propranolol is a beta-adrenergic blocker that affects carbohydrate metabolism, especially in diabetics. It may not only block the

108

development of symptoms of hypoglycemia[76] but reduce the rate of recovery from it.[77] An additional risk of the use of propranolol with myocardial disease, particularly in hypoglycemia-prone diabetics with myocardial disease, arises from the imbalance between alpha- and beta-adrenergic activity. The increased alpha function results in systolic and diastolic hypertension, reflex bradycardia, and subsequently ectopic arrhythmias, which may be fatal.[78]

The primary treatment of hypoglycemia is prevention. This is accomplished by careful history-taking and adjustment of insulin and diet. Frequently the movement or addition of a fruit or bread exchange to coincide with exercise and/or the peak hypoglycemic effect of the insulin the patient is taking will suffice. For some patients home monitoring of blood glucose is a procedure that is well worth the expense of the glucose-measuring device.[79] For difficult problems the use of the artificial beta-cell,[80] as reported by Lambert et al,[47] may make it possible to profile the patient's insulin response and make appropriate changes in conventional insulin treatment programs. For additional information on patient responses to insulin and their treatment, the reader is directed to the report by Galloway and Bressler in 1978.[4]

The treatment of insulin-induced hypoglycemia has been previously reported[81] and is recapitulated below.

Class I Alert patient with signs and/or symptoms of hypoglycemia. Treatment consists of oral carbohydrates.

1. Give 100 ml of orange juice or high carbohydrate beverage (Coca-Cola, ginger ale, or juices) every 5 to 10 minutes until symptoms and signs of hypoglycemia are clear, or give glucagon, 1 or 2 mg subcutaneously. If no improvement in 15 minutes, dose may be repeated.*

2. Observe patient for at least one hour or until next meal is taken. If patient has recognized the appearance of hypoglycemia and has treated himself, by prior instruction he will have placed himself near someone who is aware of his condition.

Class II Patient has failed to respond satisfactorily to oral carbohydrate and is either in coma or cannot or will not cooperate in oral administration of carbohydrates.

1. Give glucagon, 1 or 2 mg subcutaneously, if this has not been done. Glucagon can also be given intravenously or intramuscularly. If glucagon has been administered twice as in Class I with no effect, give 20 ml of 50% dextrose in water intravenously. In using glucagon the physician must recognize two important facts. First, nausea, often resulting in vomiting, is a very common complication of glucagon

---

*Glugacon (prepared by Eli Lilly and Company) is supplied as a dry, lyophilized powder in 1- and 10-mg ampoules with diluting fluid included in the package. If kept refrigerated, the 10-mg ampoule has a shelf life in excess of three months after reconstitution.

treatment. Second, the chances for a successful response diminish with the length of time the hypoglycemic reaction has been in progress.[82,83]

2. If neither glucagon nor hypertonic glucose is available, epinephrine, 0.5 ml of 1:1000 solution, may be administered subcutaneously. Dose may be repeated in 15 minutes. In absence of this medication or means for injection, an emergency procedure is 1 teaspoon of honey applied between the teeth and the cheek with the finger. Successive applications may be required, and care must be taken to avoid aspiration.

3. When possible, draw a blood sugar as soon as feasible after administration of glucagon or before administration of intravenous glucose.

4. If patient is unconscious, keep airway open and protect tongue against biting. Remove all pillows.

5. Observe patient carefully. Upon recovery (should occur within 5 to 10 minutes after administration of intravenous glucose and within 15 minutes of administration of glucagon), ascertain cause of the hypoglycemia, if possible.

6. If hypoglycemia is an isolated episode, insulin dosage is not changed. If two reactions have occurred in a 48-hour period, insulin dose usually must be reduced.

Class III   Patient has failed to respond to the above treatments, or is known to have renal disease with mild to marked azotemia, or has evidence of heart, liver, or cerebrovascular disease. These patients must be hospitalized and initial treatment should be carried out, preferably in an emergency or intensive care unit.

1. Do blood glucose, blood urea nitrogen, and hematocrit studies immediately. Blood for electrolytes (Na, Cl, K, CO_2) and remainder of hemogram may be drawn at this time, but ordinarily need not be run on emergency basis.

2. Give 50 gm of 50% dextrose in water intravenously immediately. In children the maximum dose is 0.25 gm/kg, or 0.5 ml/kg of a 50[6] solution.

3. Follow this with continuous drip of 10% dextrose in water. Have intravenous run at 20 drops/min.

4. Place patient in lateral, recumbent position with bed rails up and restraints, if necessary.

5. Record intake and output of fluids.

6. Take vital signs every 30 minutes.

7. Give hydrocortisone, 100 mg, immediately and every eight hours.

If the patient relapses into hypoglycemia with 10% dextrose running at 1.33 ml/min (2000 ml and 200 gm of glucose per 24 hours), depending upon age and the nutritional and cardiovascular status of

110

the patient, we either increase the rate of infusion to 2 ml/min or leave the rate the same but add 100 to 200 ml of 50% dextrose solution to the 10% dextrose. Because the tendency to hypoglycemia may persist for several days, this constant infusion of hypertonic dextrose should not be discontinued until there is satisfactory evidence that the blood sugar will be maintained without the addition of dextrose for at least three hours. Our practice is to keep the vein open using a slow drip of isotonic saline and observe the patient carefully during the period when carbohydrate is withheld. Before the intravenous feeding is discontinued, not only do we require that there are no clinical signs of hypoglycemia, but we insist that the blood sugar be normal or elevated.

REFERENCES

1. Cahill, G.F., Jr., Etzwiler, D.D., and Freinkel, N. Blood glucose control in diabetes. *Diabetes* 25:237–239, 1976.

2. Tchobroutsky, G. Relation of diabetic control to development of microvascular complications. *Diabetologia* 15:143–152, 1978.

3. Bressler, R., and Galloway, J.A. Insulin treatment of diabetes mellitus. *Med Clin North Am.* 55:861–876, 1971.

4. Galloway, J.A., and Bressler, R. Insulin treatment in diabetes. *Med Clin North Am.* 62:663–680, 1978.

5. Kahn, C.R., and Rosenthal, A.S. Immunologic reactions to insulin: insulin allergy, insulin resistance, and the autoimmune insulin syndrome. *Diabetes Care* 2:283–295, 1979.

6. Chance, R.E. Amino acid sequences of proinsulins and intermediates. *Diabetes* 21:461–467, 1972.

7. Galloway, J.A., Root, M.A., Chance, R.E. et al. New forms of insulin. Edited by L.J. Kryston and R.A. Shaw. In *Endocrinology and Diabetes.* New York: Grune & Stratton, 1975, pp 329–342.

8. Root, M.A., Chance, R.E., and Galloway, J.A. Immunogenicity of insulin. *Diabetes* 21:657–660, 1972.

9. Wentworth, S.M., Galloway, J.A., Davidson, J.A. et al. The use of the purified insulins in the treatment of patients with insulin lipoatrophy. Presented at the International Diabetes Federation Meeting, Vienna, Austria, September 13, 1979.

10. Bloom, S.R., Adrian, T.E., Barnes, A.J. et al. Autoimmunity in diabetics induced by hormonal contaminants of insulin. *Lancet* 1:14–17, 1979.

11. Galloway, J.A. Clinical results with new insulin preparations. Juvenile Diabetes Foundation's International Workshop on Insulin, New York, May 4–6, 1978, pp 79–81.

12. Wright, A.D., Walsh, C.H., Fitzgerald, M.G. et al. Very pure porcine insulin in clinical practice. *Br Med J* 1:25–27, 1979.

13. Podolsky, S. Lipoatrophic diabetes and miscellaneous conditions related to diabetes mellitus. Edited by A. Marble, P. White, R.F. Bradley, and L.P. Krall. In *Joslin's Diabetes Mellitus,* 11th Edition. Philadelphia: Lea & Febiger, 1971, pp 722–746.

14. Kumar, D., Miller, L.V., and Mehtalia, S.D. Use of dexamethasone in treatment of insulin lipoatrophy. *Diabetes* 26:296–299, 1977.

15. deShazo, R.D., Levinson, A.I., Boehm, T. et al. Severe persistent biphasic local (immediate and late) skin reactions to insulin. *J Allergy Clin Immunol.* 59:161–164, 1977.

16. Bucholtz, H.K. Insulin allergy: an approach to therapy. *South Med J.* 69:1118–1120, 1976.

17. Mattson, J.R., Patterson, R., and Roberts, M. Insulin therapy in patients with systemic insulin allergy. *Arch Intern Med.* 135:818–821, 1975.

18. Shore, R.N., Shelley, W.B., and Kyle, G.C. Chronic urticaria from isophane insulin therapy. *Arch Dermatol.* 111:94–97, 1975.

19. Feinglos, M.N., and Jegasothy, B.V. "Insulin" allergy due to zinc. *Lancet* 1:122–124, 1979.

20. Cudworth, A.G. "Type I diabetes mellitus." Review article. *Diabetologia* 14:281–291, 1978.

21. Corcoran, A.C. Note on rapid desensitization in a case of hypersensitiveness to insulin. *Am J Med Sci.* 196:359–361, 1938.

22. Marble, A. Allergy and diabetes. Edited by E.P. Joslin, H.F. Root, P. White, and A. Marble. In *The Treatment of Diabetes Mellitus,* 10th Edition. Philadelphia: Lea & Febiger, 1959, pp 395–406.

23. Cockel, R., and Mann, S. Insulin allergy treated by low-dosage hydrocortisone. *Br Med J.* 3:722, 1967.

24. Berson, S.A., Yalow, R.S., Bauman, A. et al. Insulin I[131] metabolism in human subjects: demonstration of insulin binding globulin in circulation of insulin treated subjects. *J Clin Invest.* 35:170–190, 1956.

25. Chance, R.E., Root, M.A., and Galloway, J.A. The immunogenicity of insulin preparations. *Acta Endocrinol.* 83(suppl 205):185–196, 1976.

26. Bolinger, R.E., Stephens, R., Lukert, B. et al. Galvanic skin reflex and plasma free fatty acids during insulin reactions. *Diabetes* 13:600–605, 1964.

27. Bolinger, R.E., Morris, H., McKnight, F.G. et al. Disappearance of I[131]-labeled insulin from plasma as a guide to management of diabetes. *N Engl J Med.* 270:767–770, 1964.

28. Dixon, K., Exon, P.D., and Malins, J.M. Insulin antibodies and control of diabetes. *Q J Med.* 44:543–553, 1975.

29. Wehner, H., Huber, J., and Kronenberg, K.H. The glomerular basement membrane of the rabbit kidney on long-term treatment with heterologous insulin preparations of different purity. *Diabetolgia* 9:255–263, 1973.

30. Yue, D.K., and Turtle, J.R. Antigenicity of "Monocomponent" pork insulin in diabetic subjects. *Diabetes* 24:625–632, 1975.

31. Ludvigsson, J., and Heding, L.G. C-peptide in children with juvenile diabetes. *Diabetologia* 12:627–630, 1976.

32. Smelo, L.S. Insulin resistance. *Proc Am Diabetes Assoc.* 8:75–111, 1948.

33. Genuth, S.M. Insulin secretion in obesity and diabetes: an illustrative case. *Ann Intern Med.* 87:714–716, 1977.

34. Akre, P.R., Kirtley, W.R., and Galloway, J.A. Comparative hypoglycemic response of diabetic subjects to human insulin or structurally similar insulins of animal source. *Diabetes* 13:135–143, 1964.

35. Oakley, W., Field, J.B., Sowton, G.E. et al. Action of prednisone in insulin-resistant diabetes. *Br Med J.* 1:1601–1606, 1959.

36. Field, J.B. Chronic insulin resistance. *Acta Diabetol Lat.* 7:220–241, 1970.

37. Davidson, J.K., and DeBra, D.W. Immunologic insulin resistance. *Diabetes* 27:307–318, 1978.

38. Diaz-Pereda, L., Yang, T.-I., and Knowles, H. Long term use of intravenous insulin because of failure of subcutaneous insulin treatment. *Trans Am Clin Climatol Assoc.* (in press).

39. Paulsen, E.P., Courtney, J.W., III, and Duckworth, W.C. Insulin resistance caused by massive degradation of subcutaneous insulin. *Diabetes* 28:640–645, 1979.

40. Villalpando, S., and Drash, A. Circulating glucagon antibodies in children who have insulin-dependent diabetes mellitus. *Diabetes* 28:294–299, 1979.

41. Faulk, W.P., Tomsovic, E.J., and Fudenberg, H.H. Insulin resistance in juvenile diabetes mellitus. *Am J Med.* 49:133–139, 1970.

42. Saudek, C.D., Boulter, P.R., Knopp, R.H. et al. Sodium retention accompanying insulin treatment of diabetes mellitus. *Diabetes* 23:240–246, 1974.

43. Bleach, N.R., Dunn, P.J., Khalafalla, M.E. et al. Insulin edema. *Br Med J.* 2:177–178, 1979.

44. Zerbe, R.L., Vinicor, F., and Robertson, G.L. Plasma vasopressin in uncontrolled diabetes mellitus. *Diabetes* 28:503–508, 1979.

45. Spark, R.F., Arky, R.A., Boulter, P.R. et al. Renin, aldosterone and glucagon in the natriuresis of fasting. *N Engl J Med.* 292:1335–1340, 1975.

46. Galloway, J.A., Nelson, R.L., Spradlin, C.T. et al. The bioavailability of regular insulin in normal fasted subjects—the effect of mixing with NPH and Lente, of depth, and of method of administration. Presented at the American Diabetes Association Meeting, Los Angeles, June, 1979.

47. Lambert, A.E., Buysschaert, M., and Lambotte, L. Use of an artificial pancreas as a tool to determine subcutaneous insulin doses in juvenile diabetes. *Diabetes Care* 2:256–264, 1979.

48. Fatourechi, V., Molnar, G.D., and Service, F.J. et al. Growth hormone and glucose interrelationships in diabetes: studies with insulin infusion during continuous blood glucose analysis. *J Clin Endoc Metab.* 29:319–327, 1969.

49. Feldman, J.M., Plonk, J.W., and Bivens, C.H. The role of cortisol and growth hormone in the counter-regulation of insulin-induced hypoglycemia. *Horm Metab Res.* 7:378–381, 1975.

50. Unger, R.H. Pancreatin glucagon in health and disease. *Adv Intern Med.* 17:265–288, 1971.

51. Palmer, J.P., Henry, D.P., Benson, J.W. et al. Glucagon response to hypoglycemia in sympathectomized man. *J Clin Invest.* 57:522–525, 1976.

52. Benson, J.W., Jr., Johnson, D.G., Palmer, J.P. et al. Glucagon and catecholamine secretion during hypoglycemia in normal and diabetic man. *J Clin Endocrinol.* 44:459–464, 1977.

53. Christensen, N.J. Catecholamines and diabetes mellitus. *Diabetologia* 16:211–224, 1979.

54. Garber, A.J., Cryer, P.E., Santiago, J.V. et al. The role of adrenergic mechanisms in the substrate and hormonal response to insulin-induced hypoglycemia in man. *J Clin Invest.* 58:7–15, 1976.

55. Ensinck, J.W., Walter, R.M., Palmer, J.P. et al. Glucagon responses to hypoglycemia in adrenalectomized man. *Metabolism.* 25:227–232, 1976.

56. DeFronzo, R.A., Andres, R., Bledsoe, T.A. et al. A test of the hypothesis that the rate of fall in glucose concentration triggers counterregulatory hormonal responses in man. *Diabetes* 26:445–452, 1977.

57. Travis, L.B. Over control of juvenile diabetes mellitus. *South Med J.* 68:767, 1975.

58. Rosenbloom, A.L., Giordano, B.P. Chronic overtreatment with insulin in children and adolescents. *Am J Dis Child* 131:881–885, 1977.

59. Gale, E.A.M., and Tattersall, R.B. Unrecognised nocturnal hypoglycaemia in insulin-treated diabetics. *Lancet* 1:1049–1052, 1979.

60. Greenblatt, M., Murray, J., and Root, H.F. Electroencephalographic studies in diabetes mellitus. *N Engl J Med.* 234:119–121, 1946.

61. Molnar, G.W., and Read, R.C. Hypoglycemia and body temperature. *JAMA.* 227:916–921, 1974.

62. Ramos, E., Zorilla, E., and Hadley, W.B. Fever as a manifestation of hypoglycemia. *JAMA.* 205:590–592, 1968.

63. Sussman, K.E., Crout, J.R., and Marble, A. Failure of warning in insulin-induced hypoglycemic reactions. *Diabetes* 12:38, 1963.

64. Somogyi, M. Exacerbation of diabetes by excess insulin action. *Am J Med.* 26:169–191, 1959.

65. Bloom, M.E., Mintz, D.H., and Field, J.B. Insulin-induced posthypoglycemic hyperglycemia as a cause of "brittle" diabetes. *Am J Med.* 47:891–903, 1969.

66. Bray, G.A. The overweight patient. *Adv Intern Med.* 21:292–308, 1976.

67. Panksepp, J., Pollack, A., Krost, K. et al. Feeding in response to repeated protamine zinc insulin injections. *Physiol Behav.* 14:487–493, 1975.

68. Millikan, C.H. The pathogenesis of transient focal cerebral ischemia. *Circulation* 32:438–450, 1965.

69. Libby, P., Maroko, P.R., and Braunwald, E. The effect of hypolgycemia on myocardial ischemic injury during acute experimental coronary artery occlusion. *Circulation* 51:621–626, 1975.

70. Bradley, R.F. Cardiovascular disease. Edited by A. Marble, P. White, R.F. Bradley, and L.P. Krall. In *Joslin's Diabetes Mellitus,* 11th Edition. Philadelphia: Lea & Febiger, 1971, pp 417–477.

71. Page, M. McB., and Watkins, P.J. Provocation of postural hypotension by insulin in diabetic autonomic neuropathy. *Diabetes* 25:90–95, 1976.

72. Koivisto, V.A., and Felig, P. Effects of leg exercise on insulin absorption in diabetic patients. *N Engl J Med.* 298:79–83, 1978.

73. Walsh, C.H., and Malins, J.M. Menstruation and control of diabetes. *Br Med J.* 2:177–179, 1977.

74. Asplin, C.M., Hartog, M., and Goldie, D.J. Change of insulin dosage, circulating free and bound insulin and insulin antibodies on transferring diabetics from conventional to highly purified porcine insulin. *Diabetologia* 14:99–105, 1978.

75. Arky, R.A., Veverbrants, E., and Abramson, E.A. Irreversible hypoglycemia. *JAMA.* 206:575–578, 1968.

76. Podolsky, S., and Pattavina, C.G. Hyperosmolar nonketotic diabetic coma: a complication of propranolol therapy. *Metabolism.* 22:685–693, 1973.

77. Abramson, E.A., Arky, R.A., and Woeber, K.A. Effects of propranolol on the hormonal and metabolic responses to insulin-induced hypoglycaemia. *Lancet* 2:1386–1389, 1966.

78. Lager, I., Glohme, G., and Smith, U. Effect of cardioselective and non-selective β-blockade on the hypoglycaemic response in insulin-dependent diabetics. *Lancet* 1:458–462, 1979.

79. Tattersall, R.B. Home blood glucose monitoring. *Diabetologia* 16:71–74, 1979.

80. Clemens, A.H., Chang, P.H., and Myers, R.W. The development of biostator, a glucose controlled insulin infusion system (GCIIS). *Horm Metab Res [Suppl].* 7:23–33, 1977.

81. Galloway, J.A. Treatment of hypoglycemia secondary to hypoglycemic agents. *Mod Treat.* 3:412–426, 1966.

82. Galloway, J.A. The pharmacology and clinical use of glucagon. Edited by P.J. Lefebvre, and R.H. Unger. In *Glucagon: Molecular Physiology, Clinical and Therapeutic Implications*. New York: Pergamon Press, 1972, pp 299–318.

83. MacCuish, A.C., Munro, J.F., and Duncan, L.J.P. Treatment of hypoglycaemic coma with glucagon, intravenous dextrose, and mannitol infusion in a hundred diabetics. *Lancet* 2:946–949, 1970.

6 The Oral Hypoglycemic Agents

Thomas W. Boyden, MD

The first sulfonylureas were introduced for clinical use more than 20 years ago. There are currently four sulfonylurea oral hypoglycemic agents (OHA) in common use. Daily insulin injections carry an aura of fear, are bothersome, and frequently cause hypoglycemic episodes. Unfortunately, many physicians and patients have considered the OHA as "oral insulins" without the negative features of injected insulin. Despite the availability of the OHA, people with diabetes mellitus still die from premature cardiovascular disease and renal disease, and suffer from the effects of microangiopathy at a rate that appears unchanged since the introduction of insulin and antibiotics. A separate issue of drug accelerated cardiovascular toxicity has been raised by the University Group Diabetes Program (UGDP). This chapter is a review of what is known about the OHA and should help the physician decide whether an OHA is appropriate therapy for certain patients with diabetes. For a more detailed review of these drugs, the reader is referred to articles by Shen and Bressler[1] and Boyden and Bressler.[2]

Approximately 80% of the diabetic population are insulin-resistant as the basis for their carbohydrate intolerance. Most of these people are overweight and tend to have adult-onset disease, although young people may also have this type of diabetes. It is only this group of adult-onset diabetics that can be considered for therapy with one of the sulfonylureas. Individuals with insulin-deficient diabetes mellitus do not respond to the sulfonylurea OHA. Typical juvenile onset diabetes mellitus and most thin adults with diabetes fall into this category.

ABSORPTION, METABOLISM, AND EXCRETION OF THE SULFONYLUREAS

The sulfonylureas are effectively absorbed from the gastrointestinal tract. The most important clinical difference between sulfonylureas is their duration of action. This is a function of the rate of absorption, rate of metabolism and excretion, and the degree of protein binding in any individual patient. (See Table 6-1).

Patients with liver disease may have prolonged or excessive hypoglycemic effects from tolbutamide and tolazamide. Chronic renal insufficiency impairs the excretion of chlorpropamide and the active form of acetohexamide, prolonging their hypoglycemic action. Individuals with either chronic liver or renal disease ought to have a specific OHA selected or a reduction in their usual dose if this form of hypoglycemic therapy is to be continued.

Daily doses of tolbutamide, tolazamide, acetohexamide, and chlorpropamide should never exceed 3.0 gm, 1.5 gm, 2.5 gm, and 1.0 gm, respectively. Amounts greater than this will not improve glucose tolerance without causing severe side effects.

MECHANISM OF ACTION OF THE ORAL HYPOGLYCEMIC AGENTS

Functioning pancreatic islets are necessary for sulfonylureas to lower blood glucose. The sulfonylureas acutely stimulate insulin release in man, experimental animals, and in vitro preparations.[3] Chronic chlorpropamide treatment of diabetic individuals significantly increases the mean immediate insulin response following glucose infusion after one week and this effect reaches its highest level in one month.[4,5] There is little change in the insulin response 20 to 60 minutes after a glucose challenge. It has been repeatedly demonstrated that short term OHA therapy results in higher insulin and lower plasma glucose levels after an oral glucose load, but with long-term therapy

Table 6-1
Hypoglycemic Agents in Use in the United States

Structure	Drug	Metabolism	Serum Half-life (hr)	Duration (hr)	Mean Effective (gm)	Dose Range (gm)
CH_3–⬡–SO_2–NH–$\overset{O}{\overset{\|}{C}}$–NH–$CH_2$–$CH_2$–$CH_2$–$CH_2$	Tolbutamide	Oxidized in liver; excreted in urine.	4-5	6-12	1.0	0.5-2.0
Cl–⬡ SO_2–NH–$\overset{O}{\overset{\|}{C}}$–NH–$CH_2$–$CH_2$–$CH_3$	Chlorpropamide	Minimally altered; primarily excreted in urine.	35	60	0.25	0.1-0.5
CH_3–⬡–SO_2–NH–$\overset{O}{\overset{\|}{C}}$–NH–N$\big\langle$ CH_2–CH_2–CH_2 / CH_2–CH_2–CH_2	Tolazamide	Liver metabolism. Metabolites excreted in urine.	6-8	10-12	.25	0.1-1.0
CH_3–$\overset{O}{\overset{\|}{C}}$–⬡–$SO_2$–NH–$\overset{O}{\overset{\|}{C}}$–NH–⬡	Acetohexamide	60% reduced in liver to hydroxyhexamide and secreted by renal tubules.	6-8	12-24	0.50	0.25-1.5

the plasma insulin levels are decreased from pretreatment levels even though glucose tolerance remains improved. There has been no demonstration that any sulfonylurea can return diabetic β-cell function to normal.[6-9] (See Figure 6-1.) In a four-year double-blind prospective study that assigned male patients with chemical diabetes to one of five drug groups (chlorpropamide, tolbutamide, acetohexamide, phenformin, placebo) plus diet therapy, there were no significant differences between the placebo group and each of the drug groups with regard to the number of subjects having changed insulin secretory dynamics.[10]

An additional explanation for the hypoglycemic effects during chronic sulfonylurea therapy may be the extrapancreatic effects of these drugs.[8,11] Normal subjects given intravenous tolbutamide can be shown to increase the peripheral utilization of ^{14}C-glucose, but this effect was not shown in diabetic subjects.[12] Chlorpropamide has been shown to potentiate the hepatic action of insulin to inhibit glucagon-stimulated hepatic glucose production in vitro.[13]

Our understanding of the chronic hypoglycemic effects of the OHA remains incomplete. Delayed reappearance of hyperglycemia is a continually evolving feature of sulfonylurea therapy of diabetes mellitus and may be partly explained by the loss of increased insulin response after several months of therapy.

INTERACTION OF THE SULFONYLUREAS WITH OTHER DRUGS AND LABORATORY TESTS

Drugs known to decrease glucose tolerance also antagonize the hypoglycemic action of insulin and the oral hypoglycemic agents.

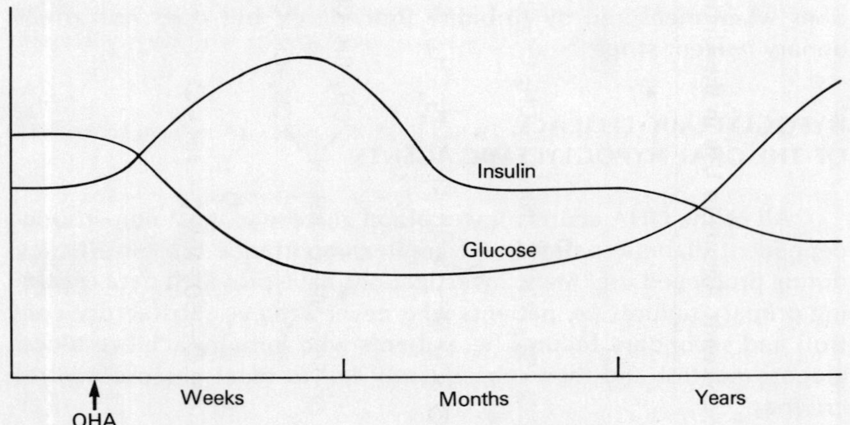

Figure 6-1 Postprandial serum insulin and glucose concentrations in response to acute and chronic therapy with an OHA in the usual insulin-resistant patient with diabetes.

These drugs include glucocorticoids in pharmacologic doses, excessive doses of thyroid hormone, thiazide diuretics, furosemide, estrogen and progestogen preparations, nicotinic acid in pharmacologic doses, and phenytoin. Drugs known to potentiate the action of the sulfonylureas are shown in Table 6-2.

Table 6-2
Potentiation of Sulfonylurea Action by Other Drugs

	Tolbutamide	Acetohexamide	Tolazamide	Chlorpropamide
MAO inhibitors	+	+	+	+
Clofibrate	?	?	?	+
Phenylbutazone	+	+		
Probenecid				+
Salicylates	?	?	?	+
Sulfonamides	+	?	?	+
Chloramphenicol	+			+
Methandrostenolone	+			
Allopurinol				?
Acetazolamide	?	?	?	?

+ indicates important potentiation of hypoglycemic effect
? indicates potential interaction to increase hypoglycemic effect

Laboratory evidence of hypothyroidism develops in a small number of patients receiving OHA. Acetohexamide has a uricosuric effect and individuals with diabetes and an elevated serum urate concentration may improve both abnormalities with this agent. Tolbutamide may produce false positive urinary protein determinations when measured by turbidity procedures, but does not affect urinary reagent strips.[14]

HYPOGLYCEMIC EFFICACY
OF THE ORAL HYPOGLYCEMIC AGENTS

All of the OHA acutely lower blood glucose in most non–insulin-dependent diabetic patients. Of greater importance is their efficacy during prolonged use. Many investigations have provided data regarding primary failures (ie, patients who never achieve satisfactory control) and secondary failures (ie, patients who initially achieve blood glucose control and then subsequently fail to meet glucose control criteria).

One of the earliest investigations of failure rates examined 200 adult-onset diabetics treated with tolbutamide over a three-year period.[15] In this study tolbutamide was used in daily doses as large as 3 gm. Failure was defined as either persistent ketonuria, persistent fasting blood sugars greater than 200 mg/dl, or persistent symptoms. Using these rather liberal indices of failure, there were 16% primary failures and a secondary failure rate of 3% per month. Viewed another way, this would mean that 50% of the initial responders will be secondary failures every two years and would predict more than 90% failures after 10 years.

A group of 2500 diabetic patients given tolbutamide were followed for five years.[16] The primary failures constituted 18% of the patients. At the end of the five years there were 22% secondary failures. Another group of 1218 subjects followed up to five years supported this 20% secondary failure rate.[17]

A literature review of 1821 patients reported over a 12-year period found the primary failure rate to range from 6.2% to 21% and the secondary failure rate from 18.6% to 31.6%.[18] A nine-year experience with 3387 patients showed that 61% had continuously satisfactory responses to tolbutamide although only 10% of the patients were actually known to be taking the drug after nine years.[19] The overall secondary failure rate was 25%, but after the first two years failure occurred in one fourth of the patients annually.

The studies presented have all shown that the best results are obtained in maturity-onset diabetics with normal or above normal body weight. Older patients and those with a shorter duration of disease also have a greater likelihood of success using sulfonylureas. In a unique study that used a placebo challenge every two years, it was found that only 21% of subjects taking tolbutamide and 31% on chlorpropamide therapy had satisfactory control after an average of 30 months.[20] Without the use of such a placebo challenge, the success rates in other series may well be overestimated in that an unspecified number of the satisfactorily controlled patients did not require the drug to maintain control.

The idea of a placebo challenge in patients receiving oral hypoglycemic agents has been advocated as a periodic screening to test the need for therapy. Hypoglycemic agents were replaced by placebo in one study of 62 diabetic patients who had previously been diet failures.[21] Most of the patients were considered to be in good to excellent control before the switch. The long-term blood sugar control remained unchanged in 31% and control worsened within six months in the remainder. A similar investigation was carried out in 50 diabetics receiving long-term chlorpropamide therapy.[22] Placebo was substituted in a single-blind fashion. Mean fasting blood glucose did not change in 54% of the patients and actually decreased in three.

Some investigations have documented absolutely no benefit in glucose tolerance with chronic OHA therapy. Male diabetics receiving diet instruction and one of the OHA or placebo were followed with annual glucose tolerance tests.[10] Comparison between the placebo group and each of the drug groups showed no significant differences between the number of subjects with normal glucose tolerance in each of the tests. Comparison between the initial test and each of the subsequent tests for each group failed to show a greater number of normal glucose tolerance tests in any group except at the first follow-up in those subjects taking chlorpropamide. Most notable has been the data from the University Group Diabetes Program.[23] After eight years of therapy, the 106 tolbutamide treated patients who appeared for the final visit had mean fasting blood glucose levels 2.3% above baseline.

Most adult-onset normal weight or overweight diabetics have normal or excessive amounts of circulating insulin. This state of insulin resistance is usually correctable by weight reduction. The standard of therapy in this diabetic population should be diet manipulation. Comparing OHA to diet therapy provides additional insight into drug efficacy. In a study that examined failure rates in patients receiving sulfonylureas or diet therapy, the 288 patients receiving sulfonylureas had 24.3% primary failures and 14.2% of the remainder failed within three years.[24] This was contrasted with 355 comparable diabetics treated with diet alone that had a failure rate of 19.5%. During recruitment for a long-term study of OHA, intensive dietary management was instituted to serve as a baseline for further comparisons and to act as an exclusion criterion.[25] Fifty-seven patients were seen by a dietician monthly and instructed on weight reduction diets as well as restricting carbohydrate to 40% of the total calories. At the end of six months the mean weight loss was 8.2 kg and only six patients (10.5%) qualified for OHA (ie, FBG > 200 mg/dl).

One final consideration has been the use of oral antidiabetic drugs in the prophylactic treatment of asymptomatic diabetes. When 42 adult, asymptomatic diabetic patients were enrolled in a randomized double-blind study with either tolbutamide or placebo, there was no reduction to normal in the repeat three-hour glucose tolerance tests done after 14 months of treatment.[26] Comparing 350 asymptomatic diabetics randomly assigned into tolbutamide, phenformin, and placebo groups, the difference in the sum of glucose tolerance values of the placebo and the tolbutamide groups was not statistically significant after 78 months although the tests were performed after stopping the drugs for three days.[27] In these prophylactic treatment attempts of asymptomatic adult-onset diabetes, there was no improvement in glucose tolerance in either the tolbutamide or the phenformin group. There was also no difference in the frequency of overt diabetes between placebo and tolbutamide, or in the incidence of mortality from all causes or from cardiovascular disease.

122

The available data regarding the long-term efficacy of the OHA is disappointing. Primary failure rates conceivably could be minimized by judicious patient selection. But the secondary failure rates indicate that these drugs are not as reliable as insulin for the treatment of this disease. By itself, the lack of chronic hypoglycemic efficacy may not justify abandoning these drugs. However, there does not appear to be any justification for treating the asymptomatic individual with mild to moderate carbohydrate intolerance in hopes of preventing deterioration of the diabetic state.

EFFECTS OF THE ORAL HYPOGLYCEMIC AGENTS ON SERUM LIPID CONCENTRATIONS

Diabetic individuals frequently have hyperlipidemia and premature atherosclerosis. Any drug used to lower blood sugar may alter lipid metabolism and interest in the effects of the OHA on plasma lipids continues. There are multiple conflicting reports about changes in plasma lipids occurring in patients taking OHA.

The OHA did not change the serum concentrations of triglycerides or cholesterol in four separate studies of diabetic patients.[28-31] More recently a prospective four-year study in male chemical diabetic subjects demonstrated no significant changes in serum cholesterol or triglycerides using sulfonylureas or phenformin.[10] In contrast, there are at least three investigations that reported a reduction in the serum concentration of cholesterol following therapy with OHA.[32-34]

Plasma concentrations of high density lipoprotein cholesterol (HDL-C) correlate inversely with the risk of developing ischemic heart disease and peripheral vascular disease. The plasma HDL-C concentration appears to be a better predictor of these events than either plasma cholesterol or triglyceride concentration. Patients with diabetes receiving various treatments have been examined for their plasma HDL-C concentrations. HDL-C levels in those patients who were treated with OHA were significantly lower than diabetic patients treated with diet or with insulin, or a control population.[35,36] This relationship was valid regardless of the degree of glucose control as reflected by the measurement of hemoglobin A_{1c} concentrations.

TOXICITY OF THE ORAL HYPOGLYCEMIC AGENTS

Clinical Safety

There are numerous side effects associated with the use of oral hypoglycemic drugs. In a series of 9168 patients taking tolbutamide, the overall frequency of side effects was 3.2%.[37] These reactions primarily consisted of hematologic, cutaneous, and gastrointestinal problems. Sulfonylurea-induced hypothyroidism occurs in a small percentage of patients.

Chlorpropamide can cause water intoxication and symptomatic dilutional hyponatremia.[38] It exerts its antidiuretic action both by increasing release of antidiuretic hormone and by augmenting the hormone's renal effects. Chlorpropamide, and to a lesser extent the other sulfonylureas, may provoke an Antabuse-like reaction to ethanol.

All of the sulfonylureas cause severe hypoglycemia. In a review of 473 episodes of drug-induced hypoglycemia, it was found that 220 cases could be attributed to a single sulfonylurea.[39] Chlorpropamide, the longest acting agent, was responsible in over half of the cases. There was a fatality rate of 11% and irreversible brain damage or other serious sequelae in another 5%. Most studies have implicated hepatic or renal insufficiency as a prerequisite for hypoglycemia when the sulfonylureas are used at conventional doses, but this is not always the case. Symptoms may appear suddenly after long, uneventful therapy. Factitious hypoglycemia induced with a sulfonylurea is being more frequently recognized.

Animal Studies

In general, people with diabetes show an increased morbidity and mortality from all cardiovascular diseases. The UGDP raised the possibility that the OHA might accelerate cardiovascular disease in persons with diabetes.[40] Subsequent to the UGDP clinical study several animal investigations have attempted to look at various aspects of cardiac disease related to the administration of the OHA. The chronic effects of tolbutamide on the coronary arteries of Rhesus monkeys fed an atherogenic diet has been studied.[41] After 18 months the animals were sacrificed and the coronary arteries examined for the frequency and severity of atheromatous lesions. Lesions in the three main coronary arteries were nearly twice as frequent and three times as severe in the tolbutamide-treated animals as in the control animals. Using alloxan-diabetic dogs, cardiac hemodynamics were examined in untreated controls and those treated with 250 mg/day of tolbutamide.[42] After one year, treated diabetic dogs had a significantly higher left ventricular end-diastolic pressure (LVEDP) and an abnormal response to acute volume expansion when compared to untreated controls and normals. Tolbutamide did improve glucose tolerance but appeared to cause reduction of left ventricular function and also altered the myocardial morphology beyond that seen in untreated diabetic dogs.

124

At serum concentrations of drug attained clinically, tolbutamide, tolazamide, chlorpropamide, and acetohexamide have been shown to increase contractility in rabbit atria and to increase the rate and slope of depolarization in Purkinje fibers.[43]

THE UNIVERSITY GROUP DIABETES PROGRAM

The University Group Diabetes Program (UGDP) was begun in order to determine whether or not control of blood glucose helps to prevent or delay vascular disease in non–insulin-dependent diabetic patients. Over 800 patients were randomly assigned to each of five treatment groups: placebo, a standard dose of tolbutamide (1.5 gm/-day), a fixed dose of insulin, a variable dose of insulin, or a standard dose of phenformin (100 mg/day). The patients were followed for over eight years at 12 treatment centers. Analysis of the results for the first four treatment groups led to the conclusion that the combination of diet and tolbutamide was no more effective than diet alone in prolonging life. In fact, tolbutamide plus diet was less effective than diet alone or diet plus insulin with regard to cardiovascular mortality.[40] There was an excess cardiovascular mortality of nearly 1% per year in the tolbutamide group compared to diet alone or diet plus insulin.

An analysis of the nonfatal events in the UGDP patients treated with tolbutamide also provides no evidence of benefit associated with the long-term use of this drug.[23] The mean fasting blood sugar was 2.3% above baseline at the end of follow-up for the tolbutamide group. Specifically, there were no significant differences in serum cholesterol, body weight, blood pressure, digitalis use, renal impairment, retinal changes, or nonfatal myocardial infarctions between the tolbutamide plus diet group and the diet only group. Although the total occurrence of fatal and nonfatal myocardial infarctions was not different among the treatment groups, the results showed that myocardial infarctions were more likely to be fatal for patients in the tolbutamide-treated group. These observations are consistent with the observation that sulfonylurea drugs may produce an enhanced inotropic effect on myocardium.[43]

There have been many critics of the UGDP. A special committee of the Biometric Society reviewed the biostatistical aspects of the UGDP and could find no evidence that the baseline differences arising from randomization contributed in any important way to the adverse effects of tolbutamide.[44] The bulk of the mortality in the tolbutamide group has been alleged to four clinics and suggested that this represented a special clinic effect. But the Biometric Society's report concluded that the excess mortality is not in fact confined to a few clinics. A major cardiovascular risk factor, smoking history, was not included in the baseline risk factors. Control of hypertension and blood lipids were also unmonitored variables. By random assignment of patients to different treatment groups, these and other relevant cardiovascular variables would tend to be evenly distributed among all the groups. An FDA team has audited the UGDP study and confirmed the original conclusions.[45] There were some errors and discrepancies found by the audit team, but none appeared to invalidate the conclusions about tolbutamide.

OTHER HUMAN STUDIES
WITH THE ORAL HYPOGLYCEMIC AGENTS

Considerably more attention has been given to patients receiving the OHA since the publication of the UGDP results. None of the subsequent investigations has been as expensive, as detailed, as careful, or as large.

A six-year prospective study of 186 newly diagnosed adult-onset diabetics showed that the 71 patients treated with OHA had a greater frequency of myocardial infarctions than the 115 patients on diet therapy alone.[46] This study requires caution in its interpretation because the patients were allocated to treatment on the basis of their blood sugar responses, that is, those with the worst carbohydrate tolerance were given OHA.

A group of 184 diabetic patients with acute myocardial infarcts, documented by ECG and enzyme changes, was examined for mortality.[47] On admission, 27 patients were being treated with diet only, 90 were taking OHA (mean duration of treatment, 5.7 years) and 67 patients were receiving insulin (mean duration of treatment, 12.9 years). In-hospital mortality was 15% in the diet group, 40% in the OHA group, and 37% in those taking insulin. The mortality rate was slightly higher in the OHA group even though the insulin-treated patients had a higher incidence of hypertension, angina, congestive heart failure, and retinopathy. It was also reported that 12% of the patients taking OHA had primary ventricular fibrillation, compared to 3% in the insulin group and 7% of the diet group. Small numbers of patients and nonrandom assignment to treatment poses problems in interpreting this data.

The 248 patients in the Bedford study[48] with borderline diabetes have been considered comparable to the UGDP group. They were treated with placebo or 1 gm of tolbutamide daily. The patients were matched for age and sex only. Their data on cardiovascular events included a variety of changes that were not mutually exclusive: angina, intermittent claudication, worsening of ECG changes, cerebrovascular accidents, or death. Baseline inequalities (other than sex and age), lack of blind evaluation procedures, likely duplications in cardiovascular events, and the low dose of tolbutamide make the findings of fewer cardiovascular events in the tolbutamide group open to serious question.

A retrospective analysis of survival in over 6000 diabetics enrolled at the Joslin Clinic revealed that 20% could be considered as a pure tolbutamide group, 38% as a pure insulin group, 15% as a diet group, and the remainder as a combination group.[49] In general, patients with the mildest disease were given diet alone and those with the worst glucose tolerance were treated with insulin. The overall probability of death was greater for the insulin group than for the tolbutamide group, but the probability of death from atherosclerotic heart disease was higher in the tolbutamide group. Even within individual cardiovascular risk factor categories the probability of death from cardiovascular causes was greater for patients receiving tolbutamide than for those in any other treatment group. This statistical review found results consistent with those of the UGDP. Specifically, there was no indication that long-term tolbutamide treatment reduced the likelihood of death from cardiovascular disease.

The Coronary Drug Project Research Group recently reported on the prognostic importance of plasma glucose levels and of OHA use after myocardial infarctions in men.[50] In men with baseline hyperglycemia there was evidence of an increased mortality in users of OHA compared to nonusers.

The UGDP project is probably one of the most expensive and technologically advanced therapeutic trials ever completed. Because of its complexity and its findings the study has been repeatedly dissected and occasionally attacked. The analysis by a committee of the Biometric Society and the FDA audit attest to the validity of the UGDP methods and conclusions. The probability that the OHA cause excessive cardiovascular mortality remains valid.

RECOMMENDATIONS FOR THE USE
OF ORAL HYPOGLYCEMIC AGENTS

There is no evidence that the OHA can return carbohydrate tolerance to normal or prevent diabetic complications. People with asymptomatic carbohydrate intolerance ought to be observed for the development of overt diabetes. Overweight individuals should be counselled to lose weight. Achieving normal body weight in the obese, insulin-resistant subject is the only means known to regain normal carbohydrate tolerance. In addition, the majority of persons identified as having glucose intolerance without overt diabetes do not go on to develop diabetes and exposing this population to the hazards of drug administration does not seem justified.

The more important decision is whether or not the OHA should be used to treat individuals with obvious insulin-resistant diabetes mellitus. Those who would favor the use of OHA for these patients find many objectionable aspects of the UGDP study design or analysis, and correctly point out the flaws in the smaller and retrospective analyses. The definitive study examining efficacy and safety of the OHA has not been done, and probably will not be done. Those who argue against using the OHA attest to the validity of the clinical studies, as well as the animal data, suggesting that the OHA have cardiovascular toxicity and little chronic hypoglycemic efficacy.

For the symptomatic maturity-onset diabetic who cannot physically administer insulin injections, who cannot achieve substantial weight loss, and whose need for control is of relatively short duration, the OHA are useful and have predictable glucose lowering effects. None of the clinical studies have suggested any cardiovascular toxicity with short-term use of the OHA. But this special situation can only account for a small percentage of all adult-onset diabetics.

Patients with diabetes are usually not candidates for short-term therapy and the suitability of the OHA for chronic administration must be determined by the individual physician for each patient. If the decision is made to use an OHA, one of the shorter acting preparations is preferable. This should minimize the chances of drug-induced hypoglycemia and hyponatremia, and allow periodic short-term cessation of therapy to monitor the need for continued drug administration. The patients who have achieved a sustained weight reduction would be expected to remain asymptomatic without drugs. Those who become symptomatic when an OHA is stopped deserve intensive dietary instruction or consideration for insulin therapy.

REFERENCES

1. Shen, S.W., and Bressler, R. Clinical pharmacology of oral antidiabetic agents. *N Engl J Med.* 296:493–497; 787–793; 1977.

2. Boyden, T.W., and Bressler, R. Oral hypoglycemic agents. *Adv Intern Med.* 24:53–70, 1979.

3. Widstrom, A., and Cerasi, E. On the action of tolbutamide in normal man. *Acta Endocrinol.* 72:506–518, 1973.

4. Hecht, A. Gershbert, H., and Hulse, M. Effect of chlorpropamide treatment on insulin secretion in diabetics: its relationship to the hypoglycemic effect. *Metabolism* 22:723–733, 1973.

5. Chu, P.C., Conway, M.J., Krouse, H.A. et al. The pattern of response of plasma insulin and glucose to meals and fasting during chlorpropamide therapy. *Ann Intern Med.* 68:757–769, 1968.

6. Barnes, A.J., Crowley, M.F., Barbien, J.K.T. et al. Effect of short and long term chlorpropamide treatment on insulin release and blood glucose. *Lancet* 2:69–72, 1974.

7. Boshell, B.R., Fox, O.J., Roddam, R.F. et al. The effect of sulfonylurea agents on insulin secretion and insulin reserve. Edited by W.J.H. Butterfield, and W. Van Westering. In *Tolbutamide After Ten Years*. International Congress Series No. 149. Amsterdam: Excerpta Medica, 286–297, 1967.

8. Feldman, J.M., and Lebovitz, H.E. Endocrine and metabolic effects of glybenclamide: evidence for an extrapancreatic mechanism of action. *Diabetes* 20:745–755, 1971.

9. Duckworth, W.C., Solomon, S.S., and Kitabachi, A.E. Effect of chronic sulfonylurea therapy on plasma insulin and proinsulin levels. *J Clin Endocrinol Metab*. 35:585–591, 1972.

10. Tan, M.H., Graham, C.A., Bradley, R.F. et al. The effects of long-term therapy with oral hypoglycemic agents on the oral glucose tolerance test dynamics in male chemical diabetes. *Diabetes* 26:561–570, 1977.

11. Feldman, J.M., and Lebovitz, H.E. Biological activities of tolbutamide and its metabolites. *Diabetes* 18:529–537, 1969.

12. Searle, G.L., Mortimore, G.E., Buckley, R.E. et al. Plasma glucose turnover in humans as studied with ^{14}C-glucose: influence of insulin and tolbutamide. *Diabetes* 8:167–173, 1959.

13. Blumenthal, S.A. Potentiation of the hepatic action of insulin by chlorpropamide. *Diabetes* 26:485–489, 1977.

14. Hansten, P.D. *Drug Interactions*. Philadelphia: Lea & Febiger, 1975.

15. DeLawter, D.E., Moss, J.M., Tyroler, S. et al. Secondary failure of response to tolbutamide treatment. *JAMA*. 171:1786–1792, 1955.

16. Camerini-Dávalos, R.A., and Marble, A. Incidence and causes of secondary failure in treatment with tolbutamide: experience with 2,500 patients treated up to five years. *JAMA*. 181:1–9, 1962.

17. Schöffling, K., Pfeiffer, E.F., Ditschuncit, H. et al. Funf johre sulfonylharnstoff-therapie des diabetes mellitus. *Med Welt*. 16:827–835, 1961.

18. DeLawter, D.E., Moss, J.M. Twelve years experience with oral agents in the treatment of diabetes mellitus. *Med Times*. 96:855–864, 1968.

19. Balodimos, M.C., Camerini-Dávalos, R.A., and Marble, A. Nine years' experience with tolbutamide in the treatment of diabetes. *Metabolism* 15:957–970, 1966.

20. Singer, D.L., and Hurwitz, D. Long-term experience with sulfonylureas and placebo. *N Engl J Med*. 277:450–456, 1967.

21. Tomkins, A.M., and Bloom, A. Assessment of the need for continued oral therapy in diabetes. *Br Med J*. 1:649–651, 1972.

22. Lev-Ran, A. Trial of placebo in long-term chlorpropamide-treated diabetics. *Diabetologia* 10:197–200, 1974.

23. University Group Diabetes Program. A study of the effects of hypoglycemic agents on vascular complications in patients with adult-onset diabetes. VI. Supplementary report on nonfatal events in patients treated with tolbutamide. *Diabetes* 25:1129–1153, 1976.

24. Mehnert, H. Clinical and experimental findings after 5 years' treatment of diabetes with sulfonylureas. *Diabetes* 11(suppl):80–84, 1962.

25. Hadden, D.R., Montgomery, D.A.D., Skelly, R.J. et al. Maturity onset diabetes mellitus: response to intensive dietary management. *Br Med J*. 3:276–278, 1975.

26. Engehardt, H.T., and Vecchio, T.J. The long-term effect of tolbutamide glucose tolerance in adult, asymptomatic, latent diabetes. *Metabolism* 14:885–890, 1965.

27. Feldman, R., Crawford, D., Elashoff, R. et al. Oral hypoglycemic drug prophylaxis in asymptomatic diabetes. Edited by W.J. Malaisse, J. Pirart, and J.

Vallance-Owen. In *Diabetes, Proceedings of the Eighth Congress of the International Diabetes Federation, Brussels.* New York: Elsevier North-Holland, 1973, pp 574–587.

28. Bowers, C.Y., Muldrey, J.E., and Hamilton, J.G. Blood lipid and glucose levels of patients with diabetes mellitus treated with chlorpropamide. *Am J Med Sci.* 247:676–681, 1964.

29. Schwartz, M.J., Mirsky, S., and Schaefer, L.E. The effect of phenformin hydrochloride on serum cholesterol and triglyceride levels of the stable adult diabetic. *Metabolism* 15:808–822, 1966.

30. Belknap, B.H., Amaral, J.A.P., and Bierman, E.L. Plasma lipids and mild glucose intolerance. I. The response of plasma triglycerides to high carbohydrate feeding and the effect of tolbutamide therapy. Edited by W.J.H. Butterfield, and W. Van Westerling. In *Tolbutamide After Ten Years.* Augusta, Mich.: Brook Lodge Symposium, 1967, pp 159–170.

31. Belknap, B.H., Bagdad, J.D., Amaral, J.A.P. et al. Plasma lipids and mild glucose intolerance. II. A double-blind study of the effect of tolbutamide and placebo in mild adult diabetic outpatients. Edited by W.J.H. Butterfield, and W. Van Westerling. Augusta, Mich.: Brook Lodge Symposium, 1967, pp 171–176.

32. Shipp, J.C., and Munroe, J.F. Effects of sulfonylurea compounds on hyperlipemia and hypercholesterolemia in patients with minimal impairment of glucose tolerance. *Diabetes* 11(suppl):69, 1962.

33. Morris, J.H., West, D.A., and Bolinger, R.E. Effect of oral sulfonylurea on plasma triglycerides in diabetics. *Diabetes* 13:87–89, 1964.

34. Bressler, R., and Katz, R. Evaluation of tolazamide in the treatment of diabetes mellitus. *Curr Ther Res.* 7:219–225, 1965.

35. Calvert, G.D., Graham, J.J., Mannik, T. et al. Effects of therapy on plasma-high-density-lipoprotein cholesterol concentration in diabetes mellitus. *Lancet* 2:66–68, 1978.

36. Kennedy, A.L., Lappin, T.R.J., Lavery, R.D. et al. Relation of high-density lipoprotein cholesterol concentrations to type of diabetes and its control. *Br Med J.* 2:1191–1194, 1978.

37. O'Donovan, C.J. Analysis of long-term experience with tolbutamide (Orinase) in the management of diabetes. *Curr Ther Res.* 1:69, 1959.

38. Moses, A.M., Howanitz, J., and Miller, M. Diuretic action of three sulfonylurea drugs. *Ann Intern Med.* 78:541–544, 1973.

39. Seltzer, H.S. Drug-induced hypoglycemia: a review board on 473 cases. *Diabetes* 21:955–966, 1972.

40. University Group Diabetes Program. A study of hypoglycemic agents on vascular complications in patients with adult-onset diabetes. II. Mortality results. *Diabetes* 19(suppl):789–830, 1970.

41. Borensztajn, J., Getz, G.S., Glagor, S. et al. A study of the chronic effects of tolbutamide in the Rhesus monkey. *Senate Hearings* 28:13560–13566, 1975.

42. Wu, C.F., Haider, B., Ahmed, S.S. et al. The effects of tolbutamide on the myocardium in experimental diabetes. *Circulation* 55:200–205, 1977.

43. Lasseter, K.D., Levery, G.S., Palmer, R.F. et al. The effect of sulfonylurea drugs on rabbit myocardial contractility, canine Purkinje fiber automaticity and adenyl cyclase activity from rabbit and human heart. *J Clin Invest.* 51:2429–2434, 1972.

44. Report of the Committee for the Assessment of Biometric Aspects of Controlled Trials of Hypoglycemic Agents. *JAMA.* 231:583–608, 1975.

45. Audit confirms conclusions of UGDP study on oral diabetic drugs. *FDA Drug Bull.* 8:34–36, 1978–79.

46. Boyle, D., Bhatea, S.K., Hadden, D.R. et al. Ischaemic heart-disease in diabetics, a prospective study. *Lancet* 1:338–339, 1972.

47. Soler, N.G., Bennett, M.A., Lamb, P. et al. Coronary care for myocardial infarction in diabetics. *Lancet* 1:475–477, 1974.

48. Keen, H. Factors influencing the progress of atherosclerosis in the diabetic. *Acta Diabetol Lat.* 1(suppl):444–462, 1971.

49. Kanarek, P.H. Assessing survival in a diabetic population. *Senate Hearings* 28:13393–13401, 1975.

50. Coronary Drug Project Research Group. The prognostic importance of plasma glucose levels and of the use of oral hypoglycemic drugs after myocardial infarctions in men. *Diabetes* 26:453–465, 1977.

7 The Value of Control of the Blood Glucose Level in Patients with Diabetes Mellitus

Rubin Bressler, MD

Controversy has existed for many years over the gain-risk aspects of rigid control of the blood glucose in patients with diabetes mellitus. The proponents of rigid control contend that correction of the metabolic abnormalities of the diabetic state will delay or prevent the development of vascular complications.[1-5] Opponents of this thesis have raised a number of serious problems faced by patients and physicians in the attainment of good blood glucose control.[6-8] They also have questioned whether diabetic vascular complications are a consequence of the metabolic disorder or a separate and distinct manifestation of a disease state affecting both the blood glucose (metabolism) and the vascular system.[1,2,6] The problem of diabetic control includes the following considerations:

1. Patient errors in carrying out prescribed regimens (diet; activity; insulin dose, type, and timing).
2. Periodic testing of urine and occasionally blood (or both) are inadequate assessments of diabetic control.

131

3. Insulin schedules are fixed whereas there is variability of activity and diet. Regimentation is difficult and imperfect (social-psychologic problems).
4. Methods for blood glucose control are imperfect. Insulin delivery systems are insensitive and crude, and as yet drugs are not available for control of gluconeogenesis (lipolysis, glucagon, growth hormone, proteolysis).
5. Dangerous hypoglycemia with risks of mental deterioration.
6. Emotional problems deriving from the obligatory regimentation necessary for rigid blood glucose control. This results in socioeconomic problems in the adult and problem of family and peer-group acceptance in the pediatric population.

Although it has not been ascertained that more precise quantitative regulation of blood glucose (closer simulation of physiologic control) affords protection against the multiple complications of diabetes mellitus, many investigators and practitioners advocate a regimen affording, as much as is possible, physiologic control of blood glucose without wide fluctuations.[1-5] In this chapter, the evidence on which this viewpoint is based will be reviewed.

BLOOD SUGAR CONTROL AND DIABETIC COMPLICATIONS: SOME INVESTIGATIVE APPROACHES IN ANIMALS AND HUMANS

The University Group Diabetes Program

Opponents of rigid control consider that the University Group Diabetes Program (UGDP) has already shown that control of blood glucose does not afford protection against microvascular lesions.[9,10] The UGDP was begun in order to determine whether or not control of blood glucose helps to prevent or delay vascular disease in non–insulin-dependent diabetic patients. Over 800 patients were randomly assigned to each of five treatment groups: placebo, a standard dose of tolbutamide (1.5 gm/day), a fixed dose of insulin, a variable dose of insulin, or a standard dose of phenformin (100 mg/day). The patients were followed for over eight years at 12 treatment centers. Analysis of the study revealed no protective effects of any of the therapeutic regimens against cardiovascular deaths.[10] However, only one of the five forms of therapy resulted in blood glucose lowering (variable dose of insulin). Although the study failed to demonstrate any benefit of blood glucose control on reduction of cardiovascular mortality, it should be noted that the patients studied exhibited minimal initial hyperglycemia and the blood glucose reductions achieved were small (ie, under 20%).[6,9] Moreover, the same data have been interpreted as showing a beneficial effect of control of the blood glucose on cardiovascular mortality.[11] A comparison of the placebo vs insulin-variable group has been carried out via reevaluation of the UGDP data.

The cardiovascular mortality found in the two groups occurred in a setting of different fasting blood glucose (FBG) responses. The FBG levels in the variable-insulin treated group was significantly lower than that of the placebo group. These data would imply little benefit of blood glucose lowering on the natural history of diabetic cardiovascular deaths. However, the conclusions drawn from the data in this study have been called into question because of the inclusion of postulated inappropriate subjects.[11]

Since the UGDP study was designed to assess the effects of blood glucose control on cardiovascular deaths it was considered important to eliminate patients who died early in the study (less than one year) and dropouts or patients who changed their medications. These considerations were not dealt with in the published results of the UGDP study.[11] Additional criticisms of this report include inequities in the insulin-variable group. This group was found to contain a disproportionate number of subjects who were 70 years of age or older and had either diastolic blood pressures > 110 mm Hg or fasting blood glucose levels ⩾ 150 mg/dl.[11]

When the subjects with these baseline inequities (age, diastolic blood pressure, FBG) are excluded from the analysis in order to render all groups comparable at baseline, a beneficial effect of control of blood glucose on cardiovascular deaths is evident. The data of Table 7-1 show that the frequency of cardiovascular deaths in the insulin-variable group was only 25% of that of the placebo group and around 30% of that of the standard-dose insulin group. The insulin-variable group was the only group that achieved a significant fall in blood glucose.[9] If subjects with baseline fasting blood glucoses up to 200 mg/dl are included in the analysis (instead of 150 mg/dl) there were still over twice as many cardiovascular deaths in the placebo group as in the insulin-variable group (15.9% vs 6.7%).[11]

Subjects in the insulin-variable group could not be considered to have received optimal therapy since they were all treated with a single daily dose of lente insulin (intermediate duration of action).

These data would lend support to the value of control of the blood glucose in regard to lowering the frequency of cardiovascular deaths in diabetic subjects.

Table 7-1
Cardiovascular (CV) Deaths in Subjects Who Did Not Change Medication or Drop Out* and Who Were Younger than 70 Years with Diastolic Blood Pressures < 110 mm Hg and Fasting Blood Glucose Values < 150 mg/dl at Baseline

	All Subjects	CV Deaths	
		No.	%
Placebo	71	12	16.9
Insulin Standard	68	10	14.7
Insulin Variable	69	3	4.4

*Subjects who received medication different from that originally assigned or who missed four or more consecutive quarterly examinations were considered medication changes or dropouts, respectively.
From: Kilo, C., Williamson, J.R., Choi, S.C. et al. Insulin treatment and diabetic vascular complications. *JAMA.* 241:26–27, 1979. Copyright 1979, American Medical Association. Reprinted with permission.

Atherogenesis and Insulin Excess

Although not a specific feature of diabetes mellitus, atherosclerotic disease occurs in greater frequency among diabetics. Atherosclerosis is intensified in diabetic patients, and several characteristics of the diabetic state may promote atherosclerosis.[12,13] The obesity, insulin resistance, and insulin excesses (endogenous or exogenous) of diabetes mellitus may contribute to atherogenesis.[12] Excess insulin output in the obese insulin-resistant patient or excess insulin use in the insulin-dependent patient can influence atherogenesis in several ways:

1. Insulin directly stimulates arteriole wall lipid accumulation[13];
2. Insulin increases hepatic production of triglyceride-rich (very-low-density) lipoproteins[14];
3. Insulin stimulates the proliferation of arteriole wall smooth muscle cells that are involved in the pathogenesis of atherosclerotic lesions.[12,15]

These data have raised concerns over the possibility that insulin may play a role in the development of premature atherosclerosis in diabetic patients. Whereas insulin replacement may ameliorate the effects of hormonal and metabolic deficiency, its excess use due to resistance (obesity) or imperfect insulin delivery schedules (subcutaneous insulin mismatches with diet) may accelerate atherosclerosis.[12] This would represent a potential danger in the pursuit of rigid control of the blood glucose.

Animal Studies

In recent years, a number of animal studies from several laboratories have shown that control of hyperglycemia in diabetic rats, dogs, monkeys, hamsters, and mice by means of insulin therapy or islet transplantation prevents or minimizes the formation of diabetic-like lesions in kidney, nerves, and eye.[3] These studies will be discussed further.

Natural History of Diabetic Complications

Any therapeutic intervention must take into account the natural history of diabetes mellitus. Diabetic complications do not occur in all patients nor do they occur with equal degrees of severity and incapacitation. Reviews of the natural history of diabetic vascular disease seen in patients at the Joslin Clinic attest to a low complication rate among survivors of 40 years of disease. Although three fourths of the insulin-dependent patients showed retinopathy, only half of them had severe proliferative retinopathy and only 8% became blind. A similar result found in a survey in London confirms the low frequency of diabetic retinopathy as well as the low incidence of blindness.[2,16,17]

The relationship of blood glucose control to diabetic complications has focused on a number of areas. These include: prospective-epidemiologic surveys on blood glucose levels and diabetic complications, capillary basement membrane width in muscle, renal pathology of diabetes, hemoglobin A_{1c} and intravascular factors, and diabetic neuropathy.

It has become evident from a number of studies that the pathologic changes characteristic of diabetes mellitus in animals and humans may not be obligatory consequences of a genetic disease. The alterations of blood components and the renal pathologic changes may be a result of poor control of an abnormal metabolic state, ie, elevated levels of blood glucose. Evidence supporting this view exists.[3,5] However, the question of whether the metabolic control necessary involves blood glucose, hemoglobin A_{1c}, serum lipids, plasma glucagon, growth hormone, myoinositol, erythrocyte 2,3-diphosphoglyceric acid, blood viscosity, erythrocyte and/or platelet aggregation, or other unknown factors is still unanswered. Although a number of these abnormalities have been returned toward normal with treatment, none has been causally related to the pathologic changes of diabetes.

Epidemiologic studies A prospective study has been carried out in England to ascertain the quantitative relationship between the degree of abnormality of glucose tolerance and the development of diabetic retinopathy.[18] Three groups of subjects were defined by their blood glucose levels two hours after a 50-gm oral glucose challenge. The groups were: 1) blood glucose $\leq$ 120 mg/dl (normals), 2) blood glucose 120 to 199 mg/dl (borderline diabetics), and 3) blood glucose > 200 mg/dl (frank diabetics). The groups were followed and reexamined five years later. The group with frank diabetes had been referred to their physicians for therapy of the diabetes. The therapies included insulin (5), oral antidiabetic drugs (54), diet (22) or no specific therapy (24).[18,19] The data of Table 7-2 show that the prevalence of retinopathy had increased greatly among the frank diabetics. The smaller numbers of borderline diabetics with retinopathy showed lesser increases in retinal disease. The passage of time had resulted in a qualitative as well as a quantitative difference between these groups.

Table 7-2
**Frequency of Diabetic Retinopathy* in Diabetics
and Borderline Diabetics at Survey and Five Years Later**

	2-Hour Capillary Blood-Sugar Concentrations (mg/dl)				
	120	*200*	*240*	*285*	*330*
Number at survey	248	26	29	31	30
% with retinopathy					
At survey	1.3	0	3.4	15.4	8.0
5 years later	3.3	11.8	22.7	26.3	33.3

*Includes microaneurysms (small red dots) only or with hemorrhages and/or exudates.
From: Jarrett, R.J., and Keen, H. Hyperglycaemia and diabetes. *Lancet* 2:1009–1012, 1976. Reprinted with permission.

The Pima Indians of Arizona have a high incidence of non–insulin-dependent diabetes mellitus.[20] In this diabetic population, two-hour blood glucose concentrations following a 75-gm oral glucose challenge are bimodally distributed. Retinopathy and proteinuria, suggesting renal disease, were found to be virtually confined to the more hyperglycemic subgroup (2-hour blood glucose over 200 mg/dl).[20,21] The level of blood glucose seemed to predict the incidence of retinopathy and nephropathy in these studies.

The relationship of blood glucose concentrations to the incidence of cataracts has been studied in patients with diabetes mellitus and in controls.[18] Cataracts were more common in the diabetics and the incidence was higher in those diabetics with higher blood glucose ($\geq$ 220 mg/dl).[18] These data imply that cataracts are a complication of diabetes that occur more often in patients with substantial degrees of hyperglycemia.

Muscle capillary basement membrane (MCBM) width   The most direct controversy concerning the relationship of control to microvascular disease in humans centers about the several groups that have studied MCBM thickness. Siperstein and associates[22] have found no relationship between the degree of blood glucose abnormality, duration of the diabetic or prediabetic state and the width of the MCBM. These findings are in conflict with Williamson's group, which found a high correlation between MCBM width and duration of the disease.[23]

The influence of fixation and morphometric techniques in determining muscle capillary basement membrane thickness has been a central issue in this controversy.[22] Data from recent comparative studies appears to have resolved these technical questions.[23] Evaluation of studies, in light of these new findings, supports the conclusion that muscle capillary basement membrane thickening is related to the duration of decreased carbohydrate tolerance.[24-26]

The relationship between basement membrane thickening and the duration of overt diabetes mellitus has also been investigated in the renal glomerulus in a prospective study using biopsy material obtained from patients with juvenile diabetes.[27] Data from patients biopsied at the time of diagnosis and repeated 1 to 2 years later were compared with that from controls and juvenile diabetics with disease of 3½ to 5 years' duration. Using sophisticated statistical analyses of 500 to 2000 measurements per glomerulus, no significant differences were found between controls and diabetics at the onset of disease. Significant, but slight increases in capillary basement membrane (CBM) were found at repeat biopsy at 1 to 2 years whereas greater thickening of CBM were seen in the 3½- to 5-year biopsy specimens. These studies imply that human basement membrane morphology is normal at the onset of diabetes, and only shows increased thickness after several years of abnormal metabolism. However, concomitance does not prove causality. The CBM and metabolic abnormalities could be separate and distinct manifestations of a genetic or nongenetic disorder.

The CBM changes found in the extremities may not be related to the functional impairments or pathologic changes that characterize the renal complications of diabetes. In spite of MCBM changes, there does not appear to be a progressive diabetic myopathy, and the renal disease of diabetics is a complex pathologic entity that involves much more than capillaries.[3]

Renal pathology of the diabetic state   The renal pathology of diabetes is complex and encompasses more and less specific types of glomerulosclerosis (nodular > diffuse > capillary drop lesion >> exudative).[3] Information on the relationship of diabetic control to the renal pathology has derived from both animal and human studies.

138

Studies have been carried out in rats, monkeys, and dogs. Although glomerular changes have been found in several of the diabetic animal models, the characteristic specific nodular lesion was lacking. Bloodworth, however, has found nodular lesions identical to those found in human diabetes in dogs made diabetic by means of alloxan or growth hormone.[28]

The development of immunohistochemical techniques has led to a better characterization of diabetic renal pathology. Immunofluorescent analysis of renal tissues from diabetic and nondiabetic subjects revealed characteristic features in the diabetic kidneys.[29] These were readily separable from the nondiabetic specimens. The differentiating finding was an intense linear staining of extracellular membranes. The most specific aspect was the presence of albumin and IgG lining the tubular basement membrane.[29]

Alloxan diabetic rats have been studied similarly after months of hyperglycemia. The renal immunofluorescent studies revealed mesangial staining for IgG and complement (C'_3).[30]

Renal transplantation of kidneys from experimentally diabetic rats into nondiabetic recipients results within two months in the disappearance of IgG, IgM, and C'_3 from the mesangium and the arrest or reversal of glomerular mesangial thickening.[31]

Conversely, transplantation of normal rat kidneys into diabetic recipients results in deposition of immunoglobulin and complement in the mesangium and visible mesangial thickening within two months.[31]

Pancreatic islet transplantation in streptozotocin diabetic rats, whose diabetes had been present for six to eight months, resulted in a significant reduction in mesangial thickening and in the mesangial staining for IgG, IgM, and C'_3. These changes were apparent two weeks after the restoration of normal blood glucose and insulin levels. Complete regression of the light microscopic changes had not occurred at nine weeks.[32]

In man, experiments of a similar nature have given results remarkably like those obtained in experimental diabetes. A group of investigators from the University of Minnesota examined kidney tissue obtained from 12 diabetic and 17 nondiabetic patients from 2 to 12 years following renal transplantation. The frequency and intensity of IgG and albumin staining of the tubular and glomerular basement membrane and Bowman's capsule was significantly greater in the diabetic than in the nondiabetic patients. Except for some staining of the glomerular basement membranes in the nondiabetic kidneys, there was practically no overlap between the two groups. Although 9 of the 12 diabetic patients received their kidney from a living, related donor, no immunofluorescénce was observed in seven kidneys studied at the time of their transplantation into diabetic recipients.[33]

This same group studied renal-transplant tissue from 12 diabetic and 28 nondiabetic patients who had a renal graft for at least two years. Ten of the 12 kidneys studied from diabetic patients showed arteriolar hyalinosis and in six of the ten, the hyaline change involved both the afferent and efferent limb of the glomerular arterioles. One diabetic patient developed typical nodular glomerulosclerosis 35 months after transplantation. Three of the 28 kidneys studied from the nondiabetic transplant recipients had hyaline vascular changes. These occurred only in rare vessels and did not appear until five years posttransplantation and never involved both afferent and efferent arterioles. None of the blood-vessel changes were present in the kidneys transplanted into the diabetic recipients at the time of transplantation although 10 of the 12 received living, related donor grafts.[34]

Good control of the blood glucose is difficult to achieve in patients with diabetes who have received renal transplants. The relationship between poor blood glucose control and the development of characteristic diabetic pathologic changes in transplanted kidneys suggests that the renal pathology might be the result of poor blood glucose control. This possibility is strengthened by the report of the development of diabetic nephropathy in a nondiabetic kidney transplanted into a nondiabetic patient who developed diabetes upon treatment with prednisone.[35] In spite of a nondiabetic recipient and nondiabetic kidney, clinical and morphologic evidence of diabetic nephropathy developed in the transplant following steroid-induced diabetes.

Hemoglobin A_{1C} and other intravascular factors   The microvascular pathology of diabetes is frequent and fairly specific. This has led to studies on the abnormalities of intravascular factors in diabetics. Longitudinal assessment of these factors might serve as another index (in addition to blood glucose) of metabolic control and/or a prognostic guide. Some of the factors that have been studied include hemoglobin A_{1C} and platelet aggregation.

Hemoglobin A_{1C} is a minor hemoglobin component that was first characterized as a fast moving component on agar gel electrophoresis. A number of studies have shown that hemoglobin A_{1C} is elevated in diabetics. Whereas, A_{1C} comprises 3% to 6% of the hemoglobin A of normals there is a 2- to 3-fold increase in diabetics.[36,37] Moreover, a number of diabetic animal models, both genetic and nongenetic (alloxan), show elevations in A_{1C}.[38,39] The rise in hemoglobin A_{1C} seems to be a consequence of hyperglycemia.[40,41]

The increase in hemoglobin A_{1C} does not seem to be an inherited abnormality as it has been found to be elevated only in the hyperglycemic member of identical twins discordant for juvenile-onset diabetes mellitus.[42]

Hemoglobin A_{1C} is the product of the chemical condensation of hemoglobin and glucose. It differs from hemoglobin A because of the glucose moiety, which is attached to the N-terminal amino group of the beta chain by a unique ketoamine linkage formed by a rearrangement of the Schiff base. It appears, from the kinetic studies of Bunn et al, that the rate of formation of HbA_{1C} should be proportional to the time-averaged concentration of glucose within the erythrocyte.[43] Thus, the level of HbA_{1C} could be a reflection of the adequacy of blood glucose control over a sustained period of time. Furthermore, the postsynthetic glycosylation of hemoglobin A in the diabetic may be representative of similar changes in other proteins that may occur during periods of sustained hyperglycemia. The monitoring of HbA_{1C} may provide a better index of longitudinal blood glucose control and allow correlations with other pathologic changes in the kidneys and nerves.

Although no specific pathologic effects of higher levels of hemoglobin A_{1C} have been discerned, it has been shown that the release of oxygen from HbA_{1C} occurs less readily. Control of the blood glucose results in decreased levels of HbA_{1C} (Table 7-3).[41]

Table 7-3
Changes in Minor-Hemoglobin and Glucose Measurements with Control of Diabetes

	Fasting Blood Sugar (mg/dl)	Weekly Urinary Sugar*	Glucose Brackets† (mg/dl)	Hemoglobin A_{1C} (%)
Precontrol	390	85	1060	10.1
Control	77	0	718	5.8
Precontrol	280	52	1613	6.8
Control	100	14	1063	4.2
Precontrol	450	112	2716	12.1
Control	70	9	653	5.4
Precontrol	312	96	1978	10.0
Control	97	0	918	5.8
Precontrol	282	100	1959	10.2
Control	75	28	1218	7.6

*Semiquantitative (0 to 4+) urinary sugar concentration was determined four times/day, and values for seven consecutive days summed to determine weekly urinary sugar.
†Sum of blood sugar concentration measured just before and one hour after breakfast, lunch, and dinner.
Reprinted by permission from the *New England Journal of Medicine* (295:417–420, 1976).

Recent in vivo and in vitro studies on rat lens suggest a new mechanism for diabetic cataract formation secondary to hyperglycemia.[44] The glycosylation of the epsilon-amino groups of lysine in the protein of the lens is thought to increase the susceptibility of the lens to cataract formation. The basis of this chemical glycosylation is identical to that which takes place in the formation of HbA_{1C}.

Platelet aggregation in diabetics has been found to be more sensitive to stimulation by a number of agents (ADP, epinephrine, collagen) than in normal subjects.[45-47] This has been attributed to increased levels of plasma β-thromboglobulin, and increased synthesis of PGE-like material.[45,46] Institution of strict diabetic blood glucose control modifies these abnormalities.[45-47] It is difficult to ascertain whether the increased platelet sensitivity to aggregating agents is causally related to microvascular disease. Moreover, the fibrinolytic system, which is a defense mechanism against platelet occlusion of microvasculature, has been found to be decreased in diabetics.[48,49] However, it still remains to be established whether these intravascular abnormalities cause diabetic microangiopathy rather than being merely consequences of the disease.

Diabetic neuropathy A number of clinical neuropathic states have been described in diabetes. Although segmental myelin degeneration is a characteristic, lesion impairment of the microvasculature supply of nerves has also been found.

Decreased velocity of motor nerve conductive (VMNC) has been found in diabetic rats shortly after the onset of hyperglycemia resulting from streptozotocin administration. Correction of the hyperglycemia with insulin therapy normalized the VMNC when therapy was instituted soon after the onset of the hyperglycemia.

Studies in rats with chronic diabetes have shown a correlation between the reduced VMNC and a diminished concentration of free myoinositol in the nerves. Myoinositol is a major component of peripheral nerve that is supplied by diet. It has been found that glucosuric diabetic patients excrete a large fraction of dietary myoinositol whereas nondiabetics do not.[49-51]

Insulin therapy, which ameliorated the hyperglycemia in streptozotocin-diabetic rats with chronic diabetes, did not correct the impairment in VMNC, whereas dietary supplementation with myoinositol prevented the impairment of VMNC in face of continued hyperglycemia. This study suggests that hyperglycemia results in losses of myoinositol from nerve and that decreased neural myoinositol results in diminished VMNC. Correction of the hyperglycemia alone does not restore the neural myoinositol.[50,51] However, early therapy with insulin decreases loss of the myoinositol and prevents decreased VMNC from developing. Human studies are now in progress regarding myoinositol balance and VMNC. (Clements, R.S., personal communication). Reduction of the VMNC has been found to be more marked in more poorly controlled patients.[52]

RIGID CONTROL OF BLOOD GLUCOSE

If control of blood glucose (metabolic abnormalities) was a critical aspect of the development of microvascular, renal, and neurologic lesions in diabetic patients then it would be expected that close control of the blood glucose would delay or prevent these lesions. The problem is simple to formulate but experimental proof will be complex and costly.

The complications of diabetes take years to develop, which means that any meaningful prospective study would entail approximately 10 to 20 years of observation of a considerable population of patients. Other formidable problems in contemplated prospective studies include the following:

1. Need for groups of subjects matched in regard to age, sex, weight, duration of diabetes, baseline diabetic complications, race, and other disease states.
2. Although blood and urine glucose and HbA_{1C} testing are neither inordinately expensive nor complex, fluorescein angiographic studies of the retina, measurements of VMNC, urinary myoinositol, and other tests may be expensive and difficult. The need for renal biopsies is an open and difficult question.
3. Our ability or inability to rigidly control the blood glucose with current therapeutic modalities.

The factors involved in control of the blood sugar include delivery of adequate amounts of insulin at the time of food challenge, and sensitivity to the insulin (endogenous exogenous).

The labile (insulin-dependent) diabetic patient is almost totally dependent upon exogenous insulin for its anabolic and anticatabolic actions. The matching of injected insulin to ingested diet is an imperfect one, so the insulin-dependent patient experiences wide swings of blood glucose during the course of a day.[53]

However, recent studies utilizing home monitoring of blood glucose as a guide to insulin therapy have demonstrated that good control was achieved in the majority of patients using conventional insulin regimens.[54-56] No significant hypoglycemia or other complications occurred. This study suggests that an approach to normoglycemia may be possible using conventional technology.

It is obvious that prospective studies on control of the blood glucose in diabetes are difficult and may not be feasible at this time. Issues such as compliance, quantitative data on diabetic pathology, and intercurrent diseases are further considerations in this type of study.

If control of blood glucose is a critical factor in the development of microvascular disease then precise metabolic control would be expected to prevent or ameliorate retinal, renal, and neurologic sequelae of diabetes mellitus. Perfect regulation is not yet possible. The question thus becomes whether better degrees of blood glucose regulation favorably influence the course of the disease. Although studies relating to this question have not all been in total agreement, the increasing weight of evidence supports the view that more careful control of the blood glucose favorably influences the frequency and severity of the complications of diabetes.[1-4]

Retrospective Studies

A review of the published literature in 1964 found over 300 publications on the topic of control of blood glucose, representing data from 85 studies. Of these, 51 concluded that a correlation exists between degree of diabetic control and complications, 26 favored the opposite conclusion, and 8 were inconclusive. However, in 40 it was felt that there was not enough data to support the conclusions of the authors. The remaining 45 lacked random assignments of treatments and satisfactory criteria of control. In 39 of the 45, there was not adequate description of material for interpreting the results. Thus, assessment of a consensus opinion was not possible.[8,57]

The large study carried out by the Joslin Clinic Investigators supported a relationship between control and complications.[2] The study evaluated 451 patients with onset of diabetes before age 20 and a duration of 10 to 36 years. Of the 101 patients with nephropathy, only one came from the excellent/good control group. There was an absence of grade 4 retinopathy (proliferative) and only a 3% incidence of grade 3 retinopathy among the patients with excellent or good control who had had diabetes for 20 or more years compared to a 31% incidence among the fair and poor control patients of similar duration of diabetes. In some of the studies in which the influence of diabetic control on the progression of vascular disease was not demonstrated,[58] the criteria for good control more closely resembled those for the fair control group in the Joslin study, thus potentially obscuring differences between excellent/good, and fair/poor control groups.

An analysis of 149 published studies dealing with the vascular complications of diabetes was carried out.[57] The study ascertained that only 33 of these analyzed studies were suitable for critical assessment of methodology. A set of methodologic rules was proposed for this type of study. The compliance of study methodology with these rules would allow valid comparisons with other such studies.

Abnormality of the blood-retinal barrier appears to be an early change in diabetic subjects.[59] This finding has been quantitatively assessed by a newly developed technique of vitreous fluorophotometry, which measures the penetration of intravenously injected fluorescein into the vitreous.[60] A study has been carried out that sought to establish possible correlations between control of blood glucose and abnormality of vitreous fluorophotometry in a group of 77 diabetic patients. These patients all had good visual acuity, normal ophthalmologic examinations, and normal retinal vasculature by fluorescein angiography. Classification of the status of diabetic control over the year preceding the study was based on the blood glucose (less than 200 mg/dl; 50% of determinations), minimal glucosuria or ketonuria, absence of major hypoglycemic reactions, and absence of ketoacidosis.[59] The results are shown in Tables 7-4 and 7-5.

Table 7-4
Vitreous Fluorophotometry Values in Insulin-Dependent Diabetics

Metabolic Control	Vitreous Fluorophotometry — Posterior Vitreous ($\times 10^{-8}$ gm/ml; mean $\pm$ SD)				
	No. of Eyes	< 5 yr*	No. of Eyes	> 5 yr*	p values
Relatively good	10	3.6 $\pm$ 1.2	3	5.9 $\pm$ 0.8	< 0.005
Poor	11	5.5 $\pm$ 2.4	3	7.7 $\pm$ 1.5	NS
p values		< 0.025		NS	

*Duration of diabetes.
From: Cunha-Vaz, J.G., Fonseca, J.R., Abreu, J.F., et al. Detection of early retinal changes in diabetes by vitreous fluorophotometry. *Diabetes* 28:16–19, 1979. Reprinted with permission.

Table 7-5
Vitreous Fluorophotometry Values in Non–Insulin-Dependent Diabetics

Metabolic Control	Vitreous Fluorophotometry — Posterior Vitreous ($\times 10^{-8}$ gm/ml; mean $\pm$ SD)				
	No. of Eyes	< 5 yr*	No. of Eyes	> 5 yr*	p values
Relatively Good	12	4.6 $\pm$ 1.4	26	6.3 $\pm$ 1.8	< 0.01
Poor	8	8.3 $\pm$ 2.4	4	8.7 $\pm$ 3.4	NS
p values		< 0.0005		< 0.0125	

*Duration of diabetes.
From: Cunha-Vaz, J.G., Fonseca, J.R., Abreu, J.F. et al. Detection of early retinal changes in diabetes by vitreous fluorophotometry. *Diabetes* 28:16–19, 1979. Reprinted with permission.

In the insulin-dependent diabetics who had the disease for less than five years relatively good metabolic control was associated with significantly lower vitreous fluorophotometry values. In the group of patients with diabetes for over five years, there were no significant differences in vitreous fluorophotometry values between the relatively good and poor metabolic control groups. The small numbers studied in these groups leaves the issue still unresolved. In the non–insulin-dependent diabetic groups with diabetes for less than five years relatively good metabolic control resulted in significantly lower vitreous fluorophotometry values. The same results were obtained in non–insulin-dependent diabetics in relatively good control who had the disease for more than five years.[59]

Breakdown of the blood-retinal barrier appears to be the earliest detectable change to occur in the diabetic retina. The early change correlates with the status of metabolic control and with the duration of diabetes.

These types of studies have been carried out in rats with streptozotocin-diabetes. Similar abnormalities and responses to antidiabetes therapy were found.[61]

Low levels of plasma high-density-lipoprotein (HDL)-cholesterol is associated with an increased risk of coronary artery disease.[62,63] In a study carried out on 122 patients with diabetes mellitus, a significant inverse correlation was found between plasma HDL-cholesterol and HbA_{1C} concentrations.[64] In an insulin-treated subgroup improvement in control of the blood glucose (decreased levels of HbA_{1C}) was associated with a significant rise in plasma HDL-cholesterol. The study implies that improved control of the blood glucose in diabetics may diminish the risk of coronary artery disease.

Longitudinal systemic evaluations of the complications of diabetes in well-defined populations have been limited in number. Of 16 studies reported (ten prospective, six retrospective) only one study followed nephropathy, retinopathy, and neuropathy and three followed nephropathy and retinopathy. The remaining studies only followed retinopathy. Only five of these studies were of ten or more years duration.[65]

PROSPECTIVE STUDIES

Goodkin[66] in a 20-year prospective study of mortality in diabetes ascertained that mortality in patients with poor control was 2.5 times as frequent as that of patients with better blood glucose control.

A prospective study of over 4000 diabetic patients followed for up to 25 years has recently been published.[65] The incidence and prevalence of neuropathy and microangiopathy (retinal, renal) were found

146

to correlate with the duration of diabetes. Poor diabetic control was found to be associated with a higher prevalence (frequency of complication at a point in time) and incidence (frequency of appearance of a complication per time) of both microangiopathy and neuropathy particularly with severe retinopathy. The inherent severity (difficulty in achieving good blood glucose control) did not appear to play a role in the development of complications if the true duration of diabetes and the effectiveness of blood glucose control were considered. Thus, middle-aged and elderly patients with diabetes appear to develop complications with the same delay period as the younger patients in whom the onset of the disease can be more accurately dated.

Kohner and his associates[67] carried out a prospective study on the progression of diabetic retinopathy in relation to the degree of blood glucose control. Only "very good" control protected the patients from rapid progession of microaneurysm, hemorrhages and neovascularization. These findings have been confirmed.[68] Very good diabetic control has in other studies been associated with a decrease in the degree, frequency, and progression rate of proteinuria.[69,70] The degree of diabetes has also been correlated with basement membrane changes in muscle biopsies of juvenile diabetic patients. Those with excellent control had normal MCBM thickness 5 to 20 years after diagnosis, whereas, those with poor control had increased thickness in less than five years.[76] Effective control of blood glucose also significantly decreased the elevated plasma cholesterol, triglycerides, and accelerated cholesterol synthesis that occur in association with diabetic hyperglycemia.[72] This could favorably influence the accelerated course of atherosclerosis in diabetic patients.

An interesting study has been reported by Johnsson in which the effects of different therapeutic regimens on the incidence of microvascular disease was evaluated.[73] Johnsson assessed diabetic subjects treated in Sweden in two different eras of treatment. Two groups of patients were surveyed: 1) Patients treated with strict diet and multiple daily doses of regular insulin in the years 1922 to 1935, and 2) Patients treated with less rigid diets and long-acting insulin in the years 1935 to 1945.

Comparison of the incidence of retinopathy and nephropathy in these two groups, both of which had diabetes for more than 15 years, showed that retinopathy and nephropathy occurred at a lesser frequency in the 1922 to 1935 group, despite the fact that diabetes was of longer duration (8.6 years) in this group than in the second group. This study represents an impressive testimony to the value of better blood glucose control (See Tables 7-6 and 7-7.)

A prospective study was carried out in France to ascertain any relationship between blood glucose control and the progression of

Table 7-6
Blood Glucose Control

	Strict Control	Less Strict Control
Number of patients	56	104
Duration of diabetes	24.5 yr	15.9 yr
Patients with nephropathy	18 (32%)	56 (54%)

From: Johnsson, S. Retinopathy and nephropathy in diabetes mellitus: comparison of the effect of two forms of treatment. *Diabetes* 9:1–8, 1960. Reprinted with permission.

Table 7-7
Blood Glucose Control

Duration of Diabetes > 15 Years	Strict Control	Less Strict Control
Number of patients	56	57
Patients with nephropathy	5 (9%)	35 (61%)

From: Johnsson, S. Retinopathy and nephropathy in diabetes mellitus: comparison of the effect of two forms of treatment. *Diabetes* 9:1–8, 1960. Reprinted with permission.

diabetic retinopathy.[74,75] Two groups of 21 insulin-dependent diabetic patients were treated with either a single prebreakfast dose of insulin (long-acting alone or with additional intermediate- or short-acting) or with multiple daily doses of insulin (short-acting before breakfast and lunch and intermediate-acting and/or short-acting before supper). At the end of four years of the study, the data revealed a slower rate of progression in the number of retinal microaneurysms in the patients treated with divided, multiple insulin doses when compared with patients treated with a single daily injection of insulin. The study data are shown in Tables 7-8 and 7-9. Whereas the differences in fasting blood glucose levels were significant, they were not large, and normoglycemia was not achieved. However, the FBG represents a single-point blood sugar value and may not have reflected the true magnitude of blood glucose differences in the two groups of patients. The study does support a slower rate of progression of diabetic retinopathy with better degrees of blood glucose control. This study, however, must be faulted on the grounds of small numbers of patients and because subjects in each group crossed over (changed pattern of insulin use) during the course of the study.[74]

It is of interest to note that retrospective evaluations of diabetic patients surviving 20 to 40 years reveals that the majority of these patients had been treated with multiple daily doses of insulin.[76,77]

Table 7-8
Comparison of the Progression of Microaneurysms
Between Single- and Multiple-Injection Groups (mean ± SEM)

	Single-Injection Group	Multiple-Injection Group	p Value*
No. of microaneurysms			
At baseline	13 ± 3	9 ± 3	NS
At the final examination	55 ± 8	30 ± 7	< 0.05
Difference	42 ± 7	21 ± 5	< 0.02
Mean yearly increase in the number of microaneurysms	9 ± 1	3 ± 1	< 0.001

*p value is given for nonparametric test (Mann and Whitney).
From: Eschwege, E., Job, D., Guyot-Argenton, C. et al. Delayed progression of diabetic retinopathy by divided insulin administration: a further follow-up. *Diabetologia* 16:13–15, 1979. Heidelberg: Springer-Verlag. Reprinted with permission.

Table 7-9
Control of Diabetes (mean ± SEM)

	Single-Injection Group	Multiple-Injection Group	p Value
Mean fasting blood sugar (mg/100 ml)	192 ± 8	166 ± 9	< 0.05
Mean 24-hour glycosuria (gm/24 hr)	27 ± 4	24 ± 3	NS
Variation of 24-hour glycosuria from baseline (gm/24 hr)	+5 ± 4	−5 ± 3	< 0.05
Mean daily insulin dosage (units/24 hr)	45 ± 3	49 ± 4	NS

From: Eschwege, E., Job, D., Guyot-Argenton, C. et al. Delayed progression of diabetic retinopathy by divided insulin administration: a further follow-up. *Diabetologia* 16:13–15, 1979. Heidelberg: Springer-Verlag. Reprinted with permission.

SUMMARY

The controversy over whether strict control of blood glucose prevents complications in the diabetic patient will continue. The resolution of the controversy is not feasible at present because of the complexity and financial cost of a definitive prospective study and because we do not yet possess the pharmacologic agents that can accomplish the goal of strict control of the blood glucose. However, many practicing physicians and clinical investigators believe that better degrees of blood glucose control can decrease the frequency and severity of the complications of diabetes. The weight of evidence from the literature supports this view.

REFERENCES

1. Cahill, G.F., Etzwiler, D.D., and Freinkel, N. "Control" and diabetes. *N Engl J Med.* 294:1004–1005, 1976.

2. Keiding, N.R., Root, H.F., and Marble, A. Importance of control of diabetes in prevention of vascular complications. *JAMA.* 150:964–969, 1952.

3. Raskin, P. Diabetic regulation and its relationship to microangiopathy. *Metabolism.* 27:235–252, 1978.

4. Bressler, R. The controversy over blood glucose control. *Drug Ther.* 8:24–37, 1978.

5. Brownlee, M. Normoglycemia as a therapeutic goal in insulin-dependent diabetes. *Drug Ther.* (Hospital Edition) 3:13–20, 1978.

6. Siperstein, M.D., Foster, D.W., and Knowles, H.C., Jr. et al. Control of blood glucose and diabetic vascular disease. *N Engl J Med.* 296:1060–1063, 1977.

7. Bondy, P.K., and Felig, P. Relation of diabetic control to development of vascular complications. *Med Clin North Am.* 55:889–898, 1971.

8. Knowles, H.C., Guest, G.M., Lampe, J. et al. The course of juvenile diabetes treated with unmeasured diet. *Diabetes* 14:239–273, 1965.

9. Goldner, M.G., Knatterud, G.L., and Prout, T.E. A study of effects of hypoglycemic agents on vascular complications in patients with adult-onset diabetes. III. Clinical implications of UGDP results. *JAMA.* 218:1400–1410, 1971.

10. Meinert, C.L., Knatterud, G.L., Prout, T.E. et al. A study of the effects of hypoglycemic agents on vascular complications in patients with adult-onset diabetes. II. Mortality results, University Group Diabetes Program. *Diabetes* 19:(suppl 2):789–830, 1970.

11. Kilo, C., Williamson, J.R., Choi, S.C. et al. Insulin treatment and diabetic vascular complications. *JAMA.* 241:26–27, 1979.

12. Bierman, E.L., and Brunzell, J.D. Interrelation of atherosclerosis, abnormal lipid metabolism and diabetes mellitus. Edited by H.M. Katzen, and R.J. Mahler. In *Advances in Modern Nutrition: Diabetes, Obesity and Vascular Disease,* Part 1. New York: Halsted Press, 1978, pp 187–210.

13. Topping, D.L., and Mayes, P.A. The immediate effects of insulin and fructose on the metabolism of the perfused liver. *Biochem J.* 126:295–311, 1972.

14. Smith, E.B., and Slater, R.S. Relationship between low-density lipoprotein in aortic intima and serum-lipid levels. *Lancet* 1:463–469, 1972.

15. Stout, R.W. Insulin stimulation of cholesterol synthesis by arterial tissue. *Lancet* 2:467–468, 1969.

16. Hardin, R.C., Jackson, R.L., Johnston, T.L. et al. The development of diabetic retinopathy. The effects of duration and control of diabetes. *Diabetes* 5:397–405, 1956.

17. Dolger, H. Clinical evaluation of vascular damage in diabetes mellitus. *JAMA.* 134:1289–1291, 1947.

18. Jarrett, R.J., and Keen, H. Hyperglycaemia and diabetes mellitus. *Lancet* 2:1009–1012, 1976.

19. Reid, D.D., Brett, G.Z., Hamilton, P.J.S. et al. Cardiorespiratory disease and diabetes among middle aged civil servants. *Lancet* 1:469–473, 1974.

20. Bennet, P.H., Burch, T.A., and Miller, M. Diabetes mellitus in American (Pima) Indians. *Lancet* 2:125–128, 1971.

21. Steinberg, A.G., Rushforth, N.B., Bennett, P.H. et al. On the genetics of diabetes mellitus. Edited by E. Cerasi, and R. Luft. In *Nobel Symposium No. 13.* Stockholm: Almqvist and Wiksell, 1970, pp 237–264.

22. Siperstein, M.D., Raskin, R., and Burns, H. Electron microscopic quantification of diabetic microangiopathy. *Diabetes* 22:514–524, 2973.

23. Williamson, J.R., Rowold, E., Hoffman, P. et al. Influence of fixation and morphometric technics on capillary basement membrane thickening prevalence data in diabetes. *Diabetes* 25:604–613, 1976.

24. Danowski, T.S., Fisher, E.R., Khurana, R.C. et al. Muscle capillary basement membrane in juvenile diabetes mellitus. *Metabolism* 21:1125–1132, 1972.

25. Pardo, V., Perez-Stable, E., Alzamora, D.B. et al. Incidence and significance of muscle capillary basal lumina thickness in juvenile diabetes. *Am J Pathol.* 68:67–77, 1972.

26. Kilo, C., Vogler, N., and Williamson, J.R. Muscle capillary basement membrane changes related to aging and diabetes mellitus. *Diabetes* 21:881–905, 1972.

27. Osterby, R. Early phases in the development of diabetic glomerulopathy. *Acta Med Scand [Suppl].* 574:1–82, 1974.

28. Bloodworth, J.M.B. Experimental diabetic glomerulosclerosis. II. The dog. *Arch Pathol.* 79:113–125, 1965.

29. Miller, K., and Michael, A.F. Immunopathology of renal extracellular membranes in diabetes mellitus. Specificity of tubular basement membrane immunofluorescence. *Diabetes* 25:701–708, 1976.

30. Mauer, S.M., Michael, A.F., Fish, A.J. et al. Spontaneous immunoglobulin and complement deposition in glomeruli of diabetic rats. *Lab Invest.* 27:488–494, 1972.

31. Lee, C.S., Mauer, S.M., Brown, D.M. et al. Renal transplantations in diabetes mellitus in rats. *J Exp Med.* 139:793–800, 1974.

32. Mauer, S.M., Steffes, M.W., Sutherland, D.E.R. et al. Studies of the rate of regression of the glomerular lesions in diabetic rats treated with pancreatic islet transplantation. *Diabetes* 24:280–285, 1975.

33. Mauer, S.M., Miller, K., Goetz, F.C. et al. Immunopathology of renal extracellular membranes in kidneys transplanted into patients with diabetes mellitus. *Diabetes* 25:709–712, 1976.

34. Mauer, S.M., Barbosa, J., Vernier, R.L. et al. Development of diabetic vascular lesions in normal kidneys transplanted into patients with diabetes mellitus. *N Engl J Med.* 295, 916–920, 1976.

35. Doud, R., Lee, D.B.N., Waisman, J. et al. Development of a lesion resembling diabetic nephropathy in a renal homograft. *Arch Intern Med.* 137:945–947, 1977.

36. Paulsen, E.P., and Kowry, W. Hemoglobin A_{1c} in insulin-dependent and independent diabetes mellitus. *Diabetes* 25(suppl 2):890–896, 1976.

37. Rahbar, S. An abnormal hemoglobin in red cells of diabetes. *Clin Chim Acta.* 22:296–298, 1968.

38. Koenig, R.J., and Cerami, A. Synthesis of hemoglobin A_{1c} in normal and diabetic mice: potential model of basement membrane thickening. *Proc Natl Acad Sci.* 72:3687–3691, 1975.

39. Koenig, R.J., Araujo, D.C., and Cerami, A. Increased hemoglobin A_{1c} in diabetic mice. *Diabetes* 25:1–5, 1976.

40. Koenig, R.J., Peterson, C.M., Jones, R.L. et al. Correlation of glucose regulation and hemoglobin A_{1c} in diabetes mellitus. *N Engl J Med.* 295:417–420, 1976.

41. Koenig, R.J., Peterson, C.M., Kilo, C. et al. Hemoglobin A$_{1C}$ as an indicator of the degree of glucose intolerance in diabetes. *Diabetes* 25:230–232, 1976.

42. Tattersal, R.B., Pyke, D.A., Ranney, H.M. et al. Hemoglobin components in diabetes mellitus. Studies in identical twins. *N Engl J Med.* 293:1171–1173, 1975.

43. Bunn, H.F., Haney, D.N., Kamin, S. et al. The biosynthesis of human hemoglobin A$_{1C}$. Slow glycosylation of hemoglobin *in vivo. J Clin Invest.* 57:1652–1659, 1976.

44. Stevens, V.J., Rouzer, C.A., Monnier, V.M. et al. Diabetic cataract formation: potential role of glycosylation of lens crystallins. *Proc Natl Acad Sci.* 75:2918–2922, 1978.

45. Haloshka, P.V., Lurie, D., and Colwell, J.A. Increased synthesis of prostoglandin-E-like material by platelets from patients with diabetes mellitus. *N Engl J Med.* 297:1306–1310, 1977.

46. Preston, F.E., Marcola, B.H., Ward, J.D. et al. Elevated β-thromboglobulin levels and circulating platelet aggregates in diabetic microangiopathy. *Lancet* 1:238–240, 1978.

47. Peterson, C.M., Jones, R.L., Koenig, R.J. et al. Reversible hematologic sequelae of diabetes mellitus. *Ann Intern Med.* 86:425–429, 1977.

48. Fukuda, M. Blood fibrinolytic activity and fibrinogen concentration in diabetic retinopathy. *Eye, Ear, Nose, Throat Monthly* 51:266–272, 1972.

49. Clements, R.S., Reynertson, R.H., and Starnes, W.R. Myoinositol metabolism in diabetes mellitus. *Diabetes* 23(suppl 1):348, 1974.

50. Greene, D.A., Pacifico, V.D.J., and Winegrad, A.I. Effects of insulin and dietary myoinositol on impaired peripheral nerve conduction velocity in acute streptozotocin diabetes. *J Clin Invest.* 55:1326–1336, 1975.

51. Winegrad, A.I., and Greene, D.A. Diabetic polyneuropathy. The importance of insulin deficiency, hyperglycemia and alterations in myoinositol metabolism in its pathogenesis. *N Engl J Med.* 295:1416–1421, 1975.

52. Gregersen, G. Diabetic neuropathy: influence of age, sex, metabolic control, and duration of diabetes on motor conduction velocity. *Neurology* 17:972–980, 1967.

53. Molnar, G., Taylor, W., and Langworthy, A. Plasma immunoreactive insulin pattern in insulin-treated diabetes. *Mayo Clin Proc.* 47:709–719, 1972.

54. Sönksen, P.H., Judd, S.L., and Lowy, C. Home monitoring of blood glucose. *Lancet* 1:729–732, 1978.

55. Walford, S., Allison, S.P., Gale, E.A.M. et al. Self-monitoring of blood glucose. *Lancet* 1:732–735, 1978.

56. Danowski, T.S., and Sunder, J.H. Jet injection of insulin during self-monitoring of blood glucose. *Diabetes Care* 1:27–33, 1978.

57. Kaplan, M.H., and Feinstein, A.R. A critique of methods in reported studies of long-term vascular complications in patients with diabetes mellitus. *Diabetes* 22:160–174, 1973.

58. Downie, E. Vascular disease in juvenile diabetic patients of long duration. *Diabetes* 8:383–387, 1959.

59. Cunha-Vaz, J.G., Fonseca, J.R., Abreu, J.F. et al. Detection of early retinal changes in diabetes by vitreous fluorophotometry. *Diabetes* 28:16–19, 1979.

60. Waltman, S.R., Oestrich, C.A., Krupin, T. et al. Quantitative vitreous fluorophotometry: a sensitive technique for measuring early breakdown of the blood retinal barrier in young diabetic patients. *Diabetes* 27:85–87, 1979.

61. Waltman, S.R., Oestrich, C.A., Hanish, S. et al. Blood-retinal barrier in

152

experimental diabetes. Presented at the spring meeting of the Association of Research in Vision and Ophthalmology, April 1977.

62. Miller, G.J., and Miller, N.E. Plasma-high-density-lipoprotein concentration and development of ischemic heart-disease. *Lancet* 1:16–19, 1975.

63. Berg, K., Hørresen, A.L., and Dahlén, G. Serum-high-density-lipoprotein and atherosclerotic heart-disease. *Lancet* 1:499–501, 1976.

64. Calvert, G.D., Mannik, T., Graham, J.J. et al. Effects of therapy on plasma high-density-lipoprotein-cholesterol concentration in diabetes mellitus. *Lancet* 2:66–68, 1978.

65. Pirart, J. Diabetes mellitus and its complications: a prospective study of 4400 patients observed between 1947 and 1973. *Diabetic Care* 1:168–188, 1978.

66. Goodkin, G. Mortality factors in diabetes: a 20 year mortality study. *Occup Med.* 17:716–721, 1975.

67. Kohner, E.M., Fraser, T.R., Joplin, G.F. et al. The effect of diabetic control on diabetic retinopathy. Edited by M.F. Goldberg, and S.L. Fine. In *Symposium on the Treatment of Diabetic Retinopathy.* Washington, DC: 1968, pp 119–128.

68. Miki, E., Fukuda, M., Kuzuya, T. et al. Relation of course of retinopathy to control of diabetes, age and therapeutic agents in diabetic Japanese patients. *Diabetes* 18:773–780, 1969.

69. Miki, E., Kuzuya, T., Ide, T. et al. Frequency, degree and progression with time of proteinuria in diabetic patients. *Lancet* 1:922–924, 1972.

70. Takazadura, E., Nakamoto, Y., Hayakawa, H. et al. Onset and progression of diabetic glomerulosclerosis: a prospective study based on serial renal biopsies. *Diabetes* 24:1–9, 1975.

71. Jackson, R., Guthrie, R., Esterly, J. et al. Muscle capillary basement membrane changes in normal and diabetic children. *Diabetes* 24(suppl 2):400, 1975.

72. Bennion, L.J., and Grundy, S.M. Influence of diabetic control on cholesterol metabolism in man. *Diabetes* 25(suppl 1):324, 1976.

73. Johnsson, S. Retinopathy and nephropathy in diabetes mellitus: comparison of the effect of two forms of treatment. *Diabetes* 9:1–8, 1960.

74. Job, D., Eschwege, E., Guyot-Argenton, C. et al. Effect of multiple daily insulin injection on the cause of retinopathy. *Diabetes* 25:463–469, 1976.

75. Eschwege, E., Job, D., Guyot-Argenton, C. et al. Delayed progression of diabetic retinopathy by divided insulin administration: a further follow-up. *Diabetologia* 16:13–15, 1979.

76. Ryan, J.R., Balodimos, M.C., Chazan, B.I. et al. Quarter century victory medal for diabetes: a follow-up of patients one to 20 years later. *Metabolism* 19:493–501, 1970.

77. Oakley, W.G., Pyke, D.A., Tattersall, R.B. et al. Long-term diabetes: a clinical study of 92 patients after 40 years. *Q J Med.* 43:145–156, 1974.

8 Diabetic Ketoacidosis

David G. Johnson, MD

Diabetic ketoacidosis represents an extreme form of uncontrolled diabetes mellitus. Although ketoacidosis occurs more commonly among insulin-dependent diabetics, periods of stress, such as those caused by infections, drugs, or trauma can lead to the development of ketoacidosis in otherwise non–insulin-dependent diabetics as well. The actual cause of any particular case of ketoacidosis may be obvious, for instance failure to take insulin, infection, a physical or emotional trauma. Nevertheless the precipitating event is often never determined.

It is frequently stated that ketoacidosis is the result of "absolute or relative deficiency of insulin."[1,2] This definition raises the question, "relative to what?" The concentrations of insulin found in diabetics in ketoacidosis are low relative to those that would be obtained in nondiabetic subjects with a comparable degree of hyperglycemia, but this leaves unanswered the question as to what produced the hyperglycemia. Absolute plasma insulin concentrations are usually in the low-normal or normal range (0 to 20 μU/ml) in patients with ketoacidosis.[3,4] On the other hand, concentrations of counterregulatory hormones,

154

such as norepinephrine and epinephrine,[5] glucagon,[6,7] cortisol,[8] and growth hormone[9,10] are usually elevated. Furthermore, epinephrine, glucagon, and cortisol appear to have synergistic effects in inducing hyperglycemia.[11] This could be taken to mean that the level of insulin is low relative to the high levels of counterregulatory hormones. However, the exact concentrations of insulin needed to balance various elevated levels of the individual or combined counterregulatory hormones is not known for normal man or for people with diabetes. Studies have shown that concentrations of insulin above 100 μU/ml are sufficient to counteract the action of counterregulatory hormones.[12-15] In view of the response of patients with ketoacidosis to exogenous insulin, it can be assumed that pretreatment levels of insulin were not high enough in relation to each patient's needs, regardless of the actual circulating concentrations of insulin and other hormones.

PATHOPHYSIOLOGY OF KETOACIDOSIS

Lack of insulin leads to overproduction and underutilization of glucose and ketoacids (Figure 8-1). Glucose uptake in peripheral tissues is diminished at the same time hepatic gluconeogenesis is enhanced. Free fatty acids (FFA) are released in increased amounts by peripheral tissues and converted preferentially to ketoacids in the liver. Hyperglycemia and ketoacidosis develop, with loss of glucose, ketoacids, water, and electrolytes in the urine. Anorexia and vomiting provoked by the acidosis exacerbate the dehydration and loss of electrolytes. Contraction of extracellular fluid volume activates the sympathetic nervous system.[5] Cortisol and growth hormone secretion is stimulated.[8-10] This increases insulin requirements, which, if not matched, cause worsening hyperglycemia and ketoacidosis.

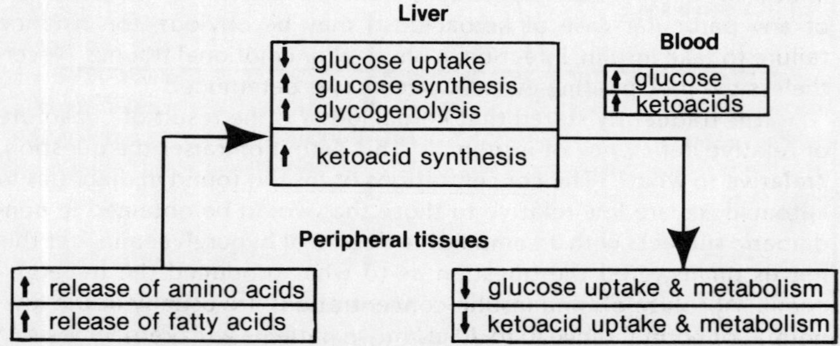

Figure 8-1   Alterations in glucose and ketoacid metabolism in diabetic ketoacidosis.

Considerable new information has accumulated regarding the hormonal and biochemical mechanisms that lead to the development of diabetic ketoacidosis. Although hepatic uptake of glucose is decreased even in milder states of diabetes mellitus, the loss of the restraining effect of insulin in patients developing ketoacidosis results in a threefold or greater increase in hepatic glucose production through gluconeogenesis.[16] Glucose uptake in peripheral tissues is also impaired as a consequence of more severe deficiency of insulin. Insulin deficiency in muscle tissue leads to decreased uptake and increased release of amino acids into the circulation, where they become available for the liver to extract and convert them to glucose.[17] The cumulative effect of all of these alterations in glucose metabolism is to create a state of starvation in spite of hyperglycemia and glucose overproduction.

As the decompensation increases in diabetic ketoacidosis, there is an increase in the release of free fatty acids from adipose tissue due to activation of hormone sensitive lipase.[2] Hepatic uptake of free fatty acids is augmented. Insulin lack causes a shift in hepatic metabolism of free fatty acids from synthesis of triglycerides and phospholipids to oxidation and generation of ketone bodies (Figure 8-2). This change in hepatic metabolism of free fatty acids appears to be mediated through increased activity of the carnitine acyltransferase system in the liver

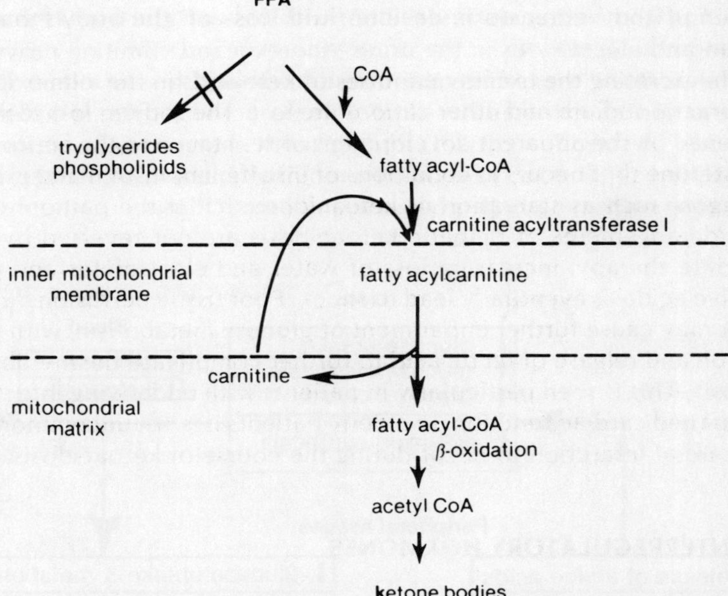

Figure 8-2 Hepatic oxidation of FFA and synthesis of ketone bodies in diabetic ketoacidosis.

156

mitochondria.[18-19] The transport of fatty acids across the inner mitochondrial membrane via a carnitine acyltransferase system is the rate-limiting step in the oxidation of fatty acids and conversion to ketone bodies. Evidence has been presented that the increase in carnitine acyltransferase activity is due to increased levels of carnitine (substrate) and decreased levels of malonyl CoA, which acts as an inhibitor of carnitine acyltransferase.[20] Glucagon secretion may play an important part in the activation of ketogenic mechanisms in the liver during ketoacidosis.[19] The end result of these changes in hepatic metabolism is a rapid increase in β-oxidation of fatty acids to acetyl CoA. The increased amounts of acetyl CoA are converted to acetoacetyl CoA and metabolized further to acetoacetate, β-hydroxybutyrate, and acetone (the "ketones" or "ketone bodies").

Insulin deficiency impairs the ability of peripheral tissues to take up and metabolize ketoacids.[21-24] Coupled with the increased production of ketoacids, this decrease in the ability of the body to clear ketoacids results in increased plasma ketone levels and metabolic acidosis. Acetoacetic and β-hydroxybutyric acid are strong organic acids (pK = 3.8) and thus are completely dissociated at body pH. As the body buffer base is consumed by hydrogen ions provided by the ketoacids, metabolic acidosis develops, as evidenced by a fall in serum bicarbonate and blood pH. The progressive metabolic acidosis causes a compensatory increase in respiration that is unable to restore a normal pH but increases insensible fluid loss and the body's energy demands.

In excreting the excess quantities of ketoacids in the kidney large amounts of sodium and other cations are lost. The sodium loss may be worsened by the apparent development of resistance to the actions of aldosterone that occurs in conditions of insufficient insulin and excess glucagon, such as starvation or ketoacidosis.[25-28] If the pathophysiologic derangements of diabetic ketoacidosis are not reversed by appropriate therapy, increasing loss of water and electrolytes and progressive acidosis eventually lead to shock. Poor tissue perfusion during shock may cause further impairment of glucose metabolism, with production and release of lactic acid to further complicate the metabolic acidosis. This is seen particularly in patients with underlying infection or impaired cardiac function. In elderly patients it is not uncommon for myocardial infarction to occur during the course of ketoacidosis.

COUNTERREGULATORY HORMONES

There is still considerable controversy as to whether secretion abnormalities of hormones other than insulin are necessary or important in the development of ketoacidosis. As mentioned earlier, elevation of the counterregulatory hormones (catecholamines, glucagon, growth hormone, and cortisol) is usually present in addition to low insulin levels.[5-10] The action of glucagon on the liver to increase gluconeogenesis and ketogenesis certainly can contribute to the overproduction of glucose and ketoacids.[6,7] Gerich and co-workers[29] have shown that infusion of somatostatin, a peptide that inhibits secretion of both insulin and glucagon, retards the development of hyperglycemia and ketoacidosis in diabetic patients after withdrawal of insulin. This implies at least a contributory role for excessive release of glucagon in the pathogenesis of ketoacidosis. However, insulin deficiency appears to be necessary for glucagon to cause significant hyperglycemia and ketoacidosis.[30-32] The effects of glucagon are limited in part because the increase in the release of hepatic glucose produced by glucagon is not maintained.[33] Studies in normal subjects given infusions of glucagon in the physiologic range have failed to stimulate ketogenesis despite adequate provision of free fatty acid.[34]

Most studies have not indicated an important role for growth hormone or cortisol in the development of ketoacidosis.[8-10] However, both of these hormones can elevate the blood glucose and increase ketone bodies in insulin-deficient diabetics.[35,36] Norepinephrine release from the sympathetic nervous system and epinephrine release from the adrenal medulla are both increased in diabetic ketoacidosis and probably contribute importantly to its development.[5] Both catecholamines activate hormone-sensitive lipase in adipose tissue, leading to mobilization of fatty acid. Exogenous administration of norepinephrine and epinephrine inhibits release of insulin by a direct action on pancreatic β-cells.[37] It is possible that norepinephrine released from nerve terminals in the pancreatic islets can inhibit insulin release in ketoacidosis.[38]

LABORATORY ABNORMALITIES

The diagnosis of ketoacidosis is usually not difficult. Even if the clinical history and examination do not suggest the diagnosis, the presence of glucose and ketones in the urine of a patient with hyperglycemia, ketonemia, and acidosis identifies the problem. It is important to distinguish between diabetic ketoacidosis and other causes of ketoacidosis such as alcoholic ketoacidosis or ingestion of toxins. The presence of moderately severe hyperglycemia (> 300 mg/dl) and ketoacidosis usually excludes these other diagnoses. On occasion the presence of ketones in the plasma and urine can be missed because most of the ketoacid is in the reduced form, β-hydroxybutyric acid.[39]

The nitroprusside reagent used to detect ketones in most laboratories does not react with β-hydroxybutyrate and reacts only 1/20 as well with acetone as acetoacetate.[40] Under these circumstances the metabolic acidosis may be misdiagnosed as lactic acidosis. During therapy with insulin, β-hydroxybutyrate is oxidized back to acetoacetate, which can lead to the seeming paradox of increasing plasma or urine ketones (by nitroprusside reaction) at a time when the actual concentrations of total ketones are falling. Plasma acetone, which determines the concentration of acetone in the breath, can remain elevated for as long as 42 hours after initiating insulin therapy.[41] This may contribute to the persistence of ketonuria that is sometimes observed for one to two days after the blood glucose and pH have returned to normal.

Elevation of several serum enzymes has been noted in patients with uncomplicated diabetic ketoacidosis.[42,43] This can be misleading, erroneously suggesting the presence of underlying disease. Serum amylase is elevated in many patients and can be attributed incorrectly to pancreatitis.[44] Fortunately, plasma lipase is usually within normal limits. It is important to recognize that even the amylase:creatinine clearance ratio may be as high in ketoacidosis as it is in pancreatitis[45] and is apparently due in part to an increase in salivary amylase.[46] Serum transaminase is often increased in diabetic ketoacidosis, particularly in patients with hepatomegaly.[47,48] Together with the elevation in creatine phosphokinase that can occur[49] the high transaminase may falsely suggest the diagnosis of myocardial infarction. The elevation in creatine phosphokinase is considered to be the result of the deficiency in phosphorus and subsequent hypophosphatemia that occurs during treatment of ketoacidosis.[1,50,51]

TREATMENT

Like most medical emergencies, the treatment of diabetic ketoacidosis should include careful monitoring of the patient and efforts to identify and treat any underlying disease, in addition to specific therapy. The main goals in the specific treatment of diabetic ketoacidosis are to replace water and electrolyte losses and to give sufficient doses of insulin to reverse the metabolic abnormalities. It should be acknowledged that opinions regarding the detailed management of diabetic ketoacidosis vary among authorities in the field. Furthermore, the exact treatment of patients with ketoacidosis should be individualized for their particular needs. In this context, "cookbook" techniques passed on uncritically from one generation of physicians to another must be condemned. The rapid advances in our understanding of ketoacidosis that have occurred in recent years were only possible when investigators began to question the scientific validity of many previous assumptions about this disorder.

Insulin Therapy

A major change in current understanding of the management of diabetic ketoacidosis is the recognition that large doses of insulin are not necessary or even desirable to correct the abnormalities of carbohydrate and lipid metabolism.[3,12-15,52-56] Whereas previously it was recommended that 50 to 200 units of insulin be given initially and repeated every two to four hours, numerous investigators have shown that doses ranging from 1.2 to 12 units/hr are adequate for most patients in diabetic ketoacidosis. It has also been demonstrated that insulin can be given by continuous intravenous infusion or by repeated intravenous, intramuscular, or subcutaneous injections with little difference in overall effect.[57] The fall in ketones may start earlier if the first dose of insulin is given by intravenous bolus, but this is a largely theoretical advantage. Regardless of the route of administration, the advantage of giving doses in the 5 to 20 units-per-hour range vs previous higher doses is the lower incidence of hypoglycemia and hypokalemia in the later stages of therapy.[3,12]

The chief objective of insulin therapy in the early treatment of diabetic ketoacidosis is to reverse the metabolic derangements producing ketoacidosis, ie, the overproduction and underutilization of ketones. Interestingly, the initial fall in blood glucose is apparently due largely to the correction of the negative fluid balance by intravenous infusion of saline rather than administration of insulin.[4,12] Nonetheless, it seems prudent to increase the dosage of insulin gradually if the blood sugar does not begin to fall after two to three hours of fluid administration. Treatment of ketoacidosis should not become a contest to see how little insulin can be given.[58] Patients may present rarely in ketoacidosis with true insulin resistance, perhaps as a result of circulating antibodies. It has also been observed that the rate of decline in the blood glucose concentration during treatment of ketoacidosis is reduced by half in the presence of infection.[12,56] Although this is not necessarily an indication for higher doses of insulin, it must be taken into account in evaluating the response to therapy.

Fluid and Electrolytes

The losses in water and electrolytes that occur in ketoacidosis are responsible for many of the morbid complications and must be given primary attention. Whereas recent information has made the selection of appropriate insulin therapy easier and more uniform, the skillful replacement of water and electrolytes remains a challenging problem.

Sodium and Water

Despite the large losses of water through glucose-induced osmotic diuresis, the serum sodium concentration in diabetic ketoacidosis is usually normal or low. This is attributable to the increased excretion of sodium in the urine and the dilution of extracellular sodium with water drawn from cells by the osmotic activity of extracellular glucose. Patients with unusually low sodium concentrations at the beginning of therapy may run an increased risk of cerebral edema.[59] The serum sodium may also be lowered factitiously by increased plasma lipoproteins, which are usually evident by the lactescent appearance of the plasma.

As a consequence of the coincident losses of both water and sodium, initial fluid replacement should normally be isotonic saline. This treatment helps to restore quickly the extracellular fluid volume, reducing the likelihood of hypovolemic shock and improving renal function. As mentioned earlier, this is the most significant factor in the initial fall in blood glucose concentrations. Most authorities recommend that one liter of isotonic saline be administered in the first hour. During the next three hours 0.5 to 1.0 liter of isotonic saline or isotonic saline alternated with half-isotonic saline should be given each hour. After assessment of the response, the infusion rate can be adjusted to deliver approximately half of the patient's estimated fluid loss within the first eight hours, followed by more gradual replacement of the remaining deficit during the next 16 hours. Since fluid losses in ketoacidosis are often equivalent to 10% to 15% of the total body weight, it is common to give 7 to 12 liters during the first 24 hours of therapy.

In elderly patients or patients with complicating illnesses it is important to monitor the central venous pressure. If shock or pulmonary congestion are present, the pulmonary capillary wedge pressure should be measured during fluid replacement. However, the time and attention required for inserting monitoring devices should not delay the pace of fluid therapy during the initial one to three hours. It is more common that initial fluid replacement is done too cautiously rather than too vigorously.

Potassium

The loss of total body potassium in diabetic ketoacidosis is profound. Deficits of 3 to 5 meq/kg body weight are common, and individual cases with losses as large as 10 meq/kg have been reported.[60-62] However, the plasma potassium concentration is usually normal or elevated before therapy. This is largely due to the coincident metabolic acidosis, which causes the hydrogen ion to shift intracellularly, resulting in potassium efflux into the extracellular space. The contraction of extracellular volume also contributes to the maintenance of serum potassium concentration. If the initial plasma potassium concentration is low, the deficit is likely to be severe and intravenous replacement therapy should be started immediately.[61] The most serious complications of hypokalemia are cardiac arrhythmias; the ECG alterations produced by changes in potassium concentration provide the best assessment of a patient's status on a minute-to-minute basis. Loss of U waves, the amplitude of T waves, P waves, and QRS changes can all be used to monitor response to therapy in cases of potassium deficiency. Serum potassium should also be measured at frequent intervals.

Within four hours after starting therapy the serum potassium begins to decrease in nearly all patients with ketoacidosis. This is due to continued urinary excretion of potassium and increased potassium uptake into cells as a result of insulin-mediated glucose uptake and partial correction of the metabolic acidosis. Some of the fall in serum potassium is simply a consequence of rehydration. Approximately 20% to 50% of administered potassium is excreted in the urine.[62] Greater amounts of potassium may be needed if bicarbonate is also administered to correct the metabolic acidosis. As stated earlier, the risk of hypokalemia is less in patients given lower doses of insulin compared to previous experience with high dose insulin therapy.[3,12]

Using repeated serum potassium determinations and monitoring the ECG, potassium should be added to the intravenous fluids as soon as the plasma concentration falls to normal levels. Although patients in renal failure have impaired ability to excrete potassium in the urine, they also require cautious potassium replacement to offset the shift of extracellular potassium into cells during therapy. Occasionally, infusion of potassium too early or too rapidly can produce hyperkalemia, which is most easily avoided by observing the ECG for the development of high or peaked T waves. Potassium is given as the chloride salt or less commonly as the phosphate salt.

Phosphate

As a consequence of increased catabolism in ketoacidosis, phosphate is released from numerous body tissues, particularly muscle. Excretion of phosphate is increased in the urine under conditions of inadequate insulin.[63-65] The impaired uptake and metabolism of glucose also impairs cellular uptake of phosphate. The end result of these processes is a large deficit in total body phosphate.[65] Like potassium, the concentration of phosphate in plasma is usually normal before initiation of treatment. As intravenous fluids and insulin reverse the ketoacidosis, plasma phosphate decreases to remarkably low levels (1.0 to 2.0 mg/dl). Levels below 0.5 mg/dl are associated with abnormalities in metabolism and organ function.[66]

Recent studies have drawn attention to how the deficiency of phosphate that occurs in ketoacidosis may adversely affect recovery. Phosphate deficiency, metabolic acidosis, and hyperglycemia are all known to impair the synthesis of 2,3-diphosphoglycerate (2,3-DPG).[67-69] As a result there is a fall in the 2,3-DPG concentration in the erythrocyte, which causes a shift in the oxygen-hemoglobin dissociation curve toward the left (Figure 8-3). This means that the affinity of hemoglobin for oxygen is increased, and the P_{50} (partial pressure of O_2 at which half of the hemoglobin has released its oxygen) is decreased. The effect of these changes is to reduce the delivery of oxygen to body tissues.

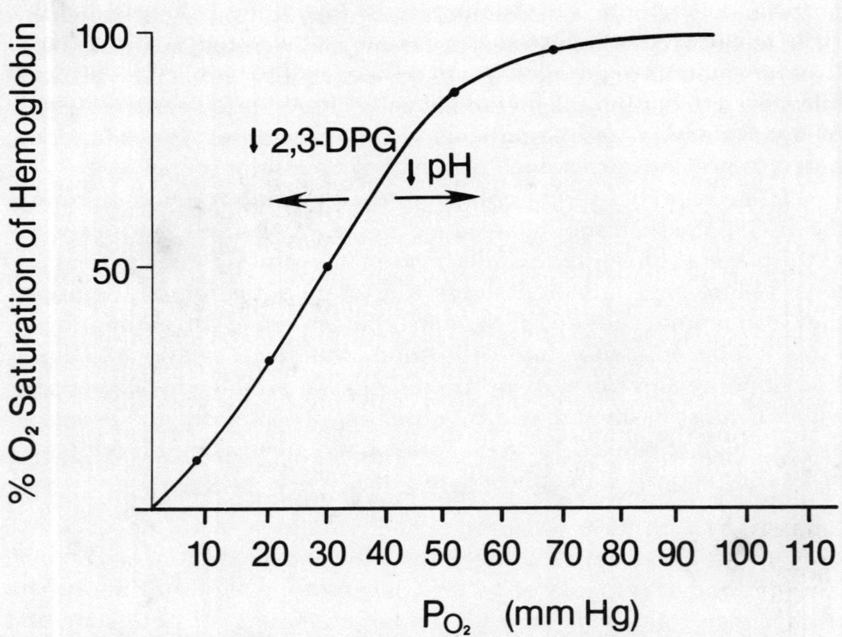

Figure 8-3 A fall in the 2,3-DPG concentration in the erythrocyte causes a shift toward the left of the oxygen-hemoglobin dissociation curve.

Part of the shift to the left in the oxygen-hemoglobin dissociation curve caused by the depressed levels of 2,3-DPG in the erythrocyte is compensated by the prior shift to the right in the curve as a result of the metabolic acidosis (the Bohr effect). As the pH rises during treatment of ketoacidosis the curve will shift further to the left. Administration of large amounts of bicarbonate can exacerbate this adverse shift of the oxygen-hemoglobin dissociation curve and further impair delivery of oxygen to tissues. As a hypothetical example, a rapid increase in the plasma pH from 7.1 to 7.4 would necessitate a threefold to fivefold increase in cardiac output to deliver an equivalent amount of oxygen to peripheral tissues.[70] In actual practice there is often no difference in oxygen transport in patients treated with bicarbonate compared to patients not given bicarbonate.[71] Phosphate deficiency has also been shown to decrease tissue sensitivity to insulin in dogs,[72] but, as mentioned before, insulin resistance is not a common problem in diabetic ketoacidosis.

Despite the theoretical importance of phosphate deficiency in diabetic ketoacidosis, there is not sufficient clinical evidence of the practical necessity of administering phosphate to recommend its routine use. Despite a fall in serum phosphate concentrations seen in children during treatment of ketoacidosis,[73] the concentration of 2,3-DPG in erythrocytes usually returns to normal within 24 hours.[71] This suggests that although phosphate administration can prevent hypophosphatemia in children,[73] it is not essential for the restoration of 2,3-DPG concentrations that occurs after treatment of hyperglycemia and metabolic acidosis.

The ratio of lactate to pyruvate varies inversely with erythrocyte 2,3-DPG concentrations.[74] This suggests that, in patients with lactic acidosis complicating ketoacidosis or in those patients with poor tissue perfusion or limited cardiac function, phosphate supplementation might be beneficial. In adults restoration of erythrocyte 2,3-DPG concentrations is definitely accelerated by phosphate administration.[64] Phosphate is usually given intravenously as the potassium salt. Rapid infusion of phosphate solutions can produce hypocalcemia. In calculating the amount of phosphate to give several factors must be considered. The average deficit of phosphate is on the order of 1 mmol/kg of body weight. Of the amount of phosphate given, approximately 30% to 95% will be retained. Finally, it is not necessary to replace the entire deficit acutely, since the phosphate concentration in the erythrocyte is regulated by the concentration of plasma phosphate rather than total body stores.[1] The large amounts of potassium and phosphate in most foods allow rapid replacement of tissue losses as soon as patients resume meals.

Bicarbonate

Few areas in the treatment of diabetic ketoacidosis have generated as much controversy as the issue of bicarbonate therapy. Probably the cause of these differences in opinion is the knowledge that bicarbonate therapy has clearly demonstrable risks and benefits. As in most therapeutic decisions that involve difficult risk:benefit ratios, the correct answer usually depends on a careful assessment of all medical aspects of the individual patient.

If the serum bicarbonate has been lost in titrating ketoacids produced in diabetic ketoacidosis, why not replace it? There are several important reasons for caution. First, as mentioned previously in the discussion of phosphate metabolism, metabolic acidosis produces a shift to the right in the oxygen-hemoglobin dissociation curve that facilitates oxygen delivery in peripheral tissues. If bicarbonate is given to "correct" the metabolic acidosis, an unfavorable shift to the left in the oxygen-hemoglobin dissociation curve can occur.

Another objection to bicarbonate administration is the adverse effect it can have on the pH of cerebrospinal fluid (CSF). As diabetic ketoacidosis develops, the peripheral chemoreceptors are stimulated, leading to an increase in ventilation. This causes a lowering of the plasma pCO_2. Since pCO_2 in the CSF and interstitial-fluid compartment of the brain equilibrate rapidly, whereas CSF bicarbonate equilibrates more slowly with plasma bicarbonate, the pH of the CSF is protected from the peripheral acidosis (Figure 8-4). If bicarbonate is administered rapidly or in large amounts to patients in ketoacidosis, there will be a decrease in the stimulation of the peripheral chemoreceptors, leading to a decrease in ventilation and an increase in pCO_2. An increase in pCO_2 of the CSF without a compensatory increase in bicarbonate causes a "paradoxical" increase in CSF acidosis.[75] Below a CSF pH of 7.2 the level of consciousness begins to decrease. Although this sequence of events has been demonstrated to occur, several arguments cast doubt on its clinical importance. First, the hyperventilation seen in diabetic ketoacidosis is not decreased suddenly with correction of systemic acidosis.[76] In cases of severe metabolic acidosis the ventilatory drive actually may be improved by administration of bicarbonate.[77] Second, study of patients in ketoacidosis has shown no great differences in the pH of CSF between patients treated with bicarbonate vs those who did not receive bicarbonate.[78] This is probably due to the ability of the body to produce endogenous bicarbonate from oxidation of ketone bodies after insulin treatment. Such a mechanism does not exist in metabolic acidosis that is not accompanied by increases in ketoacids. Third, when the pH of CSF has been measured in patients with diabetic ketoacidosis, adverse effects on the central nervous system have not been noted in the majority of patients, even when the pH was less than 7.26.[79] Finally, there are no well-documented cases where "paradoxical" CSF acidosis caused by bicarbonate therapy has led to any persistent impairment of the central nervous system or other disability.

Another objection to the use of bicarbonate is the possibility that potassium reuptake into cells will be increased too rapidly, resulting in hypokalemia. If sufficient attention is devoted to potassium replacement this does not appear to be a very strong argument against the use of bicarbonate.

If the plasma bicarbonate is normally corrected by treatment with saline and insulin alone, what is the need for intravenous administration of bicarbonate? In mild to moderately severe cases of ketoacidosis there is no obvious benefit in trying to restore the plasma bicarbonate to normal more quickly with exogenous bicarbonate. However, severe metabolic acidosis has adverse effects on the body that can be life-threatening and demand immediate relief. Kety and associates have shown that although the minute volume of respiration increases rapidly between an arterial pH of 7.2 and 7.1, there is a decrease as the pH falls below 7.1.[77] This interferes with the compensatory effect of hyperventilation on the metabolic acidosis.

Metabolic acidosis also impairs myocardial contractility and increases the risk of cardiac arrhythmias.[76] Experiments in rats have shown that the contractility of the left ventricle decreases when the

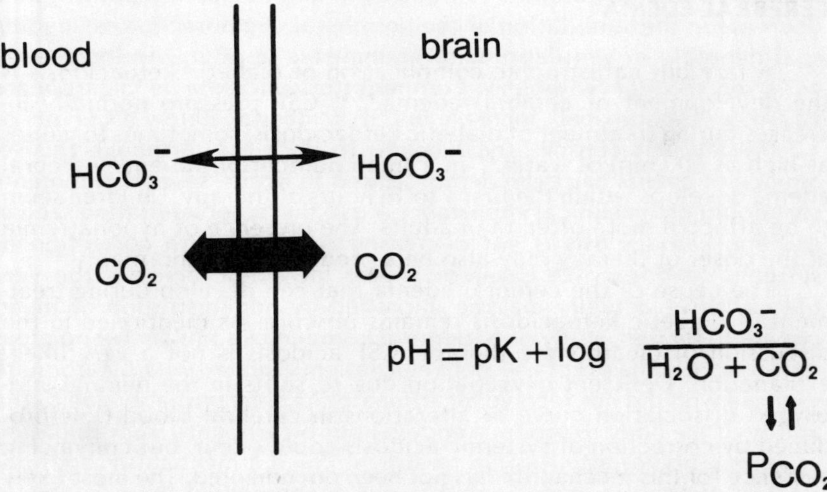

$$pH = pK + \log \frac{HCO_3^-}{H_2O + CO_2}$$

$$P_{CO_2}$$

Figure 8-4　The pH of the cerebrospinal fluid (CSF) is protected from peripheral acidosis because pCO_2 equilibrates more rapidly in the CSF and interstitial-fluid compartment, whereas CSF bicarbonate equilibrates more slowly with plasma bicarbonate.

arterial pH falls to levels 7.1 or less.[80] Ng and associates have observed decreased left-ventricular, systolic pressure with acidosis.[81] Of lesser clinical importance, Mackler et al have demonstrated reduced sensitivity to insulin in acidotic states.[82]

Studies comparing results of treating patients in moderate ketoacidosis with or without bicarbonate have, not surprisingly, found little difference. King and associates treated a series of patients without bicarbonate with satisfactory results.[76] Assal and associates treated a group of ketoacidotic patients with bicarbonate and compared their results with a previous group of patients treated at the same clinic without bicarbonate.[78] They noted a somewhat smaller decrease in CSF osmolality and a greater fall in pH of CSF in bicarbonate-treated patients.

After reviewing the evidence, Kaye wrote recently, "the bicarbonate controversy in the treatment of diabetic ketoacidosis appears to resemble many similar therapeutic dilemmas and is resolved not by 'yes' or 'no' but by asking the questions 'when' and 'how much.'"[83] He suggests that bicarbonate be given to patients when the arterial pH has fallen below 7.15. Because methods of calculating base deficit in diabetic ketoacidosis tend to exaggerate its magnitude almost twofold, replacement should be purposely incomplete.[84] It is reasonable to ignore calculations of base deficit and simply give 1 to 2 mEq of bicarbonate/kg of body weight to patients with severe acidosis (pH less than 7.1).

CEREBRAL EDEMA

A rare but catastrophic complication of diabetic ketoacidosis is the development of cerebral edema.[85,86] CSF pressure normally increases during treatment of diabetic ketoacidosis, sometimes to values as high as 600 mm of water.[87] In a small number of patients, cerebral edema develops within the first 4 to 16 hours of therapy. Children seem to be affected more often than adults. The presence of hyponatremia at the onset of therapy may also be a predisposing abnormality.[88]

The cause of the cerebral edema that can develop during treatment of diabetic ketoacidosis remains obscure. As mentioned in the discussion of bicarbonate therapy, CSF acidosis is not a very likely explanation. Deficient oxygenation due to shifts in the hemoglobin-oxygen dissociation curve or alterations in cerebral blood flow produced by correction of systemic acidosis could occur, but convincing evidence for this mechanism has not been documented. The most likely hypothesis is that hyperglycemia leads to an accumulation of "idiogenic osmoles" in brain tissue.[89,90] Although sorbitol was previously considered to be the responsible osmotic agent, the concentrations of sorbitol found in brain tissue are insufficient to account for the increase in brain osmolality.[91] Rapid lowering of the blood glucose appears to promote the development of cerebral edema.[89,92] This suggests that slower reduction of the blood glucose by avoiding excessive doses of insulin and by adding glucose to intravenous solutions when the blood glucose has fallen to 300 mg/dl may reduce the risk of cerebral edema. In the event that edema does develop, high doses of glucocorticoids or administration of intravenous mannitol have been tried, but definite proof of their efficacy is lacking.

GLUCOSE ADMINISTRATION

It is important to continue the administration of intravenous glucose solutions in the later stages of treatment of diabetic ketoacidosis to replace glycogen stores and to prevent hypoglycemia. Since insulin should be administered continuously or at hourly intervals until the ketoacidosis has disappeared, it is necessary to give sufficient glucose to counterbalance the glucose-lowering effects of the insulin. Dextrose (5%) with potassium supplementation as needed, is a convenient intravenous solution. Hypoglycemia in the later stages of treatment of ketoacidosis has become a less common problem since the advent of lower insulin dosage regimens.[3]

LACTIC ACIDOSIS

In severe diabetic ketoacidosis plasma lactate frequently is elevated.[93,94] Usually the increase in plasma lactate is only moderate and contributes little to the systemic acidosis. During insulin and fluid therapy plasma levels of lactate decline, so specific treatment is seldom indicated. In the small number of patients with significant lactic acidosis in addition to ketoacidosis, there is often coexistent shock and/or hypoxemia leading to poor tissue perfusion. The prognosis for eventual recovery is clearly worse in this group of patients. Treatment should be directed toward improving cardiac output, increasing oxygenation, and, in cases of sepsis, appropriate antibiotic therapy.

ALCOHOLIC KETOACIDOSIS

Alcoholic ketoacidosis can usually be distinguished from diabetic ketoacidosis by the absence of significant hyperglycemia.[95] In fact, many patients with alcoholic ketoacidosis are hypoglycemic, particularly if the blood alcohol is still elevated.[96] Nevertheless, moderate hyperglycemia may occur and probably constitutes an indication for insulin in addition to the parenteral administration of glucose that is the main form of therapy for this disorder.[95,97] It is important to recognize that alcoholic ketoacidosis usually occurs after discontinuation of heavy ethanol ingestion. Blood and breath alcohol concentrations are often normal or only slightly elevated. A history of gastrointestinal upset or vomiting in the period immediately prior to admission is common.

Plasma and urinary ketones are usually strikingly elevated in alcoholic ketoacidosis. As in patients with diabetic ketoacidosis, negative nitroprusside reactions are occasionally seen when most of the ketone bodies are in the form of β-hydroxybutyrate.[95,97] The plasma pH can be normal or even high in some patients with alcoholic ketosis.[95] It has been noted that alcoholic patients with diabetes are more susceptible to the development of acidosis. Although ethanol can produce lactic acidosis, high plasma lactate concentrations are seldom a significant complication in alcoholic ketoacidosis.[95,97-99]

HYPEROSMOLAR COMA

The syndrome of nonketotic hyperosmolar coma is characterized by hyperglycemia without significant ketoacidosis.[100-102] However, it must be appreciated that uncontrolled diabetes can also present as an intermediate form of decompensation with mild to moderate ketoacidosis in the presence of severe dehydration, hyperglycemia, and hypernatremia. Patients who develop hyperosmolar coma are usually insulin-independent diabetics who have sufficient insulin to prevent the excessive lipolysis and accelerated production of ketoacids that occur in ketoacidosis, but not enough insulin to control hyperglycemia. Most patients are elderly and preexistent renal disease is a common feature. The extreme dehydration that occurs in this syndrome is due to both diminished intake of water and increased excretion of water in the urine.[101] The rate of development and the magnitude of the hyperosmolality both influence the severity of CNS signs, which range from obtundation to coma.[103] Plasma osmolalities are usually greater than 340 to 350 mOsm/kg before symptoms develop. When facilities for direct measurement are not available, the plasma osmolality can be estimated by the following formula:

$$\text{osmolality in mOsm/kg} = 2(Na^+) + \frac{\text{plasma glucose in mg/dl}}{18}$$

If stupor or coma exists and the osmolality is not greater than 340 mOsm/kg other etiologies should be considered.

Complicating problems associated with hyperosmolar coma include shock, acute tubular necrosis, and vascular thromboses. The overall prognosis for recovery is worse for hyperosmolar coma than ketoacidosis, with mortality rates as high as 30% to 50%.[9,100-103]

Treatment of Hyperosmolar Coma

Ever since the syndrome of nonketotic hyperosmolar coma was recognized it has been noted that relatively small doses of insulin are usually adequate.[100-103] Since similar small amounts of insulin are now recommended for ketoacidosis as well, there is little difficulty in selecting an appropriate dosage, even in those patients who have intermediate forms of uncontrolled diabetes with aspects both of ketoacidosis and a hyperosmolar state.

The fluid therapy of hyperosmolar coma differs from ketoacidosis. It is important that hypotonic electrolyte solutions such as half-isotonic saline be used instead of isotonic solutions, except in the presence of shock. Like the treatment of ketoacidosis, initial fluid replacement should be rapid (approximately 1 liter/hr). Since the overall fluid deficit is greater in hyperosmolar coma than in ketoacidosis, the rate of infusion should usually be continued at higher levels for a longer period in treating hyperosmolar coma. Often 8 to 16 liters of fluid are required in the first 24 hours. Plasma potassium should be monitored, and replacement therapy given as required. Because of the frequent problem of organic renal disease as well as prerenal azotemia secondary to dehydration, potassium must be administered cautiously with frequent plasma potassium determinations and ECG monitoring.

REFERENCES

1. Kreisberg, R.A. Diabetic ketoacidosis: new concepts and trends in pathogenesis and treatment. *Ann Intern Med.* 88:681–695, 1978.

2. McGarry, J.D., and Foster, D.W. Regulation of ketogenesis and clinical aspects of the ketotic state. *Metabolism* 21:471–479, 1972.

3. Kitabchi, A.E., Ayyagari, V., and Guerra, S.M.D. The efficacy of low-dose versus conventional therapy of insulin for treatment of diabetic ketoacidosis. *Ann Intern Med.* 84:633–638, 1976.

4. Meinders, A.E., Koppeschaar, H.P.F., Sindram, E.D.A. et al. The influence of rehydration in uncontrolled insulin-dependent diabetes mellitus. *Neth J Med.* 21:3–10, 1978.

5. Christensen, N.J. Plasma norepinephrine and epinephrine in untreated diabetics, during fasting and after insulin administration. *Diabetes* 23:1–28, 1974.

6. Dobbs, R., Sakurai, H., Sasaki, H. et al. Glucagon: role in the hyperglycemia of diabetes mellitus. *Science* 187:544–546, 1975.

7. Unger, R.H., and Orci. L. The essential role of glucagon in the pathogenesis of diabetes mellitus. *Lancet* 1:14–16, 1975.

8. Gerich, J.E., Martin, M.M., and Recant, L. Clinical and metabolic characteristics of hyperosmolar nonketotic coma. *Diabetes* 20:228–238, 1971.

9. Cryer, P.E., and Daughaday, W.H. Diabetic ketosis: serial plasma growth hormone concentrations during therapy. *Diabetes* 19:519–523, 1970.

10. Alberti, K.G., and Hockaday, T.D. Diabetic coma: serum growth hormone before and during treatment. *Diabetologia* 9:13–19, 1973.

11. Eigler, N., Sacca, J., and Sherwin, R.S. Synergistic interactions of physiologic increments of glucagon, epinephrine, and cortisol in the dog. *J Clin Invest.* 63:114–123, 1979.

12. Alberti, K.G.M.M., Hockaday, T.D.R., and Turner, R.C. Small doses of intramuscular insulin in the treatment of diabetic coma. *Lancet* 2:515–522, 1973.

13. Kidson, W., Casey, J., Kraegen, E. et al. Treatment of severe diabetes mellitus by insulin infusion. *Br Med J.* 2:691–694, 1974.

14. Page, M.M., Alberti, K.G.M.M., Greenwood, R. et al. Treatment of diabetic coma with continuous low-dose infusion of insulin. *Br Med J.* 2:687–690, 1974.

15. Semple, P.F., White, C., and Manderson, W.G. Continuous intravenous infusion of small doses of insulin in treatment of diabetic ketoacidosis. *Br Med J.* 2:694–698, 1974.

16. Sherwin, R., and Felig, P. Pathophysiology of diabetes mellitus. *Med Clin North Am.* 62:695–711, 1978.

17. Felig, P., Wahren, J., Sherwin, R. et al. Amino acid and protein metabolism in diabetes mellitus. *Arch Intern Med.* 137:507–513, 1977.

18. McGarry, J.D., and Foster, D.W. Ketogenesis and its regulation. *Am J Med.* 61:9–13, 1976.

19. McGarry, J.D., and Foster, D.W. Hormonal control of ketogenesis. *Arch Intern Med.* 137:495–501, 1977.

20. McGarry, J.D., Leatherman, G.E., and Foster, D.W. Carnitine palmitoyl-transferase. I. The site of inhibition of hepatic fatty acid oxidation by malonyl-CoA. *J Biol Chem.* 253:4128–4136, 1978.

21. Balasse, E.O., Havel R.J. Evidence for an effect of insulin on the peripheral utilization of ketone bodies in dogs. *J Clin Invest.* 50:801–813, 1971.

22. Ruderman, N.B., and Goodman, M.N. Inhibition of muscle acetoacetate utilization during diabetic ketoacidosis. *Am J Physiol.* 226:136–143, 1974.

23. Garber, A.J., Menzel, P.H., Boden, G. et al. Hepatic ketogenesis and gluconeogenesis in humans. *J Clin Invest.* 54:981–989, 1974.

24. Sherwin, R.S., Hendler, R.G. and Felig, P. Effect of diabetes mellitus and insulin on the turnover and metabolic response to ketones in man. *Diabetes* 25:776–784, 1976.

25. DeFronzo, R.A., Cooke, C.R., Andres, R. et al. The effect of insulin on renal handling of sodium, potassium, calcium, and phosphate in man. *J Clin Invest.* 55:845–855, 1975.

26. Saudek, C.D., Boulter, P.R., and Arky, R.A. The natriuretic effect of glucagon and its role in starvation. *J Clin Endocrinol Metab.* 36:761–764, 1973.

27. Blumenthal, S.A. Observations on sodium retention related to insulin treatment of experimental diabetes. *Diabetes* 24:645–649, 1975.

28. Saudek, C.S., Boulter, P.R., Knopp, R.H. et al. Sodium retention accompanying insulin treatment of diabetes mellitus. *Diabetes* 23:240–246, 1974.

29. Gerich, J.E., Lorenzi, M., Bier, D.M. et al. Prevention of human diabetic ketoacidosis by somatostatin. *N Engl J Med.* 292:985–989, 1975.

30. Liljenquist, J.E., Bomboy, J.D., Lewis, S.B. et al. Effects of glucagon on lipolysis and ketogenesis in normal and diabetic men. *J Clin Invest.* 53:190–197, 1974.

31. Sherwin, R.S., Fisher, M., Hendler, R. et al. Hyperglucagonemia and blood glucose regulation in normal, obese, and diabetic subjects. *N Engl J Med.* 294:455–461, 1976.

32. Felig, P., Wahren, J., Sherwin, R. et al. Insulin, glucagon, and somatostatin in normal physiology and diabetes mellitus. *Diabetes* 25:1091–1099, 1976.

33. Felig, P., Wahren, J., and Hendler, R. Influence of physiologic hyperglucagonemia on basal and insulin-inhibited splanchnic glucose output in normal man. *J Clin Invest.* 58:761–765, 1976.

34. Schade, D.S., and Eaton, R.P. Modulation of fatty acid metabolism by glucagon in man. IV. Effects of a physiologic hormone infusion in normal man. *Diabetes* 25:978–983, 1976.

35. Schade, D.S., Eaton, R.P., and Standefer, J. Glucocorticoid regulation of plasma ketone body concentration in insulin deficient man. *J Clin Endocrinol Metab.* 44:1069–1079, 1977.

36. Schade, D.S., Eaton, R.P., and Peake, G.T. The regulation of plasma ketone body concentration by counter-regulatory hormones in man. II. Effects of growth hormone in diabetic man. *Diabetes* 27:916–924, 1978.

37. Porte, D. Sympathetic regulation of insulin secretion. *Arch Intern Med.* 123:252–260, 1969.

38. Johnson, D.G., Henry, D.P., Moss, J. et al. Inhibition of insulin release by scorpion toxin in rat pancreatic islets. *Diabetes* 25:198–201, 1976.

39. Marliss, E.B., Ohman, J.L., Aoki, T.T. et al. Altered redox state obscuring ketoacidosis in diabetic patients with lactic acidosis. *N Engl J Med.* 283: 978–982, 1970.

40. Nash, J., Lister, J., and Vobes, D.H. Clinical tests for ketonuria. *Lancet* 1:801–804, 1954.

41. Sulway, M.J., and Malins, J.M. Acetone in diabetic ketoacidosis. *Lancet* 2:736–740, 1970.

42. Belfiore, F., Napoli, E., and Vecchio, L.L. Increased activity of some enzymes in serum in cases of severely decompensated diabetes, with or without ketoacidosis. *Clin Chem.* 18:1403–1406, 1972.

43. Knight, A.H., Williams, D.N., Spooner, R.J. et al. Serum enzyme changes in diabetic ketoacidosis. *Diabetes* 23:126–131, 1974.

44. Knight, A.H., Williams, D.N., Ellis, G. et al. Significance of hyperamylasaemia and abdominal pain in diabetic ketoacidosis. *Br Med J.* 3:128–131, 1973.

45. Levine, R.L., Glauser, F.L., and Berk, J.D. Enhancement of the amylase-creatinine clearance ratio in disorders other than acute pancreatitis. *N Engl J Med.* 292:329–331, 1975.

46. Warshaw, A.L., Feller, E.R., and Lee, K.H. On the cause of raised serum amylase in diabetic ketoacidosis. *Lancet* 1:929–931, 1977.

47. Cryer, P.E., and Daughaday, W.H. Diabetic ketosis elevated serum glutamic-oxaloacetic transaminase (SGOT) and other findings determined by multi-channel chemical analysis. *Diabetes* 18:781–785, 1969.

48. Chen, J.C., Marster, R., and Wieland, R.G. Diabetic ketosis: interpretation of elevated serum glutamic-oxaloacetic transaminase (SGOT) by multi-channel chemical analysis. *Diabetes* 19:730–731, 1970.

49. Velez-Garcia, F., Hardy, P., Dioso, M. et al. Cysteine-stimulated serum creatine phosphokinase: unexpected results. *J Lab Clin Med.* 68:636–644, 1966.

50. Knochel, J.P., Bilbrey, G.L., Fuller, T.J. et al. The muscle cell in chronic

alcoholism: the possible role of phosphate depletion in alcoholic myopathy. *Ann NY Acad Sci.* 252:274–286, 1975.

51. Fuller, T.J., Carter, N.W., Barcenas, C. et al. Reversible changes of the muscle cell in experimental phosphorus deficiency. *J Clin Invest.* 57:1019–1024, 1976.

52. Smith, K., Martin, H.E. Response of diabetic coma to various insulin dosages. *Diabetes* 3:287–295, 1954.

53. Shaw, C.E., Hurwitz, G.E., Schmukler, M. et al. A clinical and laboratory study of insulin dosage in diabetic acidosis: comparison with small and large doses. *Diabetes* 11:23–30, 1962.

54. Genuth, S.M. Constant intravenous insulin infusion in diabetic ketoacidosis. *JAMA.* 223:1348–1351, 1973.

55. Piters, K., Goodman, J., and Bessman, A. Treatment of diabetic ketoacidosis with continuous low-dose intravenous insulin (abstract). *Diabetes* 24:396, 1975.

56. Soler, N.G., Fitzgerald, M.G., Wright, A.D. et al. Comparative study of different insulin regimens in management of diabetic ketoacidosis. *Lancet* 2:1221–1224, 1975.

57. Fisher, J.N., Shahshahnani, M.N., and Kitabchi, A.E. Diabetic ketoacidosis: low-dose insulin therapy by various routes. *N Engl J Med.* 297:238–241, 1977.

58. Reitsma, W.D. Insulin dose in the treatment of diabetic ketoacidotic coma. *Neth J Med.* 21:1–2, 1978.

59. Duck, S.C., Weldon, V.V., Pagliara, A.S. et al. Cerebral edema complicating therapy for diabetic ketoacidosis. *Diabetes* 25:111–115, 1976.

60. Beigleman, P.M. Potassium in severe diabetic ketoacidosis. *Am J Med.* 54:419–420, 1973.

61. Abramson, E., and Arky, R. Diabetic acidosis with initial hypokalemia. *JAMA.* 196:115–117, 1966.

62. Soler, N.G., Dixon, K., Bennett, M.A. et al. Potassium balance during treatment of diabetic ketoacidosis. *Lancet* 2:665–667, 1972.

63. Atchley, D.W., Loeb, R.F., Richards, D.W. Jr. et al. A detailed study of electrolyte balances following the withdrawal and re-establishment of insulin therapy. *J Clin Invest.* 12:297–326, 1933.

64. Guest, G.M., and Rapoport, S. Electrolytes of blood plasma and cells in diabetic acidosis and during recovery. *Proc Am Diabetes Assoc.* 7:97–115, 1947.

65. Seldin, D.W., and Tarail, R. The metabolism of glucose and electrolytes in diabetic acidosis. *J Clin Invest.* 29:552–565, 1950.

66. Martin, D.W., Watts, H.D., and Smith, L.H. Hypophosphatemia. *West J Med.* 122:482–489, 1975.

67. Guest, G.M., and Rapoport, S. Role of acid-soluble phophorus compounds in red blood cells. *Am J Dis Child.* 58:1072–1089, 1939.

68. Guest, G.M. Relationship of potassium and inorganic phosphorus to organic acid soluble phosphates in erythrocytes. *Lancet* 1:188–189, 1953.

69. Travis, S.F., Morrison, A.D., Clements, R.S. et al. Metabolic alterations in the human erythrocyte produced by increases in glucose concentration. *J Clin Invest.* 50:2104–2112, 1971.

70. Bellingham, A.J., Detter, J.C., and Lenfant, C. The role of hemoglobin affinity for oxygen and red-cell 2,3-diphosphoglycerate in the management of diabetic ketoacidosis. *Trans Assoc Am Physicans.* 83:113–120, 1970.

71. Munk, P., Freedman, M.H., Levison, H. et al. Effect of bicarbonate on oxygen transport in juvenile diabetic ketoacidosis. *J Pediatr.* 84:510–514, 1974.

72. Harter, H.R., Santiago, J.V., Rutherford, W.E. et al. The relative role of

calcium, phosphorus, and parathyroid hormone in glucose and tolbutamide-mediated insulin release. *J Clin Invest.* 58:359–367, 1976.

73. Lightner, E.S., Kappy, M.S., and Revsin, B. Low-dose intravenous insulin infusion in patients with diabetic ketoacidosis: biochemical effects in children. *Pediatrics* 60:681–688, 1977.

74. Alberti, K.G.M.M., Darley, J.H., Emerson, D.M. et al. 2,3-diphospho-glycerate and tissue oxygenation in uncontrolled diabetes mellitus. *Lancet* 2:391–395, 1972.

75. Posner, J.B., and Plum, F. Spinal fluid pH and neurologic symptoms in systemic acidosis. *N Engl J Med.* 277:605–613, 1967.

76. King, A.J., Cooke, N.J., McCush, A. et al. Acid-base changes during treatment of diabetic ketoacidosis. *Lancet* 1:478–479, 1974.

77. Kety, S.S., Polis, B.D., Nadler, C.S. et al. The blood flow and oxygen consumption of the human brain in diabetic ketoacidosis and coma. *J Clin Invest.* 27:500–510, 1948.

78. Assal, J.P., Aoki, T.T., Manzano, F.M. et al. Metabolic effects of sodium bicarbonate in management of diabetic ketoacidosis. *Diabetes* 23:405–411, 1974.

79. Ohman, J.L., Marliss, E.B., Aoki, T.T. et al. The cerebrospinal fluid in diabetic ketoacidosis. *N Engl J Med.* 284:283–290, 1971.

80. Opie, L.H. Effect of extracellular pH on function and metabolism of isolated perfused rat heart. *Am J Physiol.* 209:1075–1080, 1965.

81. Ng, M.L., Levy, M.N., and Zieske, H.A. Effects of changes of pH and of carbon dioxide tension on left ventricular performance. *Am J Physiol.* 213:115–120, 1967.

82. Mackler, B., Lichenstein, H., and Guest, G.M. Effects of ammonium chloride acidosis on the action of insulin in dogs. *Am J Physiol.* 166:191–198, 1951.

83. Kaye, R. Diabetic ketoacidosis—the bicarbonate controversy. *J Pediatr.* 87:156–159, 1975.

84. Zimmet, P.A., Taft, P., Ennis, G.C. et al. Acid production in diabetic acidosis: a more rational approach to alkali replacement. *Br Med J.* 3:610–612, 1970.

85. Young, E., and Bradley, R.F. Cerebral edema with irreversible coma in severe diabetic ketoacidosis. *N Engl J Med.* 276:665–669, 1967.

86. Metzger, A.L., and Rubenstein, A.H. Reversible cerebral edema complicating diabetic ketoacidosis. *Br Med J.* 3:746–747, 1970.

87. Clements, R.S., Blumenthal, S.A., Morrison, A.D. et al. Increased cerebrospinal-fluid pressure during treatment of diabetic ketosis. *Lancet* 2:671–675, 1971.

88. Martin, H.E., Smith, K., and Wilson, M.L. The fluid and electrolyte therapy of severe diabetic acidosis and ketosis. *Am J Med.* 20:376–388, 1956.

89. Arieff, A.I., and Kleeman, C.R. Studies on mechanism of cerebral edema in diabetic comas. *J Clin Invest.* 52:571–583, 1973.

90. Guisado, R., and Arieff, A.I. Neurologic manifestations of diabetic comas: correlation with biochemical alterations in the brain. *Metabolism* 24:665–679, 1975.

91. Prockop, L.D. Hyperglycemia, polyol accumulation, increased intracranial pressure. *Arch Neurol.* 25:126–140, 1971.

92. Stern, W.E., and Coxan, R.V. Osmolality of brain tissue and its relation to brain bulk. *Am J Physiol.* 206:1–7, 1964.

93. Watkins, P.J., Smith, J.S., Fitzgerald, M.G. et al. Lactic acidosis in diabetes. *Br Med J.* 1:744–747, 1969.

94. Strandgaard, S., Nielson, P.E., Bitsch, V. et al. Blood lactate and ketone bodies in diabetic ketoacidosis. *Acta Med Scand.* 190:17–20, 1971.

95. Fulop, M., and Hoberman, H.D. Alcoholic ketosis. *Diabetes* 24:785–790, 1975.

96. Heinig, R.E., Miller, P.D., and Waterhouse, C. Metabolic aspects of alcoholic ketoacidosis (abstract). *Clin Res.* 24:362, 1976.

97. Levy, L.J., Duga, J., Girgis, M. et al. Ketoacidosis associated with alcoholism in nondiabetic subjects. *Ann Intern Med.* 78:213–219, 1973.

98. Jenkins, D.W., Eckel, R.E., and Craig, J.W. Alcoholic ketoacidosis. *JAMA.* 217:177–183, 1971.

99. Cooperman, M.T., Davidoff, F., Spark, R. et al. Clinical studies of alcoholic ketoacidosis. *Diabetes* 23:433–439, 1974.

100. Nabarro, J.D.N. Hyperosmolar nonketotic diabetic coma. Edited by B.S. Leibel, and G.A. Wrenshal. In *On the Nature and Treatment of Diabetes.* New York: Excerpta Medica Foundation, 1965, pp 551–557.

101. Arieff, A.I., and Carroll, H.J. Nonketotic hyperosmolar coma with hyperglycemia: clinical features, pathophysiology, renal function, acid-base balance, plasma-cerebrospinal fluid equilibria and the effects of therapy in 37 cases. *Medicine* 51:73–94, 1972.

102. Jackson, W.P.U., and Forman, R. Hyperosmolar nonketotic diabetic coma. *Diabetes* 15:714–722, 1966.

103. Arieff, A.I., and Carroll, H.J. Cerebral edema and depression of sensorium in nonketotic hyperosmolar coma. *Diabetes* 23:525–531, 1974.

9 Infection and Diabetes Mellitus

Stanton G. Axline, MD

It has long been believed that patients with diabetes mellitus are more susceptible to infection than nondiabetic patients and that infections that do occur are more severe. Based on autopsy studies, infections of the urinary tract and soft tissue of the extremeties do appear to occur more frequently in diabetics than in nondiabetics. The increased susceptibility of diabetics to infections at other sites is considerably less certain. However, it is clear that the availability of effective antimicrobial therapy for infections has had a remarkable impact second only to the availability of insulin on the life span of the diabetic patient.

In the preinsulin era the average life span for a diabetic was 1.5 years after the diagnosis was made. In the postinsulin era before the availability of antimicrobial agents the average life span was seven years after the diagnosis. In the current postantimicrobial therapy era the life span of diabetics is nearly two-thirds that of the nondiabetic patient.

HOST DEFENSE MECHANISMS IN DIABETES MELLITUS

The mechanisms by which diabetics may exhibit increased susceptibility to certain infections have been the subject of numerous investigations. Such studies have focused on cell-mediated immunity as well as humoral aspects of host defense mechanisms. Studies of humoral immunity have shown that antibody production is normal in diabetic patients[1] and serum complement (CH50)[2] and properdin activities[3] are either normal or slightly increased. On the other hand, serum bactericidal activity against certain organisms is decreased. Balch and Watters[2] reported that serum from diabetic patients exhibited decreased bactericidal activity against *Staphylococcus albus* but not against a serum sensitive strain of *Escherichia coli*. In the group of 12 diabetics studied bactericidal activity was reduced by a mean of 50% relative to controls. The explanations for these small but statistically significant changes is not known but the authors reported that bactericidal activity was not heat-sensitive and there was no correlation between blood glucose or serum acetone concentrations and bactericidal activity.

In contrast to the few alterations in humoral immunity, multiple changes in cell-mediated immunity have been identified in diabetics. An impressive array of in vivo and in vitro data from patients and experimental animals have documented impairment of leukocyte mobilization, granulocyte adherence, leukocyte chemotaxis, phagocytosis, and bactericidal activity of polymorphonuclear leukocytes.

Leukocyte Mobilization

Sheldon and Bauer[4] reported that granulocytes from alloxan-diabetic rabbits in ketoacidosis showed delayed migration into sites of inflammation. Similar findings have been reported in diabetic patients. Brayton et al,[5] using a modified Rebuck skin window technique, found that leukocytes from diabetic patients showed diminished mobilization as compared to controls. This was felt to be an intrinsic cellular defect since it could not be correlated with uremia or ketoacidosis. Perillie et al[6] performed similar studies and found that leukocyte mobilization was diminished only in diabetics with ketoacidosis. Baciu et al,[7] in a study of juvenile-onset diabetics, found diminished leukocyte mobilization that partially improved after insulin administration. Interestingly, mobilization was again reduced by glucose infusion.

Granulocyte Adherence

Adherence of granulocytes to vascular endothelium is one of the early steps in the inflammatory process that precedes diapedesis and exudate formation in extravascular tissues. Recent studies have suggested that leukocyte adherence is diminished in diabetes. Van Oss[8] found that blood leukocytes from normal donors showed a dramatic reduction in adherence to glass coverslips when incubated in vitro with hyperglycemic (200 mg/dl) serum. More recently Bagdade et al[9] found that polymorphonuclear leukocytes from a group of untreated nonketotic diabetics with a mean fasting blood glucose of 293 mg/dl showed a reduction in their ability to adhere to nylon fibers. After insulin treatment, which resulted in a reduction in fasting blood glucose to 198 mg/dl, granulocyte adherence from these patients was improved significantly but was still somewhat less than normal. Adherence values showed an inverse linear correlation with fasting blood glucose concentrations. The authors concluded that glucose concentration was the most important factor in reducing adherence. This was suggested by 1) the observation that adherence in diabetic patients showed an inverse relationship to fasting blood glucose levels and 2) adherence of granulocytes from normal patients was reduced after incubation in hyperglycemic serum.

Leukocyte Chemotaxis

Mowatt and Baum[10] examined carefully the chemotactic activity of polymorphonuclear leukocytes and found that the chemotactic index for diabetic patients was significantly less than that for age- and sex-matched normal nondiabetic controls. There was no correlation in the diabetic patients between chemotactic index and age or sex of the patient, nor was there any correlation in the diabetic patients between the chemotactic index and the use of insulin vs oral hypoglycemic agents, fasting blood sugar, serum carbon dioxide, or blood urea nitrogen concentrations. The chemotactic index of normal patients whose leukocytes were incubated in concentrations of glucose ranging from 300 to 900 mg/dl remained within normal limits. In diabetic patients there was no correlation between the chemotaxis of polymorphonuclear leukocytes and plasma insulin concentrations. Mowatt and Baum[10] were unable to correlate the chemotactic index with any of the usual criteria employed to assess diabetic control. Specifically, they could find no further impairment of leukocyte function in patients with severe ketoacidosis than in nonacidotic diabetics. Hill et al[11] and Miller and Baker[12] reported impairment of leukocyte chemotaxis in patients with juvenile-onset diabetes. In a provocative study Molenaar et al[13] suggested that impairment of leukocyte chemotaxis may be genetic in origin. They found that the chemotactic index of insulin-treated diabetic patients as well as their nondiabetic first degree relatives

178

(parents, siblings, or children) was reduced relative to controls. There was no correlation between chemotactic index and age, sex, weight, plasma insulin concentration, insulin antibodies, or plasma glucose.

Phagocytosis

There are conflicting data regarding phagocytic activity of granulocytes in diabetics. In an early study Marble et al[14] reported that polymorphonuclear leukocytes from well-controlled diabetics showed normal phagocytosis of beta hemolytic streptococci. Cohn[15] observed that inflammatory peritoneal exudate cells from alloxan-diabetic rats phagocytized staphylococci normally. In a similar vein Briscoe and Allison[16] reported that exudate leukocytes from nonketotic diabetic rats showed normal phagocytosis of Type I pneumococci.

In contrast to the studies showing no impairment of phagocytosis in diabetes, Baciu[7] reported diminished phagocytosis in diabetics which was reversed by insulin treatment. More recently Bybee and Rogers[17] reported that circulating blood leukocytes from diabetics with ketoacidosis showed diminished phagocytosis of staphylococci. However, leukocytes from diabetics without ketoacidosis phagocytized normally. Incubation of normal leukocytes in ketotic serum did not diminish phagocytosis suggesting that the reversible impairment was cellular in origin.

In contrast to studies suggesting a cellular defect in phagocytosis associated with diabetes, several investigators have identified humoral changes that result in diminished particle uptake by diabetic leukocytes. Drachman et al[18] showed that inflammatory exudate cells from the peritoneal cavity of diabetic rats phagocytized pneumococci at a reduced rate when the assay was carried out in the presence of serum from diabetic rats. Incubation in normal rat serum reversed the impairment and, conversely, diabetic rat serum depressed phagocytosis by normal as well as diabetic leukocytes. Similarly, Bagdade et al[19] found that circulating blood leukocytes from nonketotic diabetics showed a significant reduction in phagocytosis of *Streptococcus pneumoniae* as compared to nondiabetic controls. Of special interest was their finding that after insulin treatment, which resulted in a mean drop in fasting blood sugar from 283 mg/dl to 201 mg/dl, phagocytosis of pneumococci was returned to normal. Incubation of leukocytes from nondiabetic control patients in diabetic serum resulted in a significant decrease in phagocytosis whereas incubation of leukocytes from diabetics in control serum reversed the phagocytic defect. Further, they found that addition of glucose at concentrations greater than 250 mg/dl to nondiabetic leukocytes in normal serum resulted in diminished phagocytosis. The glucose effects could not be attributed to changes in osmolarity. The latter finding is somewhat in conflict with data presented by Drachman et al[18] who found that glucose as well as equivalent molar concentrations of nonmetabolizable sugars caused a depression of phagocytosis. On this basis they suggested that the action of glucose on leukocytes was primarily osmotic.

Bactericidal Activity

Bagdade et al[19] have reported that polymorphonuclear leukocytes from diabetic patients exhibit impaired bactericidal activity against *Streptococcus pneumoniae.* In their study, eight poorly controlled nonketotic diabetic patients all showed small but significant reductions in bactericidal activity. Rate constants for leukocyte killing were reduced by a mean of 60% from controls with individual values ranging from 28% to 85%. The patients were then treated for diabetes and bactericidal activity was reassessed. Following insulin treatment, which resulted in a mean reduction in fasting blood glucose concentration from 283 mg/dl to 201 mg/dl, microbicidal activity increased by 40% but was still less than normal controls. The authors then examined the possibility that a serum factor(s) may have been responsible for altered bacterial killing. Incubation of polymorphonuclear leukocytes from control patients in the presence of diabetic serum reduced bactericidal activity, and incubation of diabetic polymorphonuclear leukocytes in the presence of control serum improved bactericidal activity. These findings demonstrated that a serum factor(s) was at least partially responsible for altered bactericidal activity. However, it is difficult to accept these findings as showing unequivocally that bactericidal activity is reduced in diabetes since the assay employed by Bagdade et al[19] did not dissociate the separate processes of phagocytosis and bacterial killing. Since the estimate of bacterial killing was influenced directly by phagocytic rate, decreased bactericidal activity may have reflected impaired phagocytosis. Indeed, the authors documented that phagocytosis for *Streptococcus pneumoniae* was reduced in the same patients in whom impaired bactericidal activity was demonstrated. Further, crossover studies showed that phagocytosis by control leukocytes was suppressed by diabetic serum and, conversely, control serum reversed impaired phagocytic activity of diabetic leukocytes. The changes in phagocytosis were identical to those seen for bactericidal activity.

Nolan et al[20] and Bagdade et al[21] examined antibacterial activity of polymorphonuclear leukocytes against *Staphylococcus aureus* using a system in which bactericidal activity could be evaluated separately from phagocytosis. In a study of 18 hyperglycemic nonketotic diabetics, 14 exhibited normal bactericidal activity. In four patients, however, bactericidal activity was reduced by a mean of 58%

relative to controls, with individual values ranging from 42% to 76%. In none of the patients was phagocytosis impaired. Of special interest were the results obtained on retesting of bactericidal activity in these four patients following treatment for diabetes. All four showed normal bactericidal activity after one or two weeks of insulin therapy. In a study of similar design, Tan et al[22] examined antibacterial activity of polymorphonuclear leukocytes for *S. aureus* in nonketotic diabetics. They found that phagocytosis or bactericidal activity or both was reduced by more than two standard deviations from normal values in 17 of 31 diabetics studied. Phagocytosis alone was reduced in 11 patients, bactericidal activity alone was reduced in three, and a combined defect was found in three patients. Neither impaired phagocytosis nor decreased bactericidal activity were correctable by normal serum. There was no clear correlation between impaired antibacterial activity and fasting blood glucose concentrations, presence of infection, or history of recurrent infections. In contrast to these results showing defective bactericidal activity in 22% of diabetics, Bybee and Rogers[17] found that none of their 27 patients with nonketotic diabetes exhibited altered bactericidal activity for *S. aureus*.

On the basis of the foregoing studies it is reasonable to conclude that some but not all patients with diabetes mellitus exhibit impaired bactericidal activity. Further, the impairment is most apparent in patients with poorly controlled diabetes and is reversible following insulin therapy. The convincing studies[20,21,22] have all employed *S. aureus* as the test organism; and it is not known if the microbicidal defect is specific for this organism or, indeed, if it is limited to bacteria. However, since there are a limited number of mechanisms for microbicidal activity, it seems likely that impaired killing activity is not specific for this organism. The specific determinants of polymorphonuclear leukocyte microbicidal dysfunction are not known at present.

SPECIFIC INFECTIONS ASSOCIATED WITH DIABETES

Urinary Tract Infection

Conflicting data are available regarding the frequency with which urinary tract infection is found in the diabetic. Bruns et al[23] reported a twofold increase in urinary tract infection in diabetics and Kass,[24] Vejlsgaard,[25] and Ooi et al[26] in separate studies, reported a nearly threefold increase. Kass reported a prevalence of 16% to 19% among diabetic women as compared to 5% to 8% in nondiabetic women.[24] At the Joslin Clinic, clinical pyelonephritis was found in 2% of men and 12% of women diabetic patients surviving for at least 20 years. In an outpatient study, Forland et al reported the prevalence of urinary tract infection as 19% in women and 2% in men.[27] On the other hand, studies by Szucs, O'Sullivan, and Pometta and their colleagues[28,29,30] have shown no substantial difference in the incidence of urinary tract infection between diabetic and control patients.

The likelihood of increased frequency of urinary tract catheterization, bladder neuropathy, bladder paresis, and intrinsic renal vascular disease all contribute to the problem of urinary tract infection in the diabetic patient.

Urethral catheterization has long been recognized as a predisposing factor for urinary tract infection, with the infection risk from a single catheterization being approximately 4%. With the use of an indwelling catheter and open drainage, urinary tract infection can be expected in 100% of patients within 48 hours; whereas with a closed sterile drainage system up to 50% of patients have remained free of urinary tract infection with catheters in place for as long as 14 days. Thus, urethral catheters should be avoided if at all possible and catheter drainage, when required, should be connected to a closed sterile drainage system.

Diabetic patients with urinary tract infections exhibit an increased incidence of pneumaturia and cystitis emphysematosis. The gas formation is nearly always by nonclostrodial organisms usually enterobacteriaceae and particularly *Escherichia coli*. Gas vesicles resulting from fermentation of glucose from within the wall or lumen of the bladder.

Renal papillary necrosis is a complication with substantial morbidity found in diabetic patients, particularly those with anatomic or functional obstructive uropathy and renal vascular disease. The disease can run a varied course from benign to very fulminant. Diagnosis can be made by intravenous pyelography and by straining the urine to obtain necrotic papillae. A prompt diagnosis and initiation of therapy consisting of relief of obstruction, use of appropriate antimicrobial agents, and careful management of the associated uremia are all important parts of the therapeutic regimen.

Neuropathy or bladder paresis, which occurs frequently in diabetics, can serve as a predisposing factor for urinary tract infection. A simple method of identifying significant bladder neuropathy is to perform a postvoiding film as part of an intravenous pyelogram. Cystometrograms may also be performed to quantitate the extent of bladder dysfunction. Possible forms of therapy to be considered for patients with a neurogenic bladder are parasympathomimetic drugs, manual suprapubic compression, and/or a transurethral resection of the bladder neck.

The principles of therapy for management of urinary tract infections, whether asymptomatic bacilluria, cystitis, or acute pyelonephritis, are essentially the same in diabetics as in nondiabetics with comparable disease. The choice of antimicrobial agents, the route of administration, and the duration of therapy should take into account the identity of the organism and its known or likely antimicrobial susceptibilities. The range of bacteria causing urinary tract infection in the diabetic is the same as that in nondiabetics. *Escherichia coli* is by far the most common cause of the first urinary tract infection. However, in patients with recurrent urinary tract infections or those who have been treated with multiple courses of antimicrobial therapy, *Pseudomonas aeruginosa,* enterobacteriaceae other than *Escherichia coli,* or enterococcus become much more common.

For uncomplicated infections patients should be treated, based on antimicrobial susceptibility tests, with the least toxic antimicrobial agent available. Drugs that should be used if possible, being relatively low in cost, are the sulfonamides: ampicillin, tetracycline, nitrofurantoin, and nalidixic acid. The more expensive oral antimicrobial agents commonly used for treatment of urinary tract infection are cephalexin, amoxicillin, and trimethoprim-sulfamethoxazole. For patients seen in an office practice oral therapy is preferred. The results of in vitro sensitivity tests correlate well with therapeutic efficacy and the usual expectation is that urine should be sterile within 24 to 48 hours after initiation of therapy. If organisms are still present at that time the physician should recognize failure and treat the patient with another antimicrobial agent based on susceptibility studies.

It is recommended frequently that urinary tract infections be treated with three or four daily doses of an antimicrobial agent for a period of 10 to 14 days. Recently, however, this conventional form of therapy has been challenged. In a study of women with lower urinary tract infection, documented by the bladder washout technique,[31] Ronald et al[32] showed that a single intramuscular 500-mg dose of kanamycin was effective curative therapy for 92% of infections. Oral antimicrobial agents given in a single high dose have also been shown to be effective in curing a high percentage of patients with lower urinary tract infections. Fang et al[33] found that patients with cystitis caused by enterobacteriaceae could be cured with a single dose of amoxicillin. Women with urinary tract infections due to sensitive organisms that were not antibody-coated[34] were randomized to treatment with a single 3-gm oral dose of 250 mg four times a day. All patients in both groups became asymptomatic within 24 to 48 hours and all were cured of their infections. There was no evidence of relapse in either group as assessed by urine cultures obtained one week and four weeks after termination of therapy. Similarly, in a study of 29 patients with lower urinary tract infections caused by sulfonamide sensitive organisms, therapy with a single oral dosage of sulphafurazole, a short-acting sulfonamide, resulted in a cure rate of 93%.[35] On the basis of these studies it seems clear that infection confined to the lower urinary tract can be treated with a single dose of an effective antimicrobial agent. Short-term therapy is a cheaper, more convenient, and acceptable alternative to a 10- to 14-day course of treatment.

If more conventional oral therapy for lower urinary tract infection is employed, sulfisoxazole is to be preferred for sensitive organisms due to its lower cost. The adult dosage of sulfisoxazole is 2 gm orally followed by 4 gm/day divided into four doses. Ampicillin is used at a dosage of 2 gm/day orally divided into four doses. Tetracyclines are administered orally at a dosage of 1 to 2 gm/day divided into four doses. Tetracyclines should not be used in patients under 12 years of age nor during pregnancy to avoid staining of teeth or enamel hypoplasia. Nitrofurantoin can be used as oral therapy for sensitive organisms at a dosage of 600 mg/day divided into four doses. Nalidixic acid can be used at a dosage of 4 gm/day orally divided into four doses.

If oral cephalosporins are employed cephalexin is preferable to cephaloglycin due to its better absorption. Cephalexin is used in adults at a dosage of 2 gm/day divided into four doses.

For patients with marked dysuria, pyridium should be used for symptomatic relief at a dosage of 600 mg/day orally divided into three doses. Therapy should be continued for a maximum of two to three days.

For patients with complicated urinary tract infections, upper tract infections, or infections of the prostate, short-term therapy is not reliably effective. In a study by Ronald et al[32] of patients with upper tract infection, as determined by the bladder washout technique, 72% of patients treated with a single dose of kanamycin had a relapse almost immediately after termination of therapy. In studies by Fang et al[33] of patients with upper tract infection 50% showed a relapse of infection within 7 days after completion of a 10-day course of amoxicillin.

It is thought that a short course of antimicrobial therapy is unable to eradicate foci of infection frequently associated with structural abnormalities of the excretory system, renal parenchyma, or the prostate. In a recent study of recurrent invasive urinary tract infections in men Gleckman et al[36] compared the efficacy of a six-week course of antimicrobial therapy with that of a more conventional two-week course. All patients enrolled in the study had infections caused by enterobacteriaceae susceptible to trimethoprim-sulfamethoxazole. In 43% of patients treated with 160 mg of trimethoprim and 800 mg of sulfamethoxazole twice a day the organism was eradicated. In contrast, among patients treated for six weeks with the same dosage of the drug combination, 89% of infections were cured. In a separate randomized double-blind clinical trial Smith et al[34] evaluated the efficacy of a 10-day vs a 12-week course of therapy with trimethoprim-sulfamethoxazole in men with recurrent invasive infection of the upper urinary tract. A cure rate of 20% was achieved in patients treated for 10 days and increased to 60% in those receiving long-term therapy. Together these studies indicate that a standard 10- to 14-day course of therapy with trimethoprim-sulfamethoxazole has a poor chance of providing a cure in men with recurrent invasive urinary tract infection. Therefore, a 6- to 12-week course of an appropriate antimicrobial agent should be employed for treatment of such urinary tract infections.

Since relapse is common in patients with upper tract infection a urine culture should be obtained two to three days after cessation of treatment. If that culture is negative, Kunin[38] has recommended that patients have a follow-up culture once a month for three months and then every three months for one year. Early relapse with the same organism, occurring within a few days to weeks after completion of therapy, suggests either renal parenchymal infection, deep bladder tissue infection, or failure of the patient to take the antimicrobial agent. A screening intravenous pyelogram should be performed in patients with relapsing infection and a urologic evaluation is recommended if structural abnormalities are identified.

If reinfection occurs following successful treatment the patient should be retreated employing the same general principles applicable to the first infection. However, if reinfection occurs repeatedly prophylaxis with nitrofurantoin, sulfisoxazole, or trimethoprim-sulfamethoxazole may be necessary. The daily dosage of nitrofurantoin for prophylaxis is 100 mg, for sulfisoxazole 500 mg, and for trimethoprim-sulfamethoxazole 1 tablet (80 mg trimethoprim and 400 mg sulfamethoxazole). Each of the drugs is administered as a single dose at bedtime.

The response to antimicrobial agents is usually of limited duration in patients with structural or neurologic abnormality of the urinary tract or with an indwelling catheter. If the underlying abnormality cannot be corrected and a chronic focus develops treatment should be limited to acute episodes of deep tissue invasion.

Gram negative-bacteremia is a particularly serious complication of urinary tract infection encountered in diabetics with recurrent upper urinary tract infection, urinary tract obstruction, neurogenic bladder changes, or following urinary tract instrumentation. Prompt antimicrobial therapy may be lifesaving and should be directed, often without the benefit of culture results, at the organisms most likely to be encountered. Bacteriostatic drugs should be avoided if possible and therapy should be continued for a minimum of 14 days. *Escherichia coli* is the most common pathogen but *Pseudomonas* species, *Enterobacter*, *Proteus, Klebsiella,* or other enterobacteriaceae are frequent causes of urinary tract infection in patients with recurrent disease or those who have been treated recently with antimicrobial agents. With the exception of *Pseudomonas aeruginosa* these organisms are likely to be sensitive to kanamycin. All of the organisms, including the pseudomonads, are likely to be sensitive to gentamicin or tobramycin. In the setting of the seriously ill patient with possible gram-negative bacteremia and the urinary tract as the most likely portal of entry, gentamicin is the single most effective drug. Gentamicin should be used at a dosage of 3 to 6 mg/kg/day, administered every eight hours intravenously or intramuscularly. Tobramycin has the same antimicrobial spectrum as gentamicin and in addition, is effective against approximately one-third of pseudomonads that are gentamicin-resistant. The dosage and interval for tobramycin therapy are identical to those for gentamicin. If kanamycin is to be employed it should be given intramuscularly or intravenously at a dosage of 10 to 15 mg/kg/day in divided dosages every 12 hours. Amikacin is the newest of the aminoglycosides available for general clinical use and has the broadest spectrum of activity among drugs of its class. Nearly all enterobacteriaceae and pseudomonads can be expected to be sensitive to amikacin but its principle therapeutic role is for treatment of disease caused by organisms resistant to gentamicin or tobramycin. The pharmacokinetics and dosage of amikacin are identical to those of kanamycin.

For pseudomonas infections the combination of carbenicillin with gentamicin, tobramycin, or amikacin is preferable to the use of an aminoglycoside alone. Combination therapy is recommended both to achieve a synergistic effect and to avoid development of carbenicillin-resistant organisms. Carbenicillin should not be used alone for invasive urinary tract infections. Carbenicillin should be administered at a dosage of 400 to 600 mg/kg/day at intervals of four hours. Ticarcillin is equivalent to carbenicillin and offers no substantial advantage. Other bactericidal parenteral antibiotics are ampicillin and the cephalosporins. If ampicillin is employed it should be used in a dosage of 6 to 12 gm/day intravenously. If cephalosporins are required, cephapirin or cephalothin should be administered intravenously in a dosage of 6 to 12 gm/day. If cefazolin is employed it should be given in a dosage of 4 to 6 gm/day.

Certain antimicrobial agents should not be used for treatment of urinary tract infections in patients with renal failure. These include chloramphenicol, nitrofurantoin, and nalidixic acid since these drugs are rapidly metabolized by the liver and the biologically active forms are excreted in inadequate amounts in the urine.

The aminoglycosides, penicillins, and cephalosporins can be used effectively for treatment of urinary tract infection in the presence of renal impairment. Because of the increased risk of renal toxicity tetracycline should not be used in patients with uremia. However, doxycycline, a tetracycline analogue, can be used in such a setting.

Foot Ulcers

The most common infectious problem leading to hospitalization of the diabetic patient is an infected foot ulcer. Bessman and Wagner[39] reported that 53% of admissions to their diabetic service were due to vascular-orthopedic problems, which included foot ulceration, gangrene, and osteomyelitis. Peripheral neuropathy and vascular changes leading to ischemia are the principle factors that result in soft-tissue ulcerations. These, in turn, lead to secondary infection most commonly with streptococci, staphylococci, aerobic gram-negative bacilli, and anaerobic bacteria. The infection may remain localized involving only soft tissue but frequently may result in progressive cellulitis, lymphangitis, septic thrombophlebitis, osteomyelitis, or bacteremia with secondary seeding of distant sites.

Gas formation by nonclostridial organisms is frequently seen in soft-tissue infections in diabetics and rarely seen in nondiabetics. Gas formation results from fermentation of glucose by bacteria found as part of normal fecal or upper respiratory tract flora. Gas formation may manifest itself as palpable crepitance or appears as radiolucent streaks or gas bubbles in muscle bundles or between fascial planes.

Although the phenomenon of nonclostridial gas gangrene has been recognized since 1893,[40] physicians still state that the presence of gas in soft tissue infections implies clostridial infection.[41,42] The two conditions should be differentiated since antimicrobial therapy, the extent and type of surgical treatment, and the prognosis are markedly different. Nonclostridial gas gangrene is far more common than clostridial disease among diabetics accounting for 17% of lower extremity infections in one series whereas clostridia accounted for less than 1% of such infections.[36]

Clostridial infection of the extremities is a rapidly progressive disease with marked toxicity whereas nonclostridial infection presents a much broader spectrum varying from slow progression with no signs of systemic involvement to rapid progression and clinical evidence of sepsis.[36] The antimicrobial therapy for clostridial infections is penicillin G, at doses up to 400,000 units/kg/day administered in divided dosages every two to four hours, whereas for nonclostridial infections therapy varies depending upon the causative organism or organisms. Aerobic bacteria identified by Bessman and Wagner[39] include *Staphylococcus aureus,* enterococcus, *Pseudomonas sp, E. coli, Proteus, Klebsiella,* and *Enterobacter sp.* Bacteroides was isolated only once but anaerobic culture techniques were not optimal. Polymicrobial involvement is the rule with two or more organisms isolated in 85% of patients.

Initial antimicrobial therapy should be devised to effectively treat the range of organisms described above. Although no specific recommendation can be made a cephalospin in combination with an aminoglycoside effective against *Pseudomonas aeruginosa* should be effective against all of the likely pathogens except *Bacteroides fragilis*. The dosage and route of administration for these agents are identical to those outlined for treatment of gram-negative bacteremia. If *Bacteroides fragilis* is present chloramphenicol or clindamycin are the drugs of choice. Chloramphenicol should be used at dosages of 3 to 6 gm/day administered in four divided doses and clindamycin at dosages of 1.2 to 2.4 gm/day intravenously in four divided doses.

Surgical therapy for nonclostridial gas gangrene ranges from debridement to above-knee amputation. Some form of amputation was required in 92% of cases with local bone resection, ankle disarticulation, or below-knee amputation accounting for the majority. Whereas above-knee amputation is recommended for clostridial gangrene, such extensive surgery was required in only one of 48 patients with nonclostridial gangrene.[39]

The prognosis for patients with nonclostridial gas gangrene of the extremity is quite good with a mortality rate of only 4%. In Bessman and Wagner's experience[36] 80% of patients were ambulatory at the time of discharge from the hospital.

Meticulous local foot care and avoidance of further trauma are the mainstays of therapy of diabetic foot ulcers. Although it is difficult to document that healing proceeds faster in patients with good diabetic control there is good experimental evidence that ketoacidosis impairs host defense mechanisms and thus should be avoided.

Systemic antimicrobial therapy is unlikely to be of any value for the uncomplicated chronic foot ulcer with minimal cellulitis. However, the presence of extensive adjacent soft-tissue involvement, lymphangitis, osteomyelitis, and systemic signs of infection require antimicrobial therapy. As with nonclostridial gas gangrene it is difficult to indentify a specific antimicrobial regimen as superior. Therapy should be based on the identity of the organisms isolated. As with nonclostridial gas gangrene, multiple organisms are often found in soft-tissue ulcers. Louie et al[43] reported finding an average of 5.8 organisms per ulcer and only one patient of 20 had a single organism isolated. As shown by their study, anaerobes are isolated with nearly the same frequency as aerobic organisms. The most common aerobic bacteria were *Proteus sp.*, enterococci, *Staphylococcus aureus*, streptococci (not group A or D), and *Escherichia coli*. The most commonly isolated anaerobes were *Bacteroides sp.*, peptococcus, clostridia, and propionibacteria. Similar findings have been obtained by others.[44,45]

Although multiple organisms can be identified it is difficult to determine their relative importance. Sharp et al[45] found that superficial cultures of draining lesions or purulent material gave results different from deep cultures taken from infected sites at the time of surgery. In 53% of patients organisms were identified from deep cultures that were not present in superficial cultures. It seems likely that bacterial synergism plays a role in infected diabetic gangrene.

Since anaerobes, particularly anaerobic gram-negative organisms, are fastidious in their growth requirements, optimal culture techniques should be employed in processing exudate from foot ulcers. Failure to do so may lead to an erroneous estimate of the range of causative organisms and result in inappropriate therapy and/or an unnecessary delay in starting effective antimicrobial therapy.

Mucormycosis

The relatively rare but often serious mycotic diseases collectively referred to as mucormycosis occur most frequently in patients with diabetes mellitus. All forms of the disease are characterized by extensive invasion across tissue planes, involvement of blood vessels producing thrombus, necrosis, hemorrhage, and nerve invasion.[46-48]

Mucormycosis is caused by any of several organisms of the order Mucorales.[46-49] The majority of such infections are caused by members of the family Mucoraceae, which include the genera *Mucor, Rhizopus,* and *Absidia.* The mucoraceae are ubiquitous usually saprophytic organisms that grow on bread, fruit, and in soil. Less commonly mucormycosis is caused by organisms of the families *Cunninghamellaceae, Mortierellaceae,* and *Saksenaeaaceae.*

Mucormycosis of all types is nearly always associated with a predisposing condition.[46,50] The most common form of the disease, rhinocerebral mucormycosis, has a very strong association with acidosis, most frequently due to diabetes mellitus. Evidence that acidosis is a major predisposing factor is suggested by experience with human disease[46,51] but demonstrated more convincingly by animal studies.[4] Rhinocerebral mucormycosis occurs occasionally in the well-controlled diabetic and may be the initial manifestation of diabetes.[52] Although the mechanisms by which diabetes and acidosis predispose to infection is not fully understood hyperglycemia alone is not sufficient.

Mucormycosis also occurs as a complication of allogeneic homotransplantation,[53-55] hematologic neoplasms,[56] treatment with cytotoxic agents, or extensive use of antimicrobial agents.[46] It is of interest that a substantial fraction of patients with leukemia, lymphoma, or organ transplant recipients who develop mucormycosis also have diabetes. In a consecutive series of 26 leukemia and lymphoma patients with mucormycosis, 14 (54%) had diabetes.[56] Similarly, among the first six renal transplantation patients reported in the English literature to have mucormycosis, four (67%) had diabetes.[54] It seems likely that the predisposition to mucormycosis was multifactorial in this heterogeneous group of patients. Nevertheless, the high incidence of diabetes whether juvenile-onset, maturity-onset, or steroid-induced is striking.

In rhinocerebral mucormycosis the portal of entry for the fungus seems to be the mucous membranes of the nose or paranasal sinuses. It spreads rapidly by direct extension resulting in involvement of the face, orbit, meninges, and the brain—particularly the frontal lobe.

Typically patients have a one- to seven-day history of unilateral headache, deterioration of level of consciousness, periorbital swelling and numbness, nasal stuffiness, and eye irritation with excess lacrimation.[46,57] Orbital or facial cellulitis occurs in approximately two thirds of cases.[58] Paranasal sinus involvement is often preceded by necrotic lesions of nasal mucosa and/or hard palate.[46,57] The clinical manifestations progress rapidly resulting in coma in approximately two thirds of cases as a result of central nervous system involvement.[58] Paralysis of the second through the seventh cranial nerves may occur and if the internal carotid artery is involved hemiplegia may result.

Because of the rapid progression of disease and high fatality rate in untreated patients, aggressive attempts at early diagnosis are imperative. Direct scrapings and histologic examination of samples obtained from involved areas provide the greatest diagnostic yield.[46,48,57]

Nonseptate hyphae are seen that characteristically stain well with hematoxylin and eosin, are of large size (6 to 50 μm wide) and show right-angle branching.[47] Although the three genera of mucoraceae cannot be distinguished by direct or histologic examination they can be differentiated from *Aspergillus,* which possess smaller hyphae (2 to 6μm in thickness) that stain poorly with hematoxylin and eosin and have acute angle branching septae.[47] Mucoraceae should not be confused with candida, which possess small (2 to 6 μm) septated pseudohyphae and blastospores.[47,57]

The diagnosis of mucormycosis does not depend on the demonstration of in vitro growth since premortem and postmortem cultures are positive in approximately 15% of cases.[46] Despite the low yield on culture, samples from involved sites should be cultured on Sabouraud glucose agar and incubated at room temperature and at 37°C. Furthermore, mucoraceae may be present in sputum, nasal swab specimens, and sinus aspirates from patients without mucormycosis. Other procedures useful in identifying sites of involvement include sinus radiographs, carotid arteriograms, radionuclide scanning procedures, and computer assisted tomography. Radiographs may show clouding of paranasal sinuses indicative of fluid accumulation, osteomylitis, or bony destruction.[57] Angiography of the carotid artery can identify irregular narrowing, filling defects, or occlusion.[59] Brain or bone scan will show increased uptake at sites of involvement.[60]

Pulmonary involvement with mucormycosis has typically been regarded as a disease of the immunocompromised host.[61] It is now clear, however, that there is also a strong association with diabetes mellitus. In a series of 26 leukemia and lymphoma patients with mucormycosis 21 had pulmonary involvement whereas only four had rhinocerebral disease.[56] It is of interest that more than 50% of patients with pulmonary mucormycosis also had diabetes. Pulmonary involvement may occur alone, as one of several sites of disseminated disease, or, rarely, as part of rhinocerebral disease.[46,56,57] Multiple forms of lung involvement have been described none of which is specific for the disease. Bronchopneumonia[55] or multiple infiltrates, either patchy or diffuse,[62] are more common but mass or nodular lesions,[63,64] cavitation,[64] or fungus ball[56] also occur.

Other sites of primary involvement with mucormycosis include gastrointestinal tract, burn infection, brain abscess[50] or surgical wound, renal, or prosthetic vascular graft infections. Such forms are quite rare and have no special association with diabetes mellitus.

Prevention and treatment of mucormycosis Because of the strong association of mucormycosis with acidosis, careful control of diabetes mellitus would seem to offer the greatest yield in preventing this infection in high-risk populations. Attempts to eliminate the organism or reduce the exposure of high-risk patients are likely to be of minimal value since the organism is ubiquitous in nature. However, it has been reported that hospital-acquired mucormycosis among patients with hematologic diseases was reduced concomitant to using a facility with filtered ventilation.[65]

Untreated rhinocerebral, pulmonary, or disseminated forms of mucormycosis have a mortality rate of nearly 100%. The mainstay of successful therapy includes both surgery and specific antifungal therapy. In rhinocerebral mucormycosis drainage of sinuses and thorough debridement of necrotic tissue are recommended. In extensive pulmonary mucormycosis excision of infected tissue is required. Similarly, surgical drainage or extirpation of other sites may be required. However, firm guidelines regarding the nature and extent of surgical therapy are difficult to establish.

Specific antifungal therapy involves the use of amphotericin B, the only drug with demonstrated clinical efficacy.[57] Meyer[50] has recommended an initial dose of 0.3 mg/kg in two divided doses. The amount is increased rapidly to 1.0 mg/kg/day and after approximately seven days changed to 1.2 mg/kg every other day. Based on pharmacokinetic data showing that the serum half-life of amphotericin B is approximately 30 hours and is independent of renal function, dosage intervals more frequent than every 48 hours would seem to be unnecessary. The total dosage depends upon the extent of disease, the type and timing of surgical procedures, the tolerance of the individual patient to the drug, and the patient's response. Often 30 to 40 mg/kg given over two to three months is employed.

REFERENCES

1. Lipscomb, H., Dobson, H.L., and Greene, J.A. Infection in the diabetic. *South Med J.* 52:16–23, 1959.

2. Balch, H.H., and Watters, M. Blood bactericidal studies and serum complement in diabetic patients. *J Surg Res.* 11:199–212, 1963.

3. Carlisle, H.N., and Saslaw, S. Comparison of properdin levels in general medical and hematologic patients. *Am J Med Sci.* 242:271–278, 1961.

4. Sheldon, W.H., and Bauer, H. The development of the acute inflammatory response to experimental cutaneous mucormycosis in normal and diabetic rabbits. *J Exp Med.* 110:845–852, 1959.

5. Brayton, R.G., Stokes, P.E., Schwartz, M.S. et al. Effect of alcohol and various diseases on leukocyte mobilization, phagocytosis and intracellular bacterial killing. *N Engl J Med.* 282:123–128, 1970.

6. Perillie, P.E., Nolan, J.P., and Finch, S.C. Studies of the resistance to infection in diabetes mellitus: local exudative cellular response. *J Lab Clin Med.* 59:1008–1015, 1962.

7. Baciu, I., Derevenco, V., Vitebski, V. et al. Influentia insulinei si a glucozei asupra functiei fagocitare si mobilitatii leucocitelor. *Studii Ceretari Endocrinologie.* 18:121–129, 1967.

8. Van Oss, C.J. Influence of glucose levels on the *in vitro* phagocytosis of bacteria by human neutrophils. *Infect Immun.* 4:54–59, 1971.

9. Bagdade, J.D., Stewart, M., and Walters, E. Impaired granulocyte adherence: a reversible defect in host defense in patients with poorly controlled diabetes. *Diabetes* 6:677–681, 1978.

10. Mowatt, A.G., and Baum, J. Chemotaxis of polymorphonuclear leukocytes from patients with diabetes mellitus. *N Engl J Med.* 284:621–627, 1971.

11. Hill, H.R., Sauls, H.S., Dettloff, J.L. et al. Impaired leukotactic responsiveness in patients with juvenile diabetes mellitus. *Clin Immunol Immunopathol.* 2:395–403, 1974.

12. Miller, M.E., and Baker, L. Leukocyte functions in juvenile diabetes mellitus: humoral and cellular aspects. *J Pediatr.* 81:979–982, 1972.

13. Molenaar, D.M., Palumbo, P.J., Wilson, W.R. et al. Leukocyte chemotaxis in diabetic patients and their non diabetic first-degree relatives. *Diabetes* 25(suppl 2):880–883, 1976.

14. Marble, A., White, H.J., and Fernald, A.T. The nature of the lowered resistance to infection in diabetes mellitus. *J Clin Invest.* 17:423–430, 1938.

15. Cohn, Z.A., Determinants of infection in the peritoneal cavity. II. Factors influencing the fate of *Staphylococcus aureus* in the mouse. *Yale J Biol Med.* 35:29–47, 1962.

16. Briscoe, H.F., and Allison, F., Jr. Diabetes and host resistance. I. Effect of alloxan diabetes upon the phagocytic and bactericidal efficiency of rat leukocytes for pneumococcus. *J Bacteriol.* 90:1537–1541, 1965.

17. Bybee, J.D., and Rogers, D.E. The phagocytic activity of polymorphonuclear leukocytes obtained from patients with diabetes mellitus. *J Lab Clin Med.* 64:1–13, 1964.

18. Drachman, R.H., Root, R.K., and Wood, W.B., Jr. Studies on the effect of experimental nonketotic diabetes mellitus on antibacterial defense. I. Demonstration of a defect in phagocytosis. *J Exp Med.* 124:227–240, 1966.

19. Bagdade, J.D., Root, R.K., and Bulger, R.J. Impaired leukocyte function in patients with poorly controlled diabetes. *Diabetes* 23:9–15, 1974.

20. Nolan, C.M., Beaty, H.N., and Bagdade, J.D. Further characterization of the impaired bactericidal function of granulocytes in patients with poorly controlled diabetes. *Diabetes* 27:889–894, 1978.

21. Bagdade, J.D. Phagocytic and microbicidal function in diabetes mellitus. *Acta Endocrinol.* 205(suppl 83):27–34, 1976.

22. Tan, J.S., Anderson, J.L., and Watanakunakorn, C. et al. Neutrophil dysfunction in diabetes mellitus. *J Lab Clin Med.* 85:26–33, 1975.

23. Bruns, W., Weuffen, W., Godel, E. et al. Zur haufigkeit von harnwegsinfekten bei schwangeren diabetikerinnen. *Z Intern Med.* 23:520–523, 1968.

24. Kass, E.H. Asymptomatic infections of the urinary tract. *Trans Assoc Am Physicians.* 119:56–63, 1956.

25. Vejlsgaard, R. Studies on urinary infection in diabetics. I. Bacteriuria in patients with diabetes mellitus and in control subjects. *Acta Med Scand.* 179:173–182, 1966.

26. Ooi, B.S., Chen, B.T.M., and Yu, M. Prevalence and site of bacteriuria in diabetes mellitus. *Postgrad Med.* 50:497–499, 1974.

27. Forland, M., Thomas, V., and Shelokov, A. Urinary tract infections in patients with diabetes mellitus. *JAMA.* 238:1924–1926, 1977.

28. Szucs, S., Cserhati, I., Csapo, G. et al. The relation between diabetes mellitus and infections of the urinary tract. *Am J Med Sci.* 240:186–191, 1960.

29. O'Sullivan, D.J., Fitzgerald, M.G., Meynell, M.J. et al. Urinary tract infection: a comparative study in the diabetic and general populations. *Br Med J.* 1:786–788, 1961.

30. Pometta, D., Rees, S.B., Younger, D. et al. Asymptomatic bacteriuria in diabetes mellitus. *N Engl J Med.* 276:1118–1121, 1967.

31. Fairley, K.F., Bond, A.G., Brown, R.B. et al. Simple test to determine the site of urinary tract infection. *Lancet* 2:427–428, 1967.

32. Ronald, A.R., Boutros, P., and Moutada, H. Bacteriuria localization and response to single-dose therapy in women. *JAMA.* 235:1854–1856, 1976.

33. Fang, L.S.T., Tolkoff-Rubin, N.E., and Rubin, R.H. Efficacy of single-dose and conventional amoxicillin therapy in urinary-tract infection localized by the antibody-coated bacteria technic. *N Engl J Med.* 298:413–416, 1978.

34. Thomas, V., Shelokov, A., and Forland, M. Antibody-coated bacteria in the urine and the site of urinary-tract infection. *N Engl J Med.* 290:588–590, 1974.

35. Kallenius, G., and Winberg, J. Urinary tract infections treated with single dose of short-acting sulphonamide. *Br Med J.* 1:1175–1176, 1979.

36. Gleckman, R., Crowley, R.N., and Natsios, G.A. Therapy of recurrent invasive urinary-tract infections of men. *N Engl J Med.* 301:878–880, 1979.

37. Smith, J.W., Jones, S.R., Reed, W.P. et al. Recurrent urinary tract infections in men: characteristics and response to therapy. *Ann Intern Med.* 91:554–558, 1979.

38. Kunin, C.M. *Detection, Prevention and Management of Urinary Tract Infections.* 2nd Edition. Philadelphia: Lea & Febiger, 1974.

39. Bessman, A.N., and Wagner, W. Nonclostridial gas gangrene: report of 48 cases and review of the literature. *JAMA.* 233:958–963, 1975.

40. Chiari, H. Zus Bacteriologie des septischen Emphysemas. *Prog Med Wochenschr.* 18:1–4, 1893.

41. Anderson, C.B., Marr, J., Jaffe, B.M. Anerobic streptococcal infections simulating gas gangrene. *Arch Surg.* 104:186–189, 1972.

42. Levin, M.M. Gas forming *Aeromonas hydrophilia* infection in a diabetic. *Postgrad Med.* 54:127–129, 1973.

43. Louie, T.J., Bartlett, J.G., Tally, F.P. et al. Aerobic and anaerobic bacteria in diabetic foot ulcers. *Ann Intern Med.* 85:461–463, 1976.

44. Sharp, C.S., Bessman, A.N., Wagner, F.W., Jr. et al. Microbiology of deep tissue in diabetic gangrene. *Diabetes* 25:385–392, 1976.

45. Sharp, C.S., Bessman, A.N., Wagner, F.W. et al. Microbiology of superficial and deep tissues in infected diabetic gangrene. *Surg Gynecol Obstet.* 149:217–219, 1979.

46. Baker, R.D. Mucormycosis (opportunistic phycomycosis). Edited by R.D. Baker. In *The Pathologic Anatomy of Mycoses. Human Infection with Fungi, Actinomycetes and Algae.* New York: Springer-Verlag, 1971, pp 832–918.

47. Emmons, C.W., Binford, C.H., Utz, J.P. et al. *Medical Mycology.* 3rd Edition. Philadelphia: Lea & Febiger, 1977, pp 254–255.

48. Baker, R.D. The phycomycoses. *Ann NY Acad Sci.* 174:592–605, 1970.

49. Ajello, L. Investigation of a case of zygomycosis caused by *Saksaneae vasiformis.* Mycoses newsletter. *ISHAM* 27:13, 1975.

50. Meyer, R.D. Agents of Mucormycosis and Related Species. Edited by G.L. Mandell, R.G. Douglas, and J.E. Bennett. Infectious Diseases and Their Etiologic Agents. Principles and Practice of Infectious Diseases. New York: John Wiley & Sons, Inc., 1979, pp 2008–2014.

51. Beigelman, P.M., and Warner, N.E. Thirty-two fatal cases of severe diabetic acidosis, including a case of mucormycosis. *Diabetes* 22:847–850, 1973.

52. Helderman, J.H., Cooper, H.S., and Mann, J. Chronic phycomycosis in a controlled diabetic. *Ann Intern Med.* 80:419, 1974.

53. Stinson, E.B., Bieber, C.P., Griepp, R.B. et al. Infectious complications after cardiac transplantations in man. *Ann Intern Med.* 74:22–36, 1971.

54. Hammer, G.S., Bottone, E.J., and Hirschman, S.Z. Mucormycosis in a transplant recipient. *Am J Clin Pathol.* 64:389–398, 1975.

55. Haim, S., Better, O.S., Lichtig, C. et al. Rhinocerebral mucormycosis following kidney transplantation. *Isr J Med Sci.* 6:646–649, 1970.

56. Meyer, R.D., Rosen, P., and Armstrong, D. Phycomycosis complicating leukemia and lymphoma. *Ann Intern Med.* 77:871–879, 1972.

57. Meyer, R.D., and Armstrong, D. Mucormycosis—changing status. *CRC Crit Rev Clin Lab Sci.* 4:421–451, 1973.

58. Ferry, A.P. Cerebral mucormycosis (phycomycosis). Ocular findings and review of the literature. *Surv Ophthalmol.* 6:1–24, 1961.

59. Lowe, J.T., Jr., and Hudson, W.R. Rhinocerebral phycomycosis and internal carotid artery thrombous. *Arch Otolaryngol.* 101:100–103, 1975.

60. Zwas, S.T., and Czerniak, P. Head and brain scan findings in rhinocerebral mucormycosis: case report. *J Nucl Med.* 16:925–927, 1975.

61. Bodey, G.P. Fungal infections complicating acute leukemia. *J Chronic Dis.* 19:667–687, 1966.

62. Medoff, G., and Kobayashi, G.S. Pulmonary mucormycosis. *N Engl J Med.* 286:86–87, 1972.

63. Hauch, T.W. Pulmonary mucormycosis: another cure. *Chest* 72:92–93, 1977.

64. Bartrum, R.J., Jr., Warnick, M., and Herman, P.G. Roentgenographic findings in pulmonary mucormycosis. *Am J Roentgenol Radium Ther Nucl Med.* 117:810–815, 1973.

65. Rosen, P.P., and Sternberg, S.S. Decreased frequency of aspergillosis and mucormycosis. *N Engl J Med.* 295:1319–1320, 1976.

10 Management of Diabetic Renal Disease

Stanley M. Lee, MB

Prior to the introduction of insulin therapy, the average life span of a patient with juvenile-onset diabetes was 1.2 years, and for adult-onset five years. With the availability of insulin in 1921, the whole spectrum of long-term complications of diabetes became apparent, with renal failure contributing a significant role in the overall morbidity and mortality.

End-stage renal failure remains a significant cause of death in diabetes mellitus. In those individuals developing the disease prior to the age of 40 years, approximately 35% to 40% will die from uremia, and the earlier the onset of the diabetic state, the higher the frequency of renal involvement.[1] The occurrence of end-stage renal disease in adult-onset non–insulin-dependent diabetes is much less. For all diabetics the overall incidence of renal failure is between 6% and 9%.[2] However, cardiovascular disease remains the major cause of death in diabetes. The onset of renal disease and its association with hypertension further accentuates the progression of diabetic vasculopathy.

Diabetes mellitus is now the fifth leading cause of death in the

196

United States, and its incidence or diagnosis appears to be increasing. With less stringent criteria for acceptability, more diabetics are receiving hemodialysis, and they now constitute a significant proportion of the total dialysis population. Because of their higher complication rate with dialysis and multiorgan involvement, treatment of end-stage diabetic nephropathy is both challenging and enormously expensive.

Diabetes is unique in its ability to affect several parameters of renal structure and function. Effects of diabetes on the kidney include alterations in renal function, glomerulopathy, vasculopathy, tubulointerstitial disease, autonomic neuropathy, and iatrogenic effects.

RENAL FUNCTION

In recently diagnosed, juvenile-onset diabetes, significant alterations in renal function are common. Glomerular filtration rate (GFR) is elevated, in some cases up to 30% above normal,[3] and renal plasma flow (RPF) is likewise increased, but less markedly. Renal size, volume, and calculated weight are increased in proportion to the changes in glomerular filtration rate. With initiation of insulin therapy, both glomerular filtration rate and renal size return to normal values.[4]

It has been observed that patients with diabetes of longer duration (1 to 12 years) not infrequently exhibit an increase in renal size comparable to that in newly diagnosed diabetics. This has been explained by the fact that imprecise regulation of blood glucose may result in swelling of the kidney. In this respect, abnormalities in GFR and renal size may be a reflection of the degree of glucose regulation. In reality complete normalization of renal size is rarely observed in patients with long-standing disease.

In newly diagnosed diabetics, quantitative histologic examination of the kidney has shown that the glomerulus is enlarged, and the capillary luminal volume and filtration surface is increased.[5] In that the glomeruli occupy only a small percentage of total renal mass, the volume of other structures in the kidney must also be elevated. Evidence suggesting that tubular hypertrophy takes place is deduced from the observation that maximal tubular reabsorptive capacity for glucose is increased to the same extent as the GFR.[6] Thus, glomerular-tubular balance is maintained.

The precise etiology of the increased GFR and renal mass in diabetes is not known, and has been attributed to a variety of factors including elevated circulating growth hormone, hyperglycemia per se, and other hormonal stimuli. An increased water content of the kidney probably accounts for some of the findings, but again its mechanism is undetermined.

The functional nature of the GFR alteration has been demonstrated by its ready reversibility in acute studies, where intravenous insulin administration resulted in an abrupt decline in GFR (9%) and RPF (13%) within 90 minutes.[7] These changes were felt to be mediated via the sympathetic nervous system, rather than an effect on blood glucose or circulating blood volume.

In experimental animals with diabetes, it has been shown that renal hemodynamics including blood flow to the kidney may influence the development of the glomerular lesions. Decreased renal blood flow produced by clipping the renal artery resulted in significant amelioration of immunopathologic findings characteristic of diabetic nephropathy. The unprotected kidney in this model, exposed to the full brunt of the systemic hypertension, developed a more profound glomerulopathy.[8] Thus in newly diagnosed diabetics, aggressive glucose control may reverse some of the renal hemodynamic abnormalities, and could theoretically modify the early natural history of the glomerulopathy.

GLOMERULAR LESIONS

The renal pathologic changes most commonly associated with diabetic nephropathy occur in the glomerulus. Four typical patterns may be observed. These include the capsular drop lesion, exudative lesion, diffuse glomerulosclerosis, and nodular glomerulosclerosis (Kimmelstiel-Wilson lesion).

Only the diffuse and nodular glomerulosclerosis lesions are considered typical for diabetes, and in these the glomerular mesangial region is predominantly involved. One of the earliest changes noted in diabetics of one to five years duration is an increased quantity of basement membrane-like material in the glomerular mesangial matrix.[9] Glomerulosclerosis, commonly noted after 10 to 15 years of diabetes, manifests as a progressive increase in mesangial matrix material, occasionally with mesangial cell proliferation. It may begin as a segmental lesion but ultimately involves the entire glomerulus. The affected areas gradually become sclerotic and there is associated compression and obliteration of the glomerular capillary lumina.

Nodular glomerulosclerosis (Kimmelstiel-Wilson lesion) is considered a pathognomonic feature of diabetes mellitus.[10] It appears initially at the periphery of the glomerular tuft as a hyaline mass of PAS-positive material. These nodules gradually increase in size and number, encroach upon, and finally obliterate the glomerular capillaries. Although the nodule appears to be located in the mesangium, ultrastructural examination has suggested that it originates from the endothelial cell. Despite the fact that it takes 15 to 20 years for the development of end-stage renal failure, a recent study of diabetic patients undergoing renal transplantation showed that early nodular lesions were apparent within three to four years in the transplanted kidney.[11]

Exudative lesions are composed of hyaline-like material appearing in the luminal aspect of the capillary endothelial cell. The capsular drop lesion occurs on the inside of Bowman's capsule, between the parietal epithelial cell and the basement membrane. Both these lesions are probably not specific for diabetes.

VASCULAR LESIONS

Widespread and accelerated atherosclerosis is common in diabetes, and may involve the major renal vessels and large branches. In addition to an ischemic effect on the kidney, atheromatous emboli and associated focal parenchymal infarction may occur. Renovascular hypertension may result from significant lesions of the renal arteries or branches.

Arteriolosclerosis is also a generalized phenomenon in diabetes and typically leads to subendothelial hyaline deposits in both the afferent and efferent glomerular arteriole. Involvement of both these structures is considered to be a pathognomonic feature of diabetes, and may occur with considerable rapidity, as was demonstrated in a transplant study[11] where these lesions were observed after two years in normal kidneys transplanted into diabetics. The generalized vascular disease may also be a contributing factor in the causation of renal papillary necrosis, a common event in diabetics.

TUBULOINTERSTITIAL LESIONS

Vacuolization of the tubular cells is a frequent observation and is probably a consequence of prolonged osmotic diuresis related to glycosuria. Lipid droplets in the tubular cells result from hyperlipidemia and lipiduria may occur as in the nephrotic syndrome. The presence of glycogen in tubular cells (the Armanni-Ebstein lesion) was at one time considered to be a pathognomonic feature of diabetic nephropathy, but is probably of little functional significance, and is rarely observed at this time.

In patients with frequent urinary tract infections or chronic pyelonephritis, the development of interstitial nephritis, with inflammatory cellular infiltration, fibrosis and scar formation may be observed. Established diabetic nephropathy is characterized by thickening of tubular basement membranes (TBM). Immunopathologic examination of this phenomenon reveals intense staining for albumin and IgG in the TBM and also in the membrane of Bowman's capsule.[12] This process probably results from a biochemical modification of the membrane and an alteration in its permeability characteristics. There is no evidence to suggest an immunologically mediated event. The immunopathologic appearance of the tubular basement membrane appears to be quite specific for diabetic nephropathy.

The association of urinary tract infection and diabetes remains a somewhat clouded issue. On a theoretical basis, it might be assumed that the diabetic would be more susceptible to bacterial infection, and glycosuria would provide an excellent culture medium. In addition, autopsy studies on diabetics have shown a high incidence of scarring and changes associated with chronic pyelonephritis. In diabetic patients with end-stage renal disease, often complicated by obstruction or instrumentation, the occurrence of urinary tract infection is certainly higher than in the general population. Many clinical studies have shown that the prevalence of urinary tract infection is no different between diabetic and nondiabetic men. Diabetic children also appear to have an incidence of infection similar to nondiabetics.[13] However, diabetic females appear to have a higher incidence of upper and lower urinary tract infections. Infections are frequently asymptomatic and recurrent.[14] The long-term consequences of urinary tract infection, or asymptomatic bacteriuria in the absence of obstruction or other structural abnormalities, are unknown.

Although rarely observed, diabetics are more prone to develop emphysematous pyelonephritis, where gas-producing organisms invade the renal parenchyma. Similarly, xanthogranulomatous pyelonephritis, perinephric abscess, and renal carbuncle should be included as part of the spectrum of diabetic nephropathy.

One of the more serious complications of diabetes is the occurrence of renal papillary necrosis, or necrotizing renal papillitis. While its exact etiology is not understood, it appears to result from a combination of infection and ischemia. It should be suspected in any diabetic patient who presents with symptoms of acute pyelonephritis, sepsis, shock, flank pain, or hematuria often in association with ureteral obstruction. Radiographic confirmation is required unless the sloughed papilla is passed in the urine. This clinical situation demands aggressive therapy, with antibiotics and supportive measures for peripheral vascular collapse.

BASEMENT MEMBRANE CHANGES

Thickening of capillary basement membranes is considered to be a characteristic ultrastructural feature of diabetic microangiopathy. It is an issue that is surrounded by controversy, and its significance is not completely understood. In normal individuals and in diabetics, capillary basement membrane width increases with age.[15] It is generally accepted that in age- and sex-matched populations, most diabetics exhibit significant thickening of capillaries in the microcirculation, as compared to nondiabetics. The controversy arises in regard to the exact onset of the membrane changes. One group has shown significant membrane widening to be present in prediabetics, and has emphasized the fact that hyperglycemia per se is not responsible for the membrane changes.[16] Other investigators have questioned these observations, and demonstrated normal capillary membrane width at the onset of diabetes, and a widening that was related to the duration of disease. Differences in fixation and mensuration techniques may explain some of the discordant results.[17]

Thickening of the glomerular basement membrane is characteristically observed in long-standing diabetes, and is associated with subtle alterations in its biochemical composition.[18,19] It is not known whether the thickened membrane results from an increased rate of synthesis or diminished degradation. The finding of basement membrane-like material within the glomerular mesangium in early diabetes suggested that this might represent a degradative pathway that was disrupted.

In addition to the morphologic alterations of the glomerular basement membrane, its function as the major barrier to glomerular filtration is disrupted. Proteinuria, often in the nephrotic range (3.5 gm/24 hr), is a common clinical feature and usually represents advanced diabetic nephropathy. As observed with the electron microscope, the thickening of the glomerular basement membrane is diffuse and without evidence of immune complex deposition.

NEUROPATHY

The development of autonomic or visceral neuropathy has important implications for the diabetic patient with impaired renal function. Neurogenic vesical dysfunction is often insidious at its onset, usually progressive and is associated with a variety of complications. The symptoms include an inability to completely empty the bladder and diminished bladder sensation, often with hesitancy, dribbling, and gradual distension. With progression of the problem, overflow incontinence results, and urinary stasis predisposes the patient to infection, with the risks of associated vesicoureteral reflux, hydroureter, and pyelocaliectasis. Diagnosis may be established by cystometric studies, wherein a flat pressure curve obtains and is associated with a lack of sensation until bladder capacity is reached. The important differential diagnosis in older men is prostatic hypertrophy, which may be a coexistent problem.

It has been shown that asymptomatic neurogenic bladder dysfunction occurs in up to 80% of diabetics who have other evidence of neuropathy.[20] Treatment of this condition requires urinary drainage or diversion. Bladder neck resection removes the involuntary effect of the internal sphincter, which allows bladder emptying to come under the voluntary control of the external sphincter.

INSULIN METABOLISM AND RENAL FAILURE

The development of renal insufficiency has important implications for the diabetic patient on insulin therapy.[21] The normal kidney possesses insulinase activity, and with progressive loss of functional renal tissue, the half-life of circulating insulin is prolonged. Thus, insulin requirements in general will diminish as renal failure advances.

In contrast with this situation is a functional state of insulin resistance or carbohydrate intolerance, which occurs as a result of the azotemic environment. Severe metabolic acidosis may further aggravate this phenomenon. Insulin dosage must be individualized and reevaluated periodically as renal insufficiency progresses. The patient who starts hemodialysis or undergoes renal transplantation may have a dramatic alteration in insulin requirements.

RELATED ENDOCRINE ABNORMALITIES

In association with the autonomic neuropathy of diabetes, a decreased activity of the adrenergic nervous system is frequently observed, with symptoms of postural hypotension. Sympathetic nervous activity is one of the factors responsible for stimulating renin secretion, and a disruption in this system may result in the syndrome of hyporeninemic hypoaldosteronism.[22] Occurring usually in patients with only a modest decline in renal function (serum creatinine 2 to 3 mg/100 ml), these individuals have severe, often life-threatening, hyperkalemia and renal tubular acidosis (Type IV).

This syndrome, which also occurs in nondiabetic patients, usually with chronic pyelonephritis, should be suspected when serum potassium levels appear inappropriately elevated for the degree of renal dysfunction. In some patients clinically unrecognized volume expansion is felt to be an important etiologic factor, but renin secretion shows little or no response to the usual stimuli of volume depletion or upright posture. Aldosterone levels rise following angiotensin infusion, and the syndrome is easily treated with oral mineralocorticoid replacement.[23]

CONTRAST MEDIUM INDUCED DAMAGE IN DIABETIC NEPHROPATHY

There is a very small but definable incidence of acute renal failure in nondiabetic individuals associated with the administration of radiographic contrast material. Several reports now attest to the fact that the diabetic faces a substantially higher risk of developing renal damage following exposure to contrast medium.[24] Patients with vascular disease and established renal insufficiency are perhaps most susceptible, but the risk extends to those individuals with only minimally decreased renal function (creatinine 2 to 3 mg/100 ml).[25] In some cases, damage to the kidney has been irreversible. State of hydration prior to the radiographic study is not always helpful in predicting patients at higher risk. While the pathophysiology of the renal damage is not completely understood, several factors may be responsible, including the high osmotic load within the tubular lumen, the uricosuric effect of contrast material, vascular spasm, and decreased renal blood flow.

Thus, diagnostic radiographic studies involving intraarterial or intravenous contrast material should be avoided in diabetic patients with renal insufficiency unless absolutely indicated.

NATURAL HISTORY OF DIABETIC NEPHROPATHY

Most of the data regarding the natural history of diabetic nephropathy has been obtained from studies of patients with juvenile-onset diabetes. In the older diabetic, the morbidity associated with large-vessel disease exceeds that of renal failure. In humans and experimental animals, histopathologic studies have demonstrated that changes in the kidney are occurring from the earliest stages of diabetes. However, in most patients, renal function is well maintained for many years. The incidence of proteinuria appears to increase in a linear fashion after ten years, and by 25 years, approximately 40% of juvenile-onset diabetics are affected. The mean time for onset of proteinura is 17 years. Proteinuria is almost invariably followed by declining renal function within two to three years. Azotemia is commonly associated with hypertension, and tends to advance rapidly such that end-stage renal failure usually occurs within two years. After 25 years of diabetes, the incidence of renal failure increases markedly, and tends to level out after 30 years, with approximately 40% of patients affected.

It is well established that uncontrolled hypertension tends to accelerate the course of diabetic vasculopathy, including the nephropathy and retinopathy. High blood pressure in diabetes is usually volume-dependent, with diminished plasma renin activity, but is often very difficult to control because of the propensity of these patients to develop postural hypotension.

Cigarette smoking has been shown to aggravate the course of diabetic retinopathy. It should be discouraged in patients with renal insufficiency.[26]

MANAGEMENT OF THE PATIENT
WITH NORMAL RENAL FUNCTION

Anecdotal reports and a limited number of controlled studies have suggested that close attention to blood glucose control may decrease the incidence of diabetic nephropathy or delay its onset.[27] Thus, an aggressive approach in terms of diet control and pharmacologic manipulation is warranted. The occurrence of known cardiovascular risk factors such as essential hypertension, cigarette smoking, and hyperlipidemia, exposes the diabetic patient to an increased morbidity, and these problems should be managed accordingly.

Periodic monitoring for urinary tract infection should be routinely considered, even in asymptomatic patients. In the presence of neuropathy, bladder function testing should be undertaken. Exposure to radiographic contrast media, and other nephrotoxic agents should be kept to a minimum. The occurrence of other renal diseases in the diabetic should be investigated and managed as in a nondiabetic individual.

MANAGEMENT OF THE PATIENT WITH RENAL FAILURE

With the onset of proteinuria and azotemia, no therapeutic intervention can prevent the inexorable progression towards end-stage renal failure. The decision to undertake renal replacement therapy (dialysis or transplantation) should be individualized for each patient. The combination of diabetes and renal failure often provokes azotemic symptoms at an earlier stage than in nondiabetics. In addition, the progression of diabetic retinopathy appears to accelerate with the onset of renal failure. For optimal results, therapy should be initiated just prior to the onset of symptoms. In most diabetics, serum creatinine between 5 and 10 mg/100 ml should be considered appropriate for starting dialysis or preparing for transplantation.

There are basically four therapeutic modalities presently available. These are hemodialysis, peritoneal dialysis, related donor transplantation, and cadaveric transplantation.

Hemodialysis

Early results with chronic hemodialysis in diabetes were very discouraging. The cardiovascular stress occasioned by repeated changes in blood pressure, blood volume, and anticoagulation is associated with considerable morbidity and mortality. Myocardial infarction is the most common cause of death, and cerebrovascular disease, limb ischemia, and progressive retinopathy are among the frequently encountered problems. Existing and accelerated peripheral vascular disease adds to the difficulty in maintaining adequate sites for vascular access, which, in addition, are highly susceptible to infection. In one large series of diabetic patients undergoing chronic hemodialysis, cumulative survival was 42% at two years and 25% at four years. This compares with 78% two-year and 48% four-year survival for nondiabetics.[28] Diabetics spend significantly more time as inpatients, and have a lower rehabilitation rate than nondiabetics. The older diabetic patient, with a history of arteriosclerotic cardiovascular disease, is most at risk to develop a fatal complication during hemodialysis. While it stands as a palliative form of therapy for most diabetics, hemodialysis should only be undertaken in patients who are informed regarding the potential problems and likely outcome.

Peritoneal Dialysis

Chronic peritoneal dialysis offers an alternative mode of therapy for diabetic patients with end-stage renal disease. It avoids the risks associated with rapid fluid shifts, blood pressure changes, and repeated anticoagulation. The procedure is easily performed in the home, which is preferable for patient rehabilitation. There has been only limited experience with peritoneal dialysis as a chronic therapy in diabetic patients, but in one study, survival after one year was comparable to those individuals receiving hemodialysis.[29] In addition, diabetic retinopathy and neuropathy improved in several patients, in contrast to those on hemodialysis where progression was the rule.

Whether or not chronic peritoneal dialysis will emerge as a viable option for long-term treatment will depend on the results of further studies. But it does offer an alternative, especially for patients with vascular access problems.

Kidney Transplantation

Kidney transplantation from a living, related donor is currently the optimal mode of therapy for diabetics with end-stage nephropathy. Successful rehabilitation and an acceptable life-style may be expected for most patients with a functioning allograft. Dramatic improvement in peripheral and autonomic neuropathy and a halt in the progression of retinopathy are commonly observed. Two year survival is approximately 70% in the largest series reported from the University of Minnesota,[30] which is similar to cadaveric transplantation in nondiabetics. Infection is the leading cause of death, followed by myocardial infarction. In contrast, the survival of diabetic patients undergoing cadaveric renal transplantation is only marginally better than those receiving hemodialysis, and by three years, almost 70% have died.

There are significant problems associated with transplantation in diabetics. Advanced atherosclerosis in the pelvic vessels often creates difficulty in the vascular anastomosis, and urologic complications including ureteral necrosis, bladder leaks, and neurogenic vesical dysfunction are more frequently observed than in nondiabetics. The ethics of using living, related donors for diabetic patients with a limited life expectancy should be weighed against the available options. A promising alternative therapeutic approach involves the pretreatment of potential cadaveric donors with high-dose immunosuppression. In one recent study using this technique the survival of diabetics receiving cadaveric grafts was comparable to those undergoing living, related donor transplantation.[31] Further data will be required to establish the value of this approach.

Renal replacement therapy, including dialysis and transplantation, although capable of prolonging the life of patients with end-stage diabetic nephropathy, is at best a limited compromise. Animal experiments have demonstrated that pancreatic islet cell transplantation can reverse the changes of early diabetic nephropathy,[32] and it is probable that endocrine factors apart from insulin play a significant role in modulating the metabolic environment of the diabetic. Improved methods for automated insulin administration, the development of new hypoglycemic pharmacologic agents and a broader understanding of the pathophysiology of diabetic vasculopathy may soon provide a means to prevent and reverse the natural history of this disease.

REFERENCES

1. Lundbaek, K. Nephropathy in diabetic subjects. Edited by B.S. Leibel, and G.A. Wrenshall. In *On the Nature and Treatment of Diabetes*. New York: Excerpta Medical Foundation, 1965, pp 436–446.

206

2. Balodimos, M.C. Diabetic nephropathy. Edited by A. Marble, P. White, R.F. Bradley, and R.F. Krall. In *Joslin's Diabetes Mellitus,* 11th Edition. Philadelphia: Lea & Febiger, 1971.

3. Mogensen, C.E., and Andersen, M.J.F. Increased kidney size and glomerular filtration rate in early juvenile diabetes. *Diabetes* 22:706–712, 1973.

4. Mogensen, C.E., and Andersen, M.J.F. Increased kidney size and glomerular filtration rate in untreated juvenile diabetes: normalization by insulin treatment. *Diabetologia* 11:221–224, 1975.

5. Osterby, R., and Gundersen, H.J.G. Glomerular size and structure in diabetes mellitus. I. Early abnormalities. *Diabetologia* 11:225–229, 1975.

6. Mogensen, C.E. Maximum tubular reabsorption capacity for glucose and renal hemodynamics during rapid hypertonic glucose infusion in normal and diabetic subjects. *Scand J Clin Lab Invest.* 28:101–109, 1971.

7. Mogensen, C.E., Christensen, N.J., and Gundersen, H.J.G. The acute effect of insulin on renal hemodynamics and protein excretion in diabetes. *Diabetologia* 15:153–157, 1978.

8. Mauer, S.M., Steffes, M.W., Azar, S. et al. The effects of the Goldblatt hypertension on development of the glomerular lesions of diabetes mellitus in the rat. *Diabetes* 27:738–744, 1978.

9. Osterby, R. A quantitative electron microscopic study of mesangial regions in patients with short term juvenile diabetes mellitus. *Lab Invest.* 29:99–110, 1973.

10. Kimmelstiel, P., and Wilson, C. Intercapillary lesions in the glomeruli of the kidney. *Am J Pathol.* 12:83, 1936.

11. Mauer, S.M., Barbosa, J., Vernier, R.L. et al. Development of diabetic vascular lesions in normal kidneys transplanted into patients with diabetes mellitus. *N Engl J Med.* 295:916–920, 1976.

12. Miller, K., and Michael, A.F. Immunopathology of renal extracellular membranes in diabetes mellitus. *Diabetes* 25:701–708, 1976.

13. Etzwiler, D.D. Incidence of urinary tract infections among juvenile diabetics. *JAMA* 191:81, 1965.

14. Ooi, B.S., Chen, B.I.M., Yu, M. Prevalence and site of bacteriuria in diabetes mellitus. *Postgrad Med J.* 50:497–499, 1974.

15. Kilo, C., Vogler, N., and Williamson, J.R. Muscle capillary basement membrane changes related to aging and to diabetes mellitus. *Diabetes* 21:881–905, 1972.

16. Siderstein, M.D., Unger, R.H., and Madison, L.L. Studies of muscle capillary basement membranes in normal subjects, diabetic and prediabetic patients. *J Clin Invest.* 47:1973–1999, 1968.

17. Williamson, J.R., Rowold, E., Hoffman, P. et al. Influence of fixation and morphometric techniques on capillary basement-membrane thickening prevalence data in diabetes. *Diabetes* 25:604–613, 1976.

18. Westberg, N.G., and Michael, A.F. Human glomerular basement membrane: chemical composition in diabetes mellitus. *Acta Med Scand.* 194:39–47, 1973.

19. Beisswenger, P.J., and Spiro, R.G. Studies on the human glomerular basement membrane. Composition, nature of the carbohydrate units and chemical changes in diabetes mellitus. *Diabetes* 22:180–193, 1973.

20. Ellenberg, M. Diabetic neuropathy: clinical aspects. *Metabolism* 25:1627–1655, 1976.

21. Reaven, G.M., Weisinger, J.R., and Swenson, R.S. Insulin and glucose metabolism in renal insufficiency. *Kidney Int.* 6(suppl 1):63–69, 1974.

22. Perez, G.O., Lespier, L., Jacobi, J. et al. Hyporeninemia and hypoaldosteronism in diabetes mellitus. *Arch Intern Med.* 137:852–855, 1977.

23. Sebastian, A., Schambelan, M., Lindenfeld, S. et al. Amelioration of metabolic acidosis with fludrocortisone therapy in hypereninemic hypoaldosteronism. *N Engl J Med.* 297:576–583, 1977.

24. Pillay, V.K.G., Robbins, P.C., Schwartz, F.D. et al. Acute renal failure following intravenous urography in patients with long-standing diabetes mellitus and azotemia. *Radiology* 95:633, 1970.

25. Harkonen, S., and Kjellstrand, C.M. Exacerbation of diabetic renal failure following intravenous pyelography. *Am J Med.* 63:939–946, 1977.

26. Paetkau, M.E., Boyd, T.A.S., Winship, B. et al. Cigarette smoking and diabetic retinopathy. *Diabetes* 26:46–49, 1977.

27. Johnsson, S. Retinopathy and nephropathy in diabetes mellitus. Comparison of the effects of two forms of treatment. *Diabetes* 9:1–8, 1960.

28. Shapiro, F.L., Leonard, A., and Compty, C.M. Mortality, morbidity and rehabilitation results in regularly dialyzed patients with diabetes mellitus. *Kidney Int.* 6(suppl 1):8–14, 1974.

29. Mitchell, J.C., Frohnert, P.P., Kurtz, S.B. et al. Chronic peritoneal dialysis in juvenile-onset diabetes mellitus. *Mayo Clinic Proc.* 53:775–781, 1978.

30. Kjellstrand, C.M., Shidemand, J.R., Simmons, R.L. et al. Renal transplantation in insulin-dependent diabetic patients. *Kidney Int.* 6(suppl 1):15–20, 1974.

31. Zincke, H., Woods, J.E., Palumbo, P.J. et al. Renal transplantation in patients with insulin-dependent diabetes mellitus. *JAMA.* 237:1101–1103, 1977.

32. Mauer, S.M., Steffes, M.W., Sutherland, D.E.R. et al. Studies on the rate of regression of the glomerular lesions in diabetic rats treated with pancreatic islet transplantation. *Diabetes* 24:280–285, 1975.

11 Diabetic Retinopathy: Recognition and Management

James D. Kingham, MD

Diabetic retinopathy is the leading cause of blindness in the United States today in the 20 to 65 year age group.[1] It is uncommon in diabetics under age 20 and in pregnant diabetic women,[2] and is extremely common in some American Indian tribes..[3] Controlled clinical trials have demonstrated the efficacy of certain types of treatment for diabetic retinopathy with subsequent preservation of vision, and have identified certain risk factors.[4,5] It appears that preservation of vision in the diabetic patient is predicated on early treatment, and early treatment is predicated on early detection of retinopathic changes by the primary care physician. The purpose of this chapter is to identify the changes seen in diabetic retinopathy and to provide guidelines for referral and treatment.

BASIC ANATOMY

The eye is a tough, fibroelastic, neurosensory end-organ about 25 mm in diameter. The posterior five-sixths of the eye wall is composed of dense, opaque, collagenous sclera, which serves as a supporting structure. The anterior one-sixth of the eye wall is clear collagenous cornea with a shorter radius of curvature than the sclera.

The eye wall, except for the cornea, is composed of three tunica. These are the supporting sclera, the vascular choroid, and the retina with its two component parts: the retinal pigmented epithelium, and the nonpigmented neurosensory retina (Figure 11-1).

The retina, a complex neural tissue with several component layers, derives its blood supply from two different sources. The inner retina (toward the vitreous) includes the nerve fiber layer, ganglion cell layer, inner plexiform, and inner nuclear or bipolar cell layer. These have as their blood supply, the central retinal artery and vein with an intervening capillary bed. No retinal vessels are found in retinal layers deeper (more scleral) than the inner nuclear layer. The outer retina (toward the scleral side) includes the retinal pigment epithelium, rod and cone layer, outer nuclear layer and outer plexiform layer. These have as their source of oxygen and nutrients, the blood vessel layer in the choroid known as the choriocapillaris (Figure 11-2). Oxygenation and nutrition to the outer retina occurs as a process of diffusion from and to the choriocapillaris. This duality of blood supply to the retina results in vascular lesions at different levels of retinal tissues. The

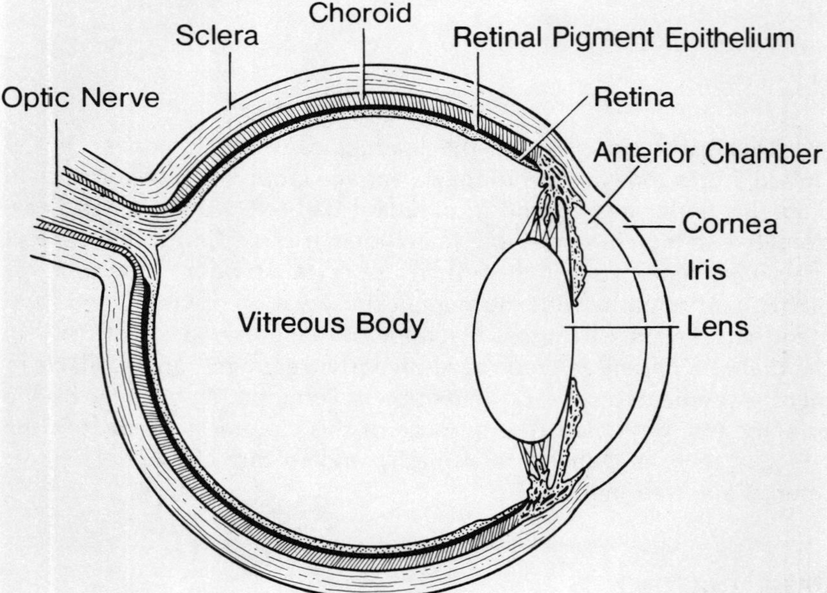

Figure 11-1 Schematic cross-section of eye to show relationship of retina to retinal pigment epithelium and choroid externally, and to vitreous internally.

microangiopathy of diabetes is manifested primarily in the retinal vascular system, thus affecting primarily the inner retina.

Seen from straight ahead, as is done ophthalmoscopically, the posterior fundus structures include the optic disc, macula, papillomacular bundle, and retinal vessels (Figure 11-3).

The blood supply of the retina, the central retinal artery and vein, are seen arising from the optic nerve head after a 12-mm course

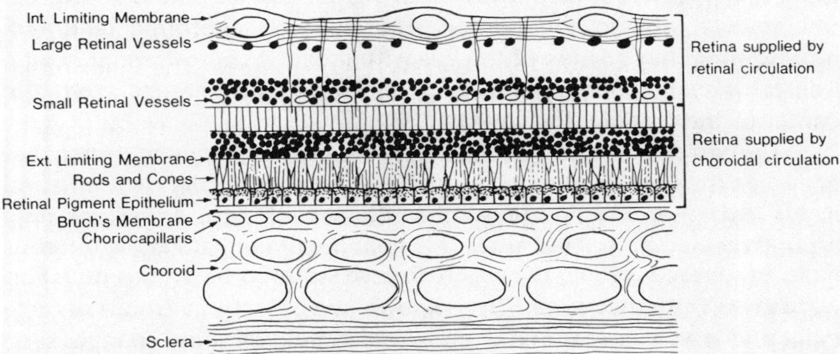

Figure 11-2 Schematic cross-section of retina to show inner half is supplied by retinal circulation, outer half is supplied by diffusion from choriocapillaris.

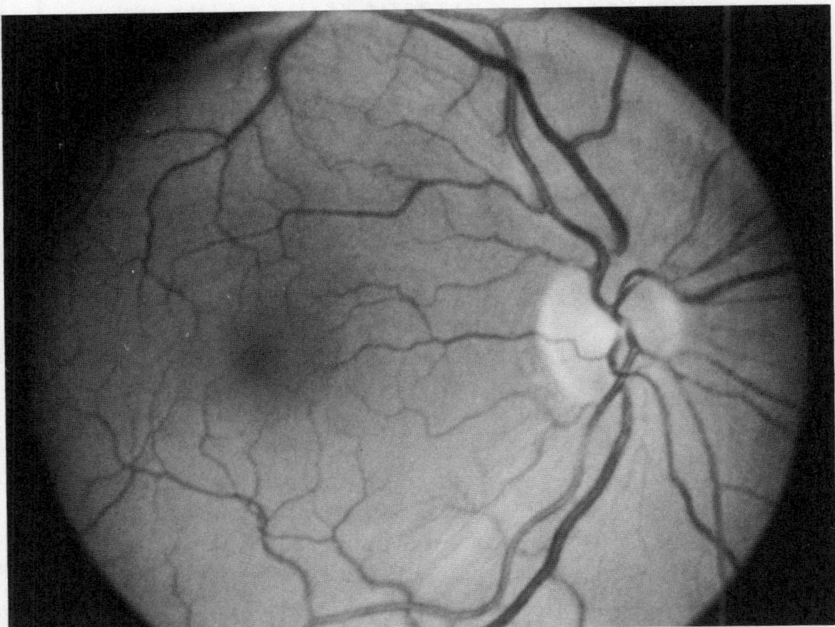

Figure 11-3 Normal posterior pole showing optic nerve head, macula with increased pigmentation, papillomacular bundle, and normal vessels with A/V ratio 2:3.

through the center of the optic nerve. They divide usually into four major branches, one pair of vessels supplying each quadrant. The temporal vessels arc above and below the macula. The nasal vessels have a more straight course toward the periphery.

The retinal tissue is thickest in the posterior pole and here has its most abundant blood supply. The major vessels lie superficially in the nerve fiber layer. Capillary networks extend deep into the inner half of the retina. Pigmentation of the retinal pigment epithelium is greatest in the macula, and in the normal state it is an anatomic landmark representing that portion of the eye with greatest central visual acuity. Central visual acuity decreases with increasing distance from the center of the macula, the fovea.

The vitreous is the jelly-like hydrated collagenous material that occupies the major volume (about 4.5 cc) of the eyeball. In youth and in health it lies firmly against the retina, with firm adhesions only around the optic disc, and anteriorly near the ora serrata at the vitreous base. In senescence and in certain disease states, the vitreous pulls forward away from the retina. This is known as a posterior vitreous detachment and is an important concept in understanding some changes seen in diabetic retinopathy.

CLINICAL APPEARANCE OF DIABETIC RETINOPATHY

Reference is made to two major types of diabetic retinopathy: proliferative and nonproliferative. Proliferative diabetic retinopathy is a response of hypoxic retina resulting in the formation of new blood vessels and accompanying fibrous connective tissue, from the surface of the optic disc, the surface of the retina, or both. It is called neovascularization or fibrovascular proliferation.

Nonproliferative diabetic retinopathy, on the other hand, is a response to hypoxic retina with changes other than neovascularization. These changes include increased vascular permeability, microaneurysms, punctate and blot hemorrhages, capillary obliteration and closure, cotton wool spots or "soft exudates," hard exudates, preretinal hemorrhages, macular edema, and generalized avascularity of the retina and optic nerve.

The earliest known retinal changes to occur in diabetes are alterations in vascular permeability and volume of flow. By vitreous and slit lamp fluorophotometry, a technique that measures the amount of fluorescein leakage from retinal vessels into the vitreous, both Cunha-Vaz[6] and Waltman[7] and their colleagues have shown as a constant finding a breakdown of the blood retinal barrier, and subsequent leakage of fluorescein. This can be demonstrated in patients with ophthalmoscopically normal fundi and is quantitatively progressive with progression of visible retinopathy. Furthermore, the amount of leakage is correlated with the degree of metabolic control and duration of diabetic disease.[6]

By slit lamp and vitreous fluorophotometry Cunha-Vaz and co-workers[8,9] have shown an increase in the volume of retinal blood flow with progression of nonproliferative diabetic retinopathy, and a return to normal levels with the development of proliferative diabetic retinopathy. The significance of an increase in retinal blood flow is not fully understood, but may be the result of, or attempt at, autoregulation of blood flow in response to decreased transit time secondary to decreased capillary and venous resistance.[10] The initiating factors of decreased capillary resistance are not known.

The earliest changes seen ophthalmoscopically in nonproliferative diabetic retinopathy are red spots in the fundus. These red spots occur first, and most typically, temporal to the macula and are microaneurysms or small punctate hemorrhages (Figure 11-4). De Venecia et al[11] have studied microaneurysms by color photography, fluorescein angiography, and precise pathologic correlation by trypsin digest technique. By color photography microaneurysms are seen as red, or sometimes white, dots in the fundus. Fluorescein angiography reveals

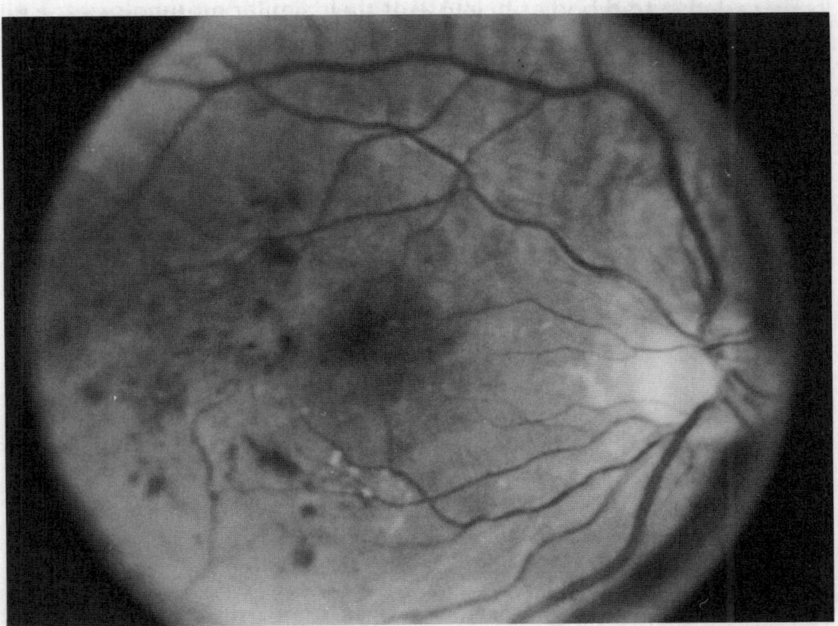

Figure 11-4 Red spots temporal to macula are blot hemorrhages and microaneurysms.

many more fluorescent dots, which correspond to microaneurysms too small for ophthalmoscopic resolution (Figure 11-5).[12] They feel, on the basis of their trypsin digest preparations, there is an evolutionary cycle to microaneurysms. The initial stage is a proliferation of endothelial cells resulting in a thin-walled microaneurysm that becomes thick-walled, hyalinized, and finally completely obliterated.[11] Some red spots in the fundus are red-blood-cell–filled microaneurysms that fail to perfuse during fluorescein angiography.

COTTON WOOL SPOTS AND CAPILLARY CLOSURE

Seen clinically, cotton wool spots are soft, fluffy-appearing, yellowish-white spots in the superficial retina of the posterior pole, frequently seen in the distribution pattern of the radial peripapillary capillary network. They are, in fact, focal edematous areas, within the nerve fiber layer, of capillary nonperfusion (Figure 11-6). These cotton wool spots, when examined by fluorescein angiography, are found to be nonfluorescent or nonperfused (Figure 11-7). Dilated capillaries of hyperfluorescence are found adjacent to atrophic, acellular capillaries.[13] Histologic study of the cotton wool spots shows them to be edematous areas with accumulations of lipid-staining, degenerating neural tissue with interrupted axons.[14] These focal accumulations have been called cytoid bodies because of their similar morphology to cell bodies.

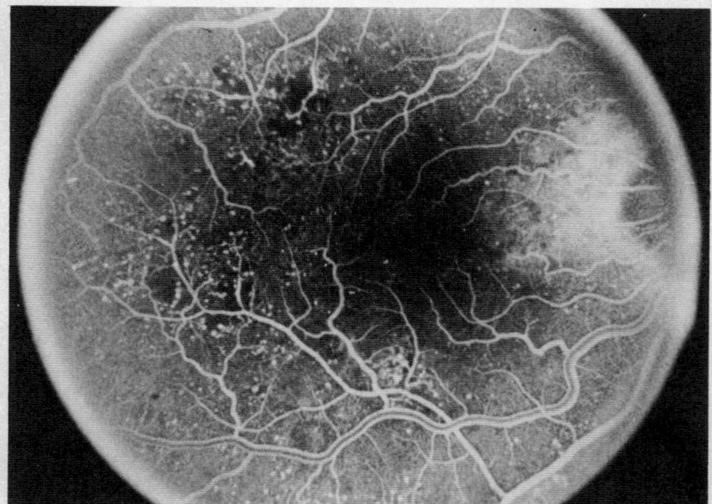

Figure 11-5   Fluorescein angiography shows multiple punctate fluorescing microaneurysms, some of which are below the limits of resolution of direct ophthalmoscopy. Perifoveal capillary free zone is about 500μ in diameter.

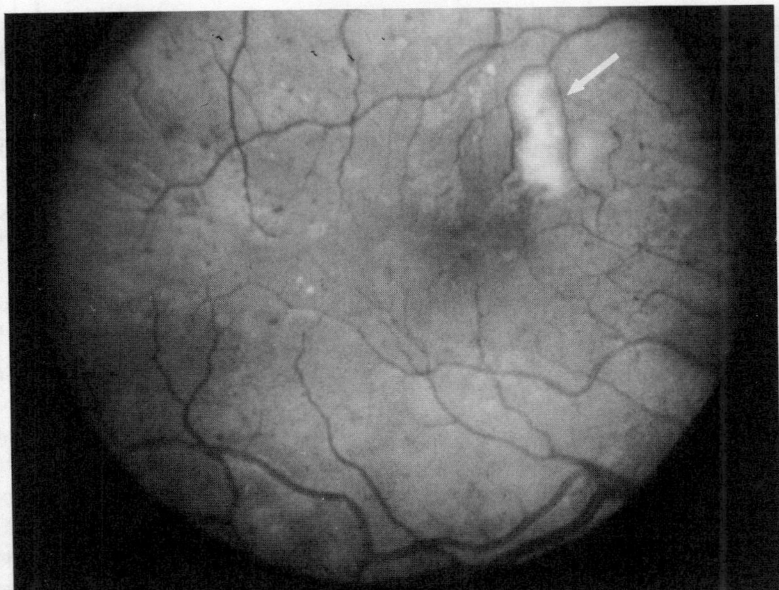

Figure 11-6 Large cotton wool spot or soft exudate is infarction of nerve fiber layer (arrow). Smaller less prominent cotton wool spot is adjacent to the large one.

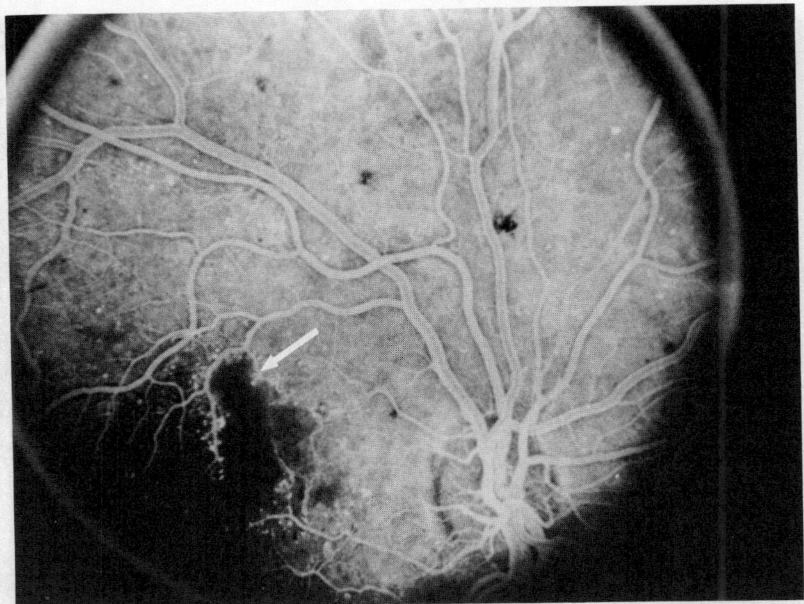

Figure 11-7 Fluorescein angiography of cotton wool spots seen in Figure 11-6. Note capillary nonperfusion, adjacent dilated capillaries, and microaneurysms surrounding the cotton wool spot. Location of arrow is identical to Figure 11-6.

Not all areas of capillary nonperfusion are recognized clinically as cotton wool spots. Some areas of retina often have a grainy or ground glass appearance with a loss of luster. Fluorescein angiography of these areas may reveal widespread absence of capillary perfusion, and there may be closure of precapillary arterioles as well.[13,15] With progression of small-vessel closure, smaller arterioles may be seen clinically as fine white lines in the fundus (Figure 11-8).

Normally, surrounding the center of the macula is the perifoveal capillary free zone of about 500μ diameter. Here the inner retinal layers are elevated to surround the fovea. The rod free center, the foveola, derives its nutrition by diffusion from the choriocapillaris. In the diabetic state the perifoveal capillaries seem to be particularly susceptible to closure.[13] This can be demonstrated by fluorescein angiography and in trypsin digest (Figure 11-9).

HARD EXUDATES AND CIRCINATE RETINOPATHY

The earliest detectable change in the diabetic retina is a breakdown of the blood retinal barrier.[7] As the duration of diabetes increases, so does vascular permeability.[6] Much of the exudative material is picked up by the vessels and transported away. Some ex-

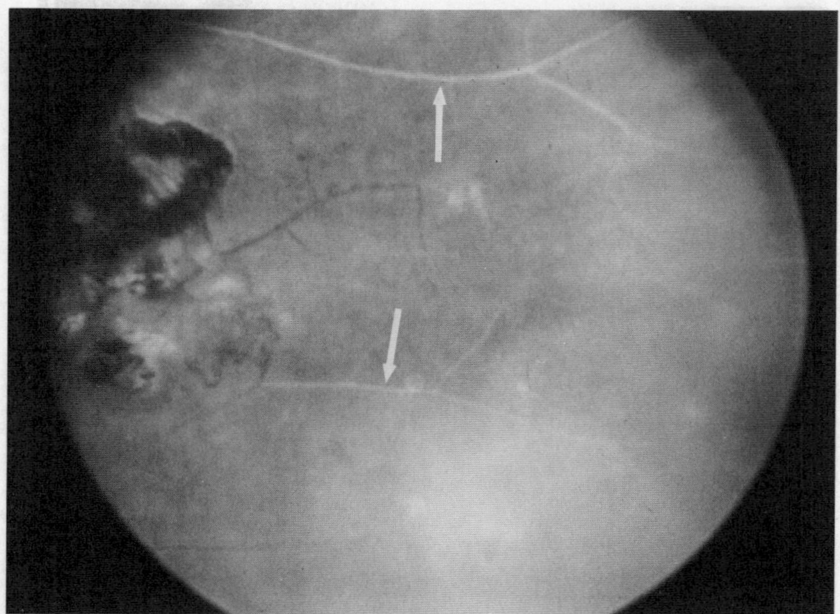

Figure 11-8 Markedly avascular retina with background showing homogenous ground glass appearance. Sheathed arterioles (arrows) are further evidence of avascularity.

udate however, finds its way into the deeper layers of the retina, the outer half where there are no retinal vessels. The exudates, rather than being carried away, persist, localized by this compact neuronal tissue, the outer plexiform layer. Seen ophthalmoscopically, these accumulations appear as discrete, well-circumscribed, reflectile, hard, waxy, yellowish spots deep in the retina (Figure 11-10). They may be punctate, medium size, or they may be massive accumulations of exudate in the macula. At times, with an identifiable epicenter of leakage seen on fluorescein angiography, they may be circinate, with the retina thickened and edematous within the center of the circinate complex.[16] Seen histologically these hard exudates are composed of exudative material, macrophages, and degenerating neural tissue.[17] Histochemically these hard exudates are nonhomogeneous accumulations of glycoproteins, lipoproteins, phospholipids, and neutral fats.[18] Resolution of these macular hard exudates by natural evolution, pharmacologic or photocoagulation intervention does not result in return of visual function.

MACULAR EDEMA

Macular edema is a significant cause of visual loss in diabetic patients.[19] It frequently occurs in adult-onset diabetes of long duration

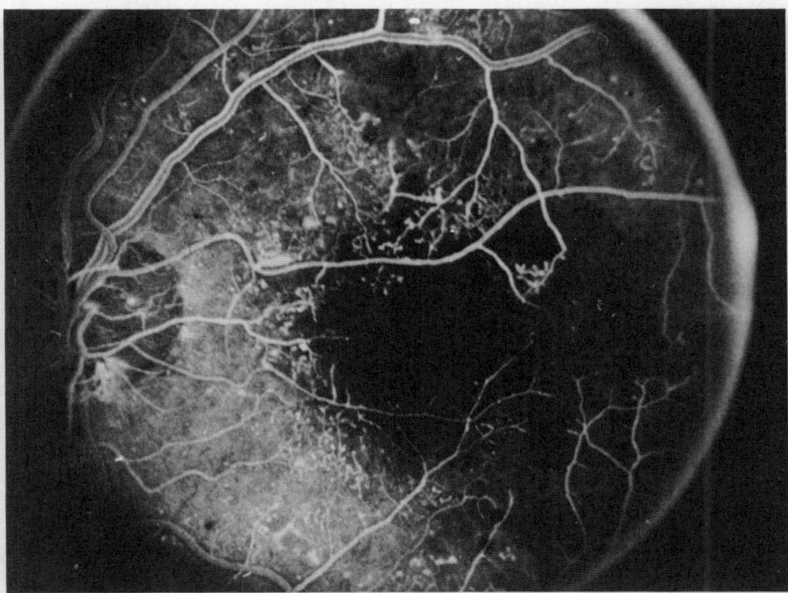

Figure 11-9 Small vessels in macula are nonperfused with fluorescein indicating capillary closure. Perifoveal capillary-free-zone has increased to two to three times its normal 500μ diameter. Small vessels adjacent to avascular retina are dilated and many microaneurysms are present.

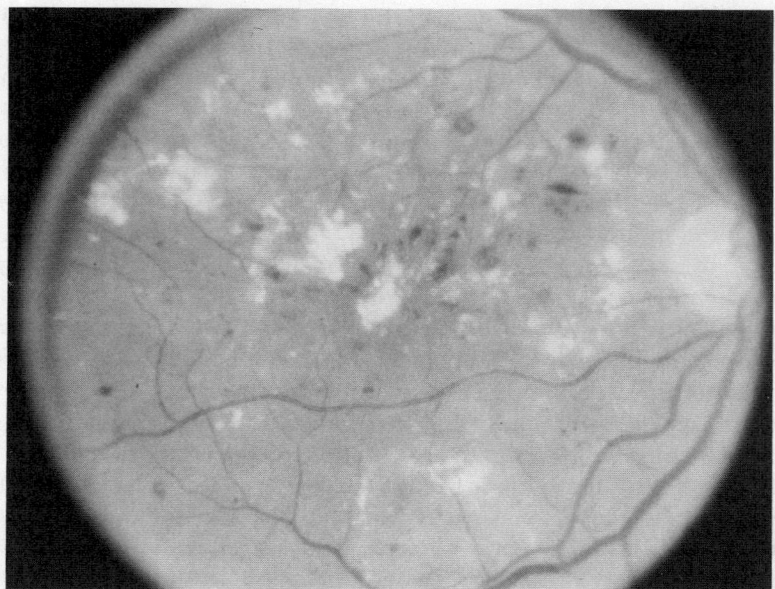

Figure 11-10 Hard exudates are yellow, waxy, reflectile accumulations of degenerating neural tissue, exudative fluid, and macrophages in the deep outer plexiform layer of the retina.

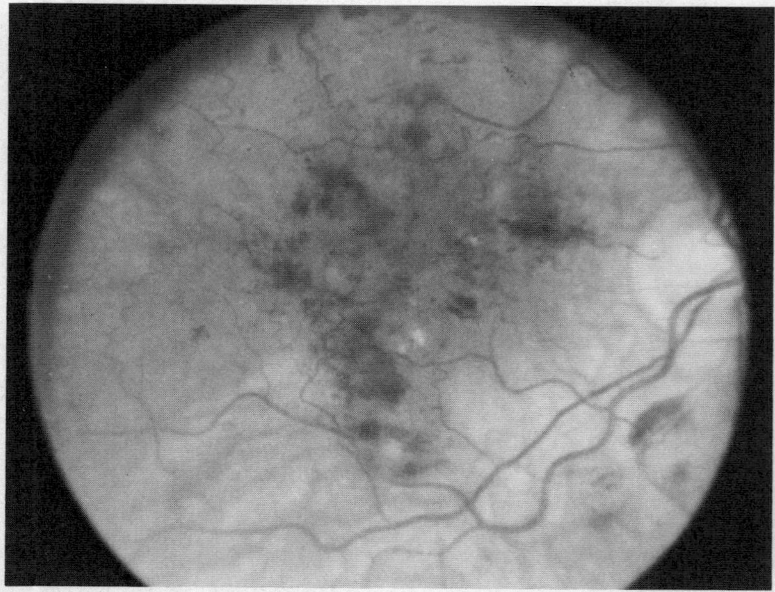

Figure 11-11 Generalized leakage of fluid from incompetent macular vessels results in macular edema and loss of granular appearance of retinal pigment epithelium in the macula.

and may cause a decrease of vision from 20/30 to 20/100 or worse.[20] The edema may be diffuse or cystoid. By ophthalmoscopy the macula loses the granular appearance of the normal retinal pigment epithelium. The retina becomes thickened, translucent, opaque, and dirty gray with an admixture of blot hemorrhages and exudates (Figure 11-11). When exudative fluid becomes loculated in the inner retinal layers, a cystoid appearance is taken on. Usually the decrease in visual acuity parallels the amount and duration of the edema.

By fluorescein angiography the leakage of fluorescein may be markedly diffuse or may be seen arising from a discrete microaneurysm as an epicenter of surrounding edematous retina. Perfusion of the capillary bed may be focally abnormal,[21] or there may be capillary perfusion with massive leakage and widespread macular edema (Figure 11-12).[22]

Classically, macular edema has been thought to develop because of leakage into the retina from incompetent retinal vasculature. Recently, however, Tso et al[23] have demonstrated in experimental animals a defect in the retinal pigment epithelium and found transport of horseradish peroxidase into the retina with a subsequent attempt to repair damaged retinal pigment epithelium. These results need to be corroborated by others and further explored.

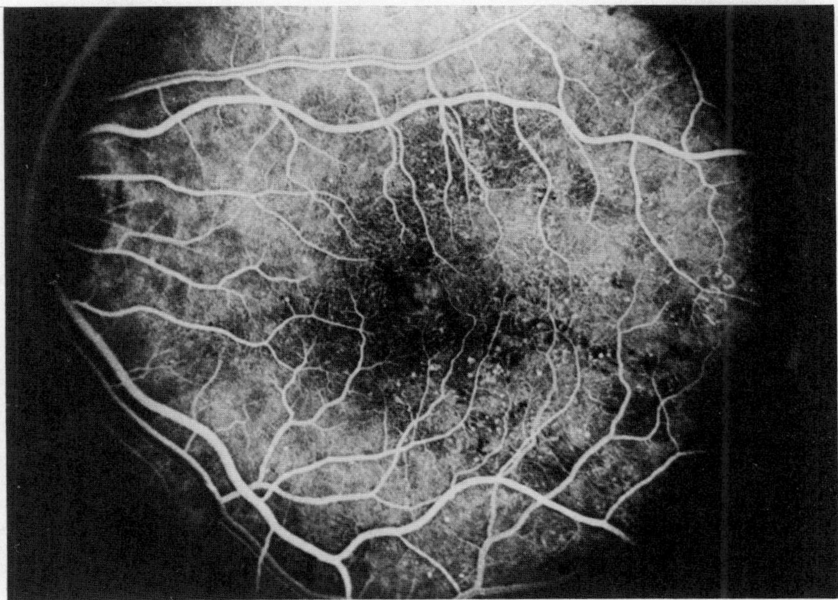

Figure 11-12A Early fluorescein angiogram of macular edema. Multiple punctate fluorescent microaneurysms are source of leakage.

PROLIFERATIVE DIABETIC RETINOPATHY

Proliferative diabetic retinopathy is the response of hypoxic retina, presumably to reestablish deprived nutritional demands, by the formation of new blood vessels (neovascularization). After neovascularization develops it proceeds through a maturation process, at times associated with intercedent events that threaten, diminish, or even destroy vision.

Neovascularization may arise from the vessels on the optic disc. Early neovascularization may be present only as fine, wispy, new vessels, just barely discernible by ophthalmoscopy. Characteristically, however, these vessels will leak fluorescein and the clinical diagnosis can be confirmed. As the neovascularization progresses the new vessels on the disc increase in height and surface area (Figures 11-13 and 11-14). They do not grow into the vitreous, but they may liberate a toxic substance that causes (or is associated with) the vitreous to detach posteriorly. The vessels then grow into the retrovitreal space and attach to the posterior surface of the vitreous.[24] Fibrous connective tissue then grows along the matrix formed by the new vessels. With further contraction of the vitreous or by maturation and contraction of the fibrous connective tissue, the fragile new vessels may be torn and bleed into the retrovitreal space with subsequent extravasation into the vitreous gel.

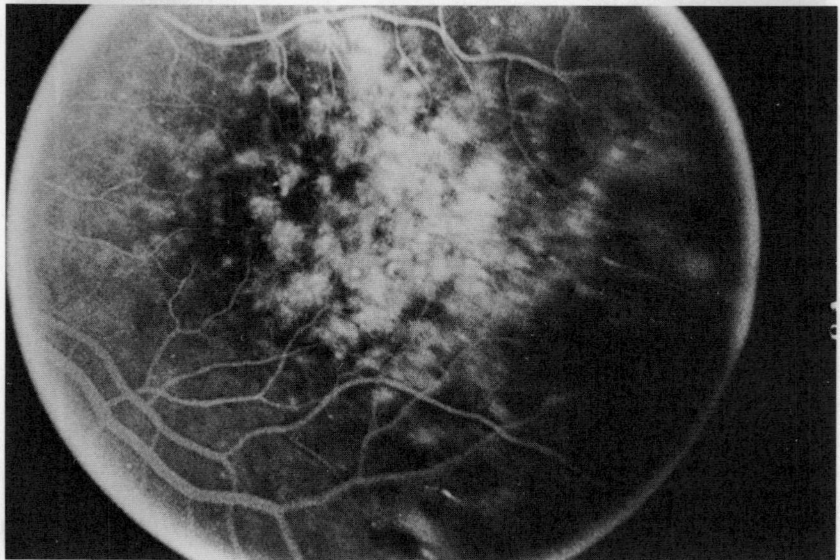

Figure 11-12B   At 77 seconds after injection, fluorescein has accumulated in the macula, indicating macula is thickened with edema.

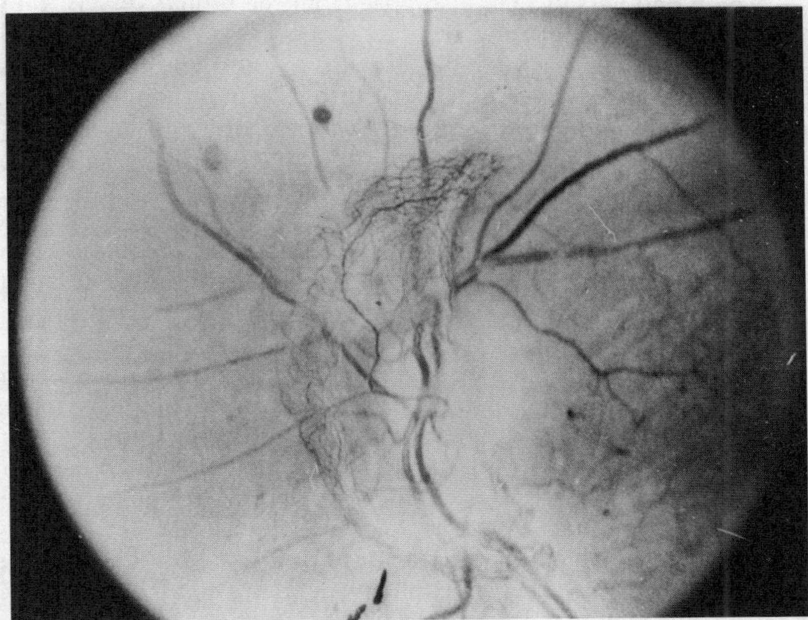

Figure 11-13 Papillovitreal neovascularization arises from the optic nerve, extends forward into vitreous cavity, and attaches to posterior surface of detached posterior vitreous.

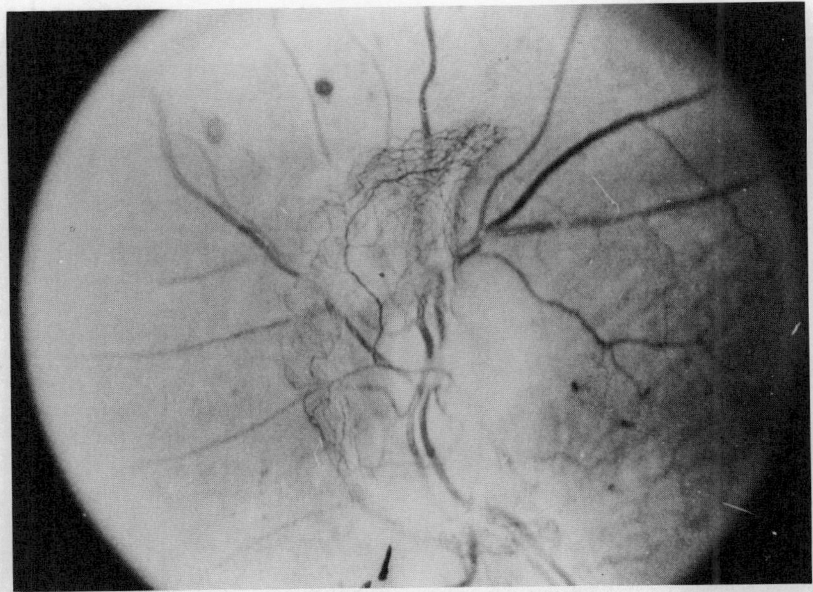

Figure 11-14 Fluorescein angiography of papillovitreal neovascularization seen in Figure 11-13. Fluorescein leaks profusely from neovascularization but not from normal vessels.

New blood vessels may also arise from the retinal vessels away from the optic disc and are referred to as new vessels elsewhere (NVE) (Figure 11-15). They have similar growth, maturation, and bleeding characteristics as new vessels on the disc (NVD). In addition, sometimes the traction from the posteriorly detached vitreous is transmitted to the retina via the new vessels and the retina becomes tractionally detached in that area (Figure 11-16).

For purposes of classification L'Esperance[25] has identified five patterns of neovascularization: 1) epipapillary neovascularization, 2) peripapillary neovascularization, 3) papillovitreal neovascularization, 4) surface retinal neovascularization, and 5) retinovitreal neovascularization.[25]

After several years, the proliferative retinopathy progresses from the wispy to the florid, through the fibrous stages, and finally becomes end-stage, involutional or burned out.[24-26] This is characterized morphologically by an absence or diminution of the vascular component and an increase in the fibrous component; narrow, attenuated, sometimes sheathed, retinal vessels; and a ground glass avascular, atrophic appearing retina, which can be demonstrated by fluorescein angiography to have large areas of capillary nonperfusion (Figures 11-17, 11-18, 11-19). Functionally, central visual acuity may be good or, because of the massive ischemia, it may be quite poor. Involutional proliferative diabetic retinopathy is probably a result of ischemia too

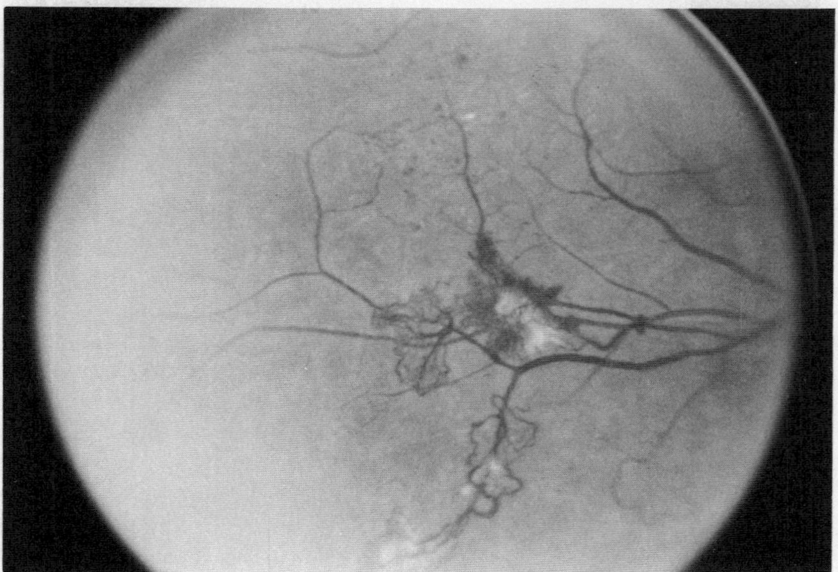

Figure 11-15 Neovascularization elsewhere arising from surface of retina away from optic disc.

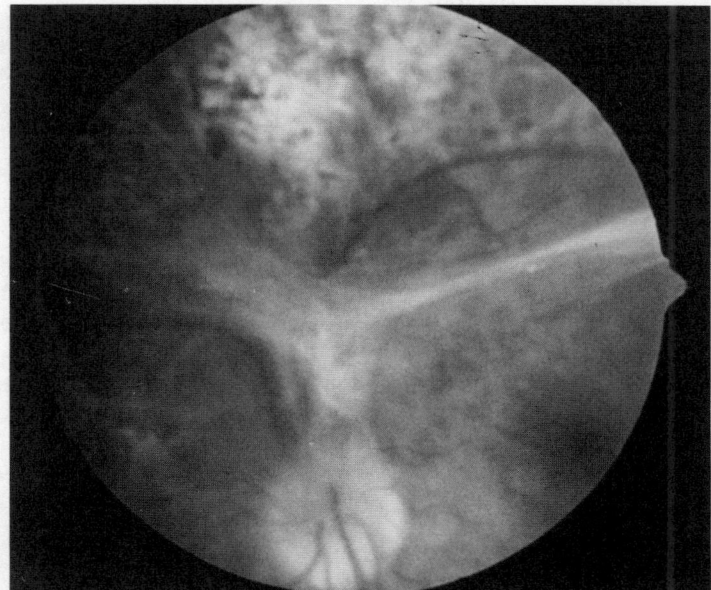

Figure 11-16 Marked fibrous component of fibrovascular proliferation has resulted in traction retinal detachment on either side of the fibrous band. When traction retinal detachment invades the macula, central vision is lost.

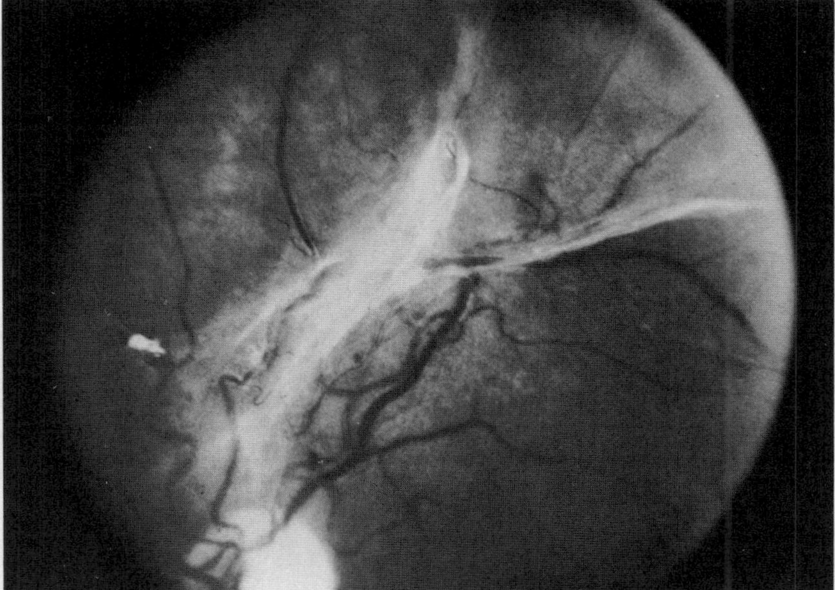

Figure 11-17 As a late stage in the evolution of neovascularization, the vascular component becomes less, and the fibrous component becomes more prominent.

severe to support vasoproliferation. It is frequently associated with decreased amplitudes of the electrooculogram and electroretinogram, color defects characteristic of optic nerve disease, visual field defects, optic atrophy, and neovascularization of the iris (rubeosis iridis).[15,26]

VISUAL EFFECTS OF DIABETIC RETINOPATHY

The visual effects of diabetic retinopathy are dependent on the type of diabetic retinopathy. Nonproliferative diabetic retinopathy, although less severe in final visual loss, affects greater numbers of people than does proliferative diabetic retinopathy. With nonproliferative diabetic retinopathy, vision loss is usually not complete and does not result in total blindness; rather it causes diminution of central visual acuity.

Intraretinal edema in the macula, hard exudates, and ischemia of the nerve fiber layer or optic nerve all contribute to diminution of central vision in nonproliferative diabetic retinopathy.

Visual loss in proliferative diabetic retinopathy is affected by preretinal hemorrhage over the macula, hemorrhage into the vitreous, traction retinal detachment affecting the macula, profound ischemia of the inner retina and optic nerve, or a combination of any or all of the

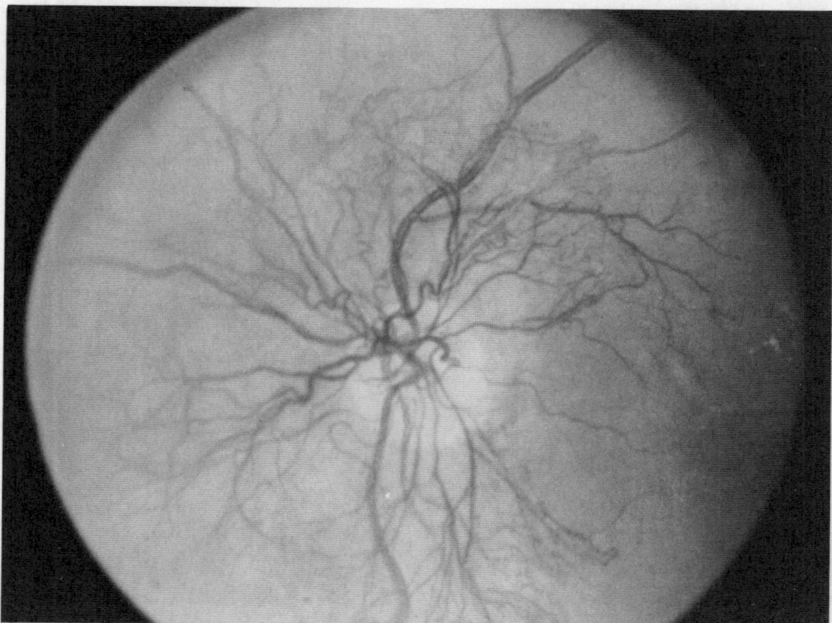

Figure 11-18   Late stage florid proliferative retinopathy.

above. As a rule, the manifestations of nonproliferative diabetic retinopathy cause loss of central vision, whereas vitreous hemorrhage or massive ischemia may cause a profound loss of all vision.

One important concept is that a diabetic patient may have excellent vision and widespread proliferative diabetic retinopathy that has remained hitherto asymptomatic, awaiting some cataclysmic event, eg, spontaneous contraction of the vitreous, minor head trauma, or Valsalva manuever. This event may initiate rupture of the small new vessels with massive vitreous hemorrhage and subsequent total loss of vision. It is for this reason that it is important for diabetics, especially juvenile-onset diabetics, to have visual acuity and funduscopic examinations by their primary care physicians during routine follow-up care for their diabetes.

INCIDENCE AND EPIDEMIOLOGY OF DIABETES AND DIABETIC RETINOPATHY

The true incidence of diabetes in the United States is not known, but published figures of 1965 and 1966 indicated that 2.8 million people had diagnosed diabetes. There were an additional 1.6 million

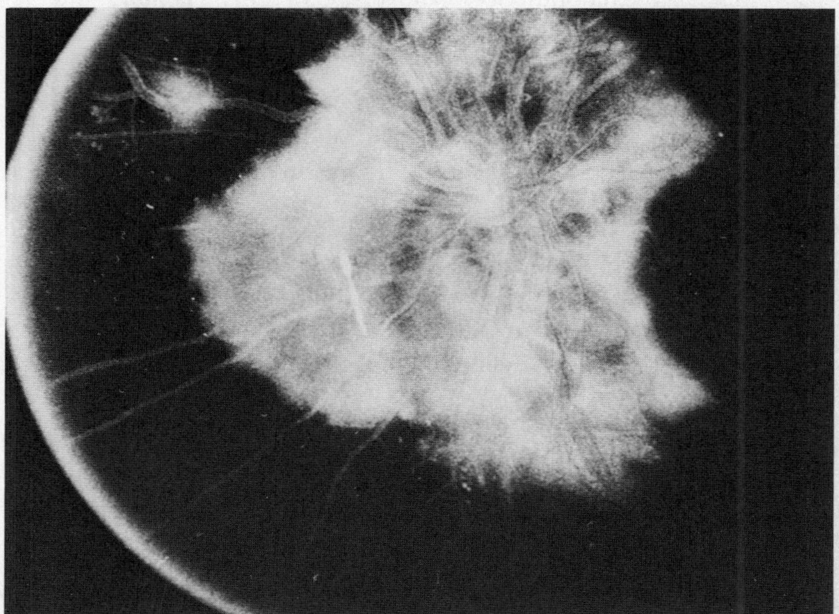

Figure 11-19   Fluorescein angiogram of florid retinopathy seen in Figure 11-18. Neovascularization fluoresces profusely while remainder of retina is nonperfused, indicating markedly avascular and compromised retina with concomitant loss of vision.

undiagnosed diabetics predicted,[27] with an incidence of about 2% of the total population. A survey of school districts in Michigan in 1976, yielded a rate of 1.6 diabetics per one thousand children.[28] Some ethnic groups, particularly the Pima and Papago Indians of Arizona,[29] and American Indians in general,[3] have a high incidence of diabetes. Indeed, in the 55 to 64 year old age group of Pima Indian women, an incidence of 70% diabetes was found.[30] In addition to being particularly tragic, the high incidence of diabetes in this closed population lends itself well to the study of diabetic retinopathy. Some study results are as follows:

- Diabetes is directly related to obesity.[30]
- Retinopathy found in Pima Indians is essentially the same as is found in non-Indian populations.[29]
- No neovascular changes were found in known diabetics with duration of less than 10 years.[29]
- The frequency of retinopathy was related to duration of diabetes. Fifty percent of those who had diabetes ten years or more had some type of retinopathy.[29]
- No significant sex difference was found in the population with retinopathy.[29]
- Of the total population 15 years and older, 5.5% had some type of retinopathy. Of these, about 7% had proliferative diabetic retinopathy.[29]
- The frequency of retinopathy was higher in those with higher glucose levels.[29]

In another epidemiologic study, the Framingham Eye Study,[31] the incidence of diabetic retinopathy was found to be 2% in the age group from 55 to 64 years, 3% from 65 to 74, and 7% from 75 to 85 years.

Diabetic retinopathy is responsible for about 10% of new blindness at all ages and almost 20% of new blindness between 45 and 74 years.[1] Women and nonwhites have a moderately increased risk of developing blindness from diabetic retinopathy, and nonwhite women have an even greater risk.[1]

After the onset of blindness caused by diabetic retinopathy, the mortality is about 15% per year at all ages. This indicates that diabetic retinopathy is but one manifestation of the microangiopathic state that exists in the overall biochemical imbalance in the diabetic patient.[32]

PREVENTION AND TREATMENT OF DIABETIC RETINOPATHY

Management of the diabetic patient to preserve vision is predicated on the type and amount of diabetic retinopathy present when first diagnosed. There is no treatment substitute for early diagnosis and management. The following management parameters seem to have some efficacy.

Treatment	Indication
Tight metabolic control	Prevention
Medical therapy	Prevention
Argon laser photo-coagulation	Nonproliferative maculopathy Proliferative retinopathy
Vitrectomy	Vitreous hemorrhage Traction retinal detachment
Pituitary ablation	Progressive florid retinopathy

Role of Metabolic Control

The actual role of control in the prevention of diabetic complications, including diabetic retinopathy, is not known and is discussed in detail elsewhere in this book (Chapter 7). Much experimental and clinical evidence, however, indicates that tight control of hyperglycemia exerts a protective influence in the prevention of diabetic retinopathy.

In a large study of diabetes of over 20 years duration, the Joslin Clinic investigators found a tenfold increase of diabetic retinopathy in patients with fair or poor control, compared to patients with good control.[33] Caird[34] has shown that patients followed for more than 12 years from one clinic had an increase in frequency of retinopathy if they consistently had a glycosuria of 2% or greater over the 12-year period. Pima Indians were shown to have increased retinopathy with higher glucose levels.[29] By vitreous fluorophotometry the amount of leakage was found to be correlated with the degree of metabolic control and duration of diabetic disease.[6]

From a prospective randomized clinical trial Job et al concluded that the use of divided daily insulin injections was effective in improving diabetic control and delaying retinal changes.[35] The validity of their statistical conclusions has been challenged by Ashikaga et al.[36] However, Job and colleagues have provided an update of their report[37] concluding that there is a slower rate of progression of microaneurysms in insulin-dependent diabetics treated with multiple daily insulin injections when compared to patients treated with a single daily injection. Also, a high number of microaneurysms is a risk factor for development of proliferative diabetic retinopathy.

The best experimental evidence for control is provided by Engerman.[38] A colony of alloxan-induced diabetic dogs was maintained for five years; one group was well-controlled, the other poorly controlled. After 60 months of diabetes, retinal capillary aneurysms, pericyte ghosts, obliterated vessels, and other microvascular abnormalities typical of diabetes were apparent histologically in each animal of the poorly controlled group. The meticulous control of the other group resulted in a statistically significant reduction in the incidence and severity of retinopathy.

Prout, in evaluating the clinical and experimental data in the literature summarizes ". . . the prudent physician should make every attempt to restore a normal physiological cellular environment in those patients with the expectation that this will offer the patient the best opportunity to minimize degenerative complications."[39]

Medical Therapy

The search for a substance that would be pharmacologically active in the prevention of diabetic retinopathy is not new. Currently, investigative emphasis in the United States is being placed on drugs that inhibit platelet aggregation. Following the report of disseminated intravascular coagulation as a complication of increased platelet aggregation in a patient with severe diabetes mellitus,[40] Dobbie et al[41] studied the role of platelets in the pathogenesis of diabetic retinopathy. They found a platelet-aggregation-enhancing activity in the plasma of diabetic patients and furthermore, found a correlation between severity of retinopathy and degree of platelet-aggregation-enhancing activity. This led them to speculate that increased platelet aggregation favors microthrombus formation, leading to the development of ischemic lesions in the retina.[41]

Colwell et al[42] described an increased sensitivity of platelets to aggregation in diabetics. This sensitivity correlates with elevated levels of von Willebrand factor, which, in turn, is influenced by growth hormone. A fundamental mechanism for increased platelet aggregation is increased prostaglandin synthethase activity, which, in turn, is affected by aspirin, a prostaglandin synthethase inhibitor. Bern, however, in a review of platelet functions in diabetes mellitus emphasized, "although tempting to assume, it is not now established that there is an etiological relationship between accelerated platelet function and the accelerated vascular disease of diabetes mellitus."[43]

Inhibition of platelet aggregation by aspirin, sulfinpyrazone, or dipyridamole in combination with aspirin is being studied in the management of stroke and myocardial reinfarction.[44] Results are not yet complete but the Canadian Cooperative Study Group has concluded that aspirin is an efficacious drug for men with stroke.[45] In another prospective study using death, or cerebal or retinal infarction as end-points, no significant difference between aspirin and placebo were found.[46]

Currently the National Eye Institute and the National Institutes of Health are sponsoring a study on the early treatment of diabetic retinopathy. One parameter will be to study the effect of aspirin, or aspirin plus dipyridamole, in altering the course of diabetic retinopathy.[47] Patients will be eligible if they have diabetic retinopathy not identified as high-risk.[5]

Perhaps some of the most exciting research in the prevention of proliferative diabetic retinopathy lies in the study of factors that inhibit neovascularization. Extract purified from cartilage has a definite inhibitory effect on corneal neovascularization. Further work has been initiated to study the retinal neovascularization inhibitory effect of cartilage, aorta, and vitreous.[48]

Laser Photocoagulation for Diabetic Maculopathy

The procedure of argon laser photocoagulation requires that a patient be seated in front of a slit lamp that is connected to the laser console (Figure 11-20). A contact lens is placed on the cornea after topical anesthesia. Laser burns are focused directly on microaneurysms or red

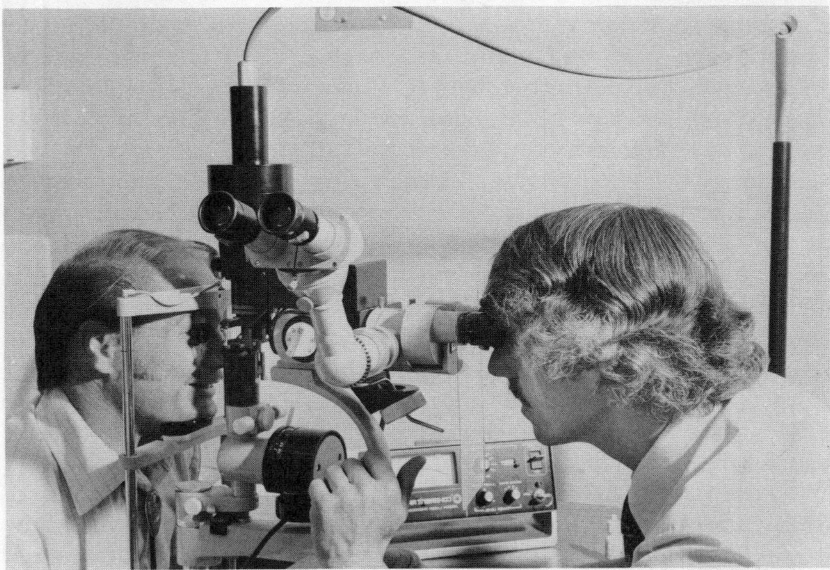

Figure 11-20 Outpatient being treated by argon laser photocoagulation. Topical anesthetic precedes placement of corneal contact lens.

spots in the posterior pole, avoiding the central 500μ, the perifoveal capillary free zone. The control module of the laser panel allows for the variables of: spot size from 50 to 1000μ, intensity from 0 to 3000 mW, and duration from 0.05 seconds to continuous burns. The laser beam is focused on the retina. The light energy of the laser beam is absorbed by the retinal pigment epithelium and converted to heat energy, which disrupts retinal pigment epithelium and the outer retinal layers, ie, photoreceptors. Generally, retinal vessels over the laser burn and subsequent scar are unaffected although some segments of capillaries within treated foci become nonfunctioning strands. This may suggest a decrease of the vascular requirement due to the reduction of metabolically active cellular elements in the retina.[49]

In diabetic maculopathy the retina is diffusely thickened with edema fluid, which is a product of incompetent retinal vasculature. At times, the source of intraretinal fluid can be localized to a discrete focus of leakage[15] or the leakage may be diffuse.[21] Furthermore, Tso et al[23] have recently reported an additional locus of leakage from the retinal pigment epithelium.

The rationale of laser photocoagulation is to dry up the source of leakage. The exact mechanism of this is not fully understood. In general, most clinicians treat microaneurysms and red spots directly, and treat diffuse edema with a diffuse type of modified retinal scatter treatment over the posterior pole (Figure 11-21).[50]

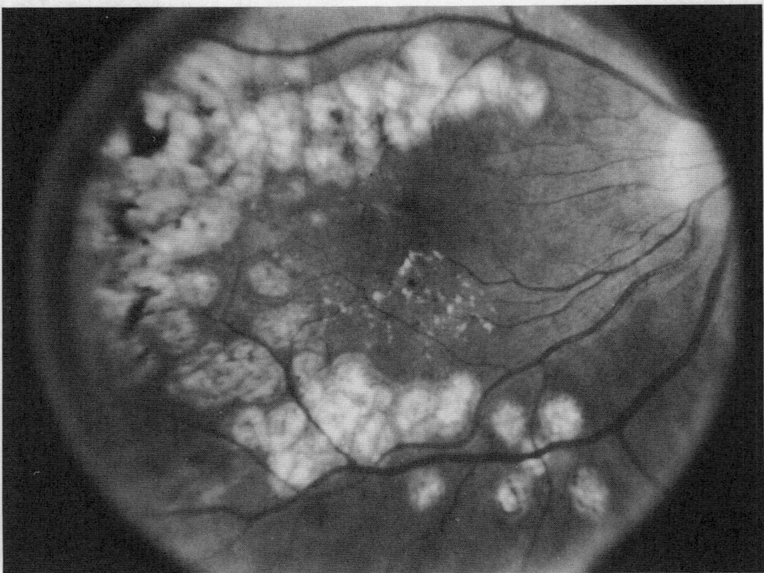

Figure 11-21 Argon laser spots to the posterior pole to dry up leaking microaneurysms that were causing macular edema. Posttreatment this macula is dry, without edema.

It appears from the figures in Table 11-1 that photocoagulation has some positive effect on final visual acuity in patients with macular edema.[18,21,51-53] Obvious shortcomings of all these studies are small treatment populations, variation in type and amount of maculopathy, dissimilarity of treated and control eyes, and short follow-up period (all less than three years).

Table 11-1
Results of Photocoagulation for Macular Edema

Study	Subject Group	Improved (%)	Same (%)	Worse (%)
Rubenstein and Myska[21]	Treated	53	43	4
	Control	7	54	39
Patz et al[19]	Treated	27	66	7
	Control	10	27	63
Marcus and Aaberg[51]	Treated	18	57	24
	Control	3	54	42
Blankenship[52]	Treated	17	60	23
	Control	3	53	43
Merin et al[53]	Treated	52	43	4
	Control	0	0	0

Laser Photocoagulation for Proliferative Diabetic Retinopathy

The exact cause of retinal neovascularization in the diabetic patient is not known, but it probably represents an ocular response to ischemic retina. What is known, however, is that untreated proliferative diabetic retinopathy leads to blindness in about 50% of patients within five years of detection (of the proliferative retinopathy).[54] Neovascularization arising from the surface of the optic disc, rather than surface retinal neovascularization, seems to be the most dangerous in the etiology of vitreous hemorrhage. In one study of patients less than 20 years of age at the time their diabetes was discovered, the interval from the discovery of diabetes to the onset of severe blindness was an average of about 17 years.[55]

Diabetic retinopathy was first treated by light coagulation by Meyer-Schwickerath in 1955.[56] Observations at that time indicated that diabetic retinopathy could be prevented or improved by the presence, or occurrence of, unilateral high myopia, optic atrophy, disseminated choroiditis, and other factors that reduce, directly or indirectly, the oxygen supply to the retina. It was felt that xenon light coagulation might simulate these conditions and reduce the metabolic activity of the retina, with subsequent regression of proliferative diabetic retinopathy. Following initial success with xenon photocoagulation, Beetham et al turned to the ruby laser, which produced a smaller, less destructive chorioretinal scar.[57] This treatment was followed immediately by the development and use of the argon laser photocoagulator,[58] which is still the principal modality of laser treatment.

Surface retinal neovascularization, not in the macula or papillomacular bundle can be treated directly with the argon laser. The technique is to whiten the retinal pigment epithelium under and around the neovascularization. Within a few weeks the neovascularization undergoes regression, involution, fibrosis, and sometimes completely disappears. Neovascularization arising from the optic disc (the type most likely to evoke vitreous hemorrhage) cannot, however, be treated in this manner. Instead, larger areas of retina are treated in a "scatter" treatment, again avoiding the macula and papillomacular bundle. It seems that this scatter treatment, which causes chorioretinal scarring, has the same effect on the developing proliferative diabetic retinopathy as does a naturally occurring chorioretinal scarring process: regression of the neovascularization (Figure 11-22).

To evaluate the efficacy of photocoagulation on final visual acuity

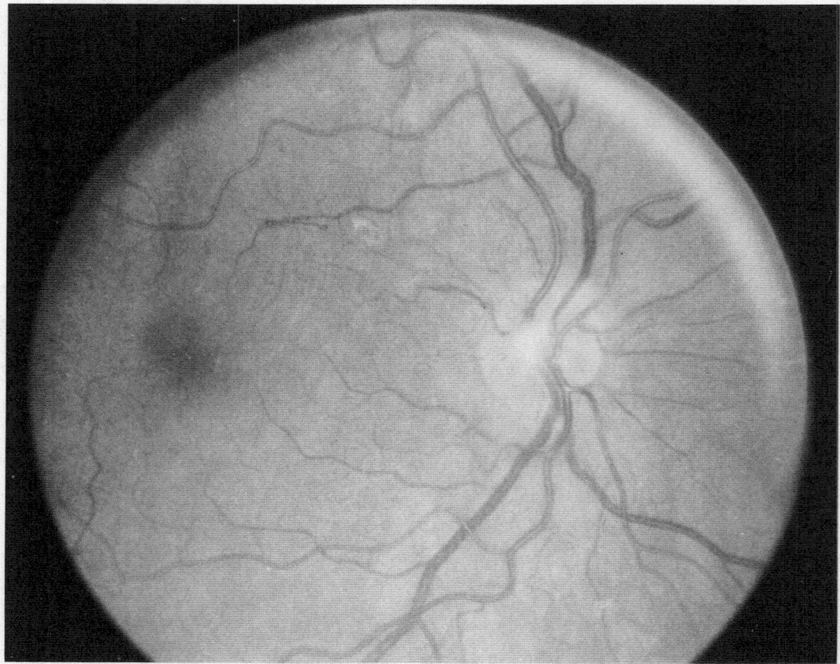

Figure 11-22A Peripapillary neovascularization present but not well seen ophthalmoscopically.

the Diabetic Retinopathy Study was begun in 1971 under the sponsorship of the National Eye Institute. This randomized, controlled, clinical trial involved more than 1700 patients enrolled in 15 medical centers. The Diabetic Retinopathy Study protocol called for:

1. Proliferative or severe preproliferative diabetic retinopathy in both eyes.
2. Visual acuity 20/100 or better in both eyes.
3. Treat one eye only with 800 to 1600 laser spots, 500μ in diameter.
4. Severe vision loss to be defined as 20/800.

At the end of two years of follow-up it was apparent that photocoagulation has a significant protective effect on visual acuity. Severe vision loss occurred in 16.3% of untreated eyes and only 6.4% in treated eyes.[4] The Diabetic Retinopathy Study Research Group was so impressed with these results after only two years that they identified four risk factors that would allow untreated eyes to be treated and remain in the study. These were: 1) presence of hemorrhage, 2) presence of new vessels, 3) new vessels on or near disc, and 4) moderate or severe new vessels.

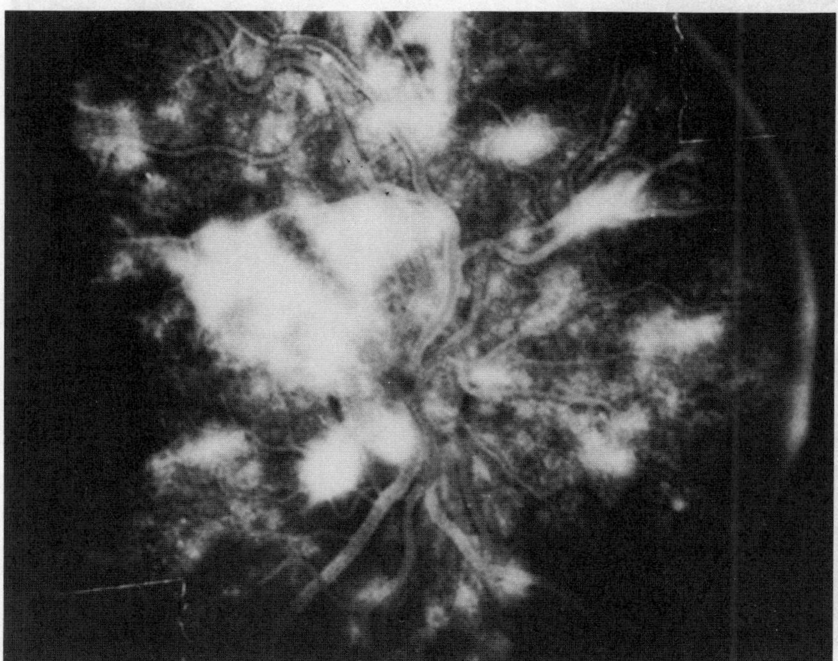

Figure 11-22B   Fluorescein angiogram accentuates peripapillary neovascularization.

They found a range of vision loss, commensurate with the number of risk factors present. The two-year incidence of severe vision loss (vision less than 20/800) in untreated eyes occurred in 3.6% with none of the four risk factors present, up to 36.9% incidence of severe vision loss if all four risk factors were present.[5]

Clearly then, argon laser photocoagulation is effective in prevention of vision loss in proliferative diabetic retinopathy. The earlier the treatment, the less risk factors present, thus less vision loss.

Complications of photocoagulation are relatively unusual and when they do occur they are frequently minimal. They include loss of visual acuity, reduction of peripheral visual field, impaired night vision, accommodative paresis, and pupillary dilation. More severe complications include severe permanent loss of vision, severe constriction of visual field, accidental foveal burn, treatment-induced retinal detachment, severe vitreous hemorrhage, or subretinal neovascularization.[50]

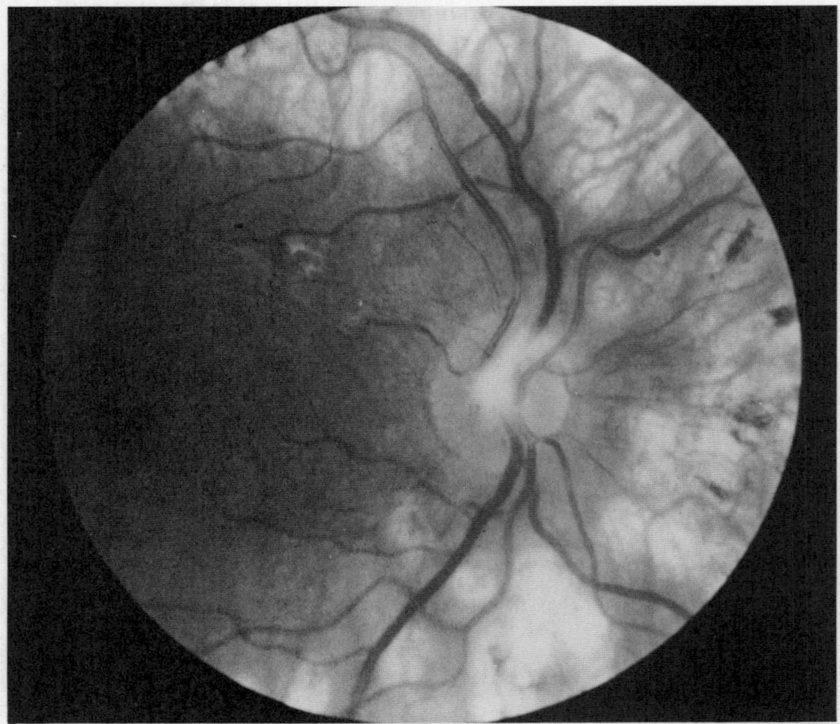

Figure 11-22C   After argon photocoagulation. Neovascularization is not present except for residual fibrous scar on disc.

Use of Vitrectomy in the Management of Complications of Diabetic Retinopathy

One of the most disabling complications of the microangiopathy of diabetes is the event of hemorrhage into the vitreous. For vitreous hemorrhage to occur it is necessary to have neovascularization present. The precipitating cause of the hemorrhage may be contraction of the vitreous gel, contraction of the fibrous component of the fibrovascular proliferation, increased intravascular pressure secondary to head position or Valsalva, or external trauma. Hemorrhage into the vitreous gel clears slowly, if at all, and breakdown products of the blood may be toxic to the retina (hemosiderosis).

Another cause of vision loss associated with proliferative diabetic retinopathy is contraction of the proliferative fibrous tissue resulting in tractional detachment of the retina. When the detachment affects the macula central vision is lost. Further contraction of the fibrous connective tissue can tear a hole in the retina, allowing a percolation of liquid vitreous into the subretinal space, resulting in a rhegmatogenous retinal detachment.

Vitrectomy is an operation developed by Machemer[59] utilizing

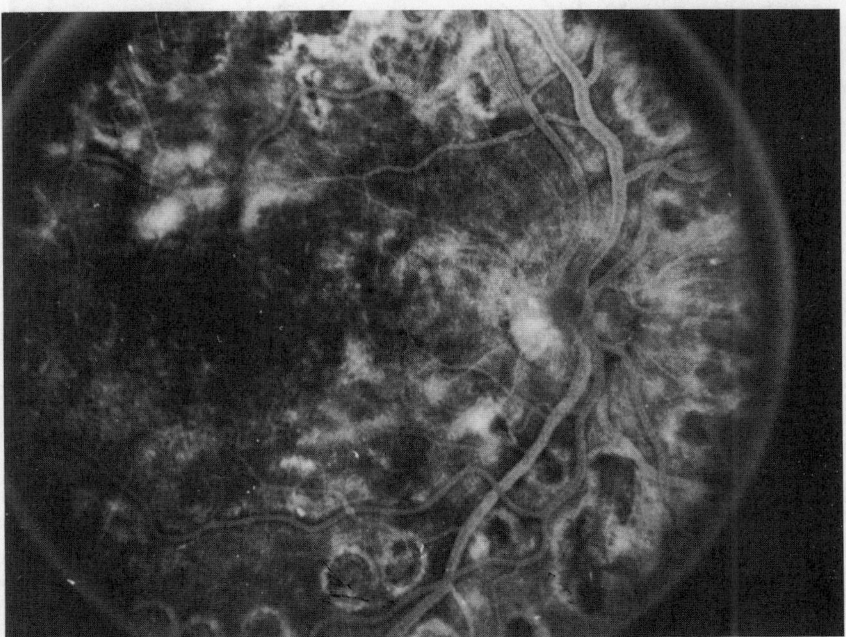

Figure 11-22D Fluorescein angiography confirms the efficacy of argon laser photocoagulation in the regression of established disc neovascularization. Minimal leakage is present. Compare with pretreatment photograph in Figure 11-22B.

special instrumentation to cut and remove vitreous and to replace the vitreous with a balanced salt solution.[60] The operation is currently performed by inserting three components into the eye through the pars plana; each of the three components of the vitrectomy instrument is the diameter of a 20 gauge needle. The first component is a short needle for infusion sutured to the sclera. The second component is a guillotine action cutting and suction device. The third component is a fiber optic light with a small hooked tip for illumination and for picking up membranes (Figure 11-23). The operation is done under visualization with an operating microscope. The primary goals of vitrectomy surgery are to remove vitreous opacities and to release vitreoretinal traction.[50]

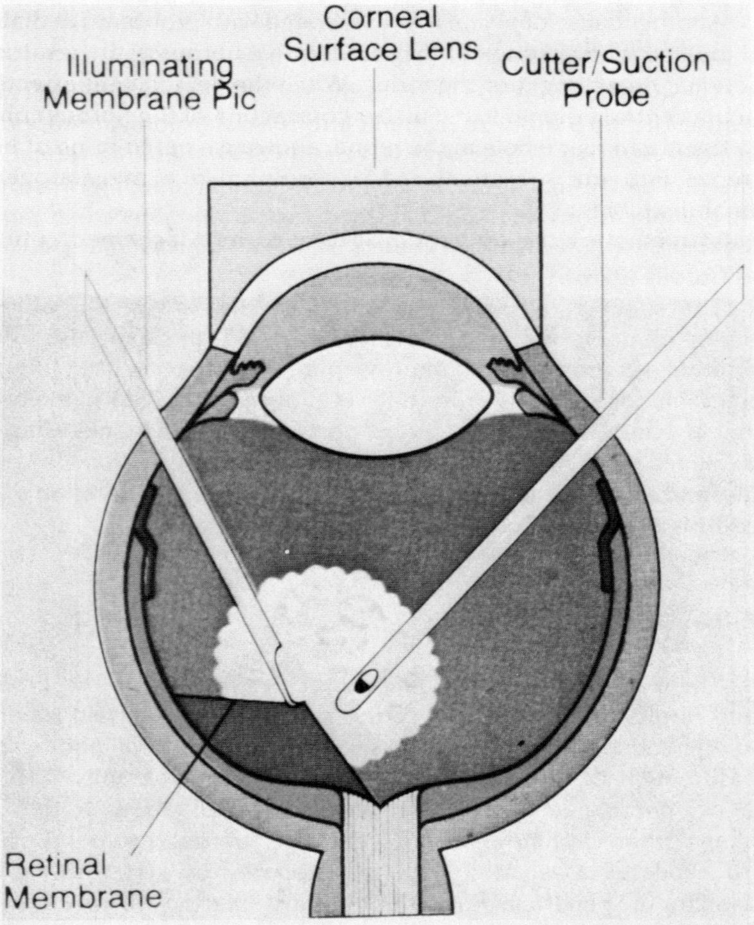

Figure 11-23   Schematic drawing of vitrectomy with fiberoptic hook and guillotine-like cutting tip. These instruments inserted into the eye, behind the iris and anterior to the retina, can remove bloody vitreous and epiretinal membranes.

Because some vitreous hemorrhages have a tendency to clear spontaneously, they are observed over a period of six to twelve months. Currently, conservative management of vitreous hemorrhage would use the following parameters as indications for vitrectomy[50]:

1. Visual acuity 20/800 or worse.
2. Presence of vitreous hemorrhage for 12 months.
3. Immediate vitrectomy if vitreous hemorrhage is coincident with retinal detachment as detected on ultrasound evaluation.
4. Vitrectomy after hemorrhage is present for six months if irreversibly poor vision is present in opposite eye.
5. Tractional retinal detachment progressing and involving, or threatening, the macula.

These indications for vitrectomy are, of necessity, conservative because the possibility of complications exists, both intraoperative and postoperative. Intraoperative complications include retinal hole formation and retinal detachment and intraocular bleeding. Postoperative complications include cataract formation, persistent corneal edema and vascularization, rubeosis iridis with neovascular glaucoma, and fibrous ingrowth.[61]

The success rate of vitrectomy includes several variables including preoperative status of the eye and the expertise of the operative surgeon. Initial improvement in visual acuity following vitrectomy for vitreous hemorrhage is about 65% to 75% in the best of surgical hands.[62] Even five years postoperatively, Blankenship and Machemer have shown that 50% have ambulatory vision.[63] Interestingly, and of visual significance, after vitrectomy, proliferation of new vessels is not usually observed.[64]

Pituitary Ablation

There is substantial evidence that destruction of the pituitary gland results in improvement of the appearance of certain lesions of diabetic retinopathy, whether assessed by serial color photographs, measurement of visual acuity, or fluorescein angiography.[65] Hemorrhages, microaneurysms, new vessels, venous irregularities, and leakage from capillaries usually improve; fibrous proliferation and hard exudates associated with maculopathy do not respond. The reason for the beneficial effects of pituitary ablation are not known but may be related to the effect of growth hormone. Reduction in growth hormone is often associated with improvement, or arrest in the deterioration of diabetic retinopathy.[65]

In a retrospective study, fourteen adolescents between ages 16 and 19 years with rapidly progressing florid proliferative diabetic retinopathy were compared.[66] Hypophysectomy was performed in eight patients with no mortality and minimal morbidity other than replacement hormone therapy (Table 11-2).

Table 11-2
Results of Pituitary Ablation

	No. of Eyes	No. Blind	Average Length Follow-up (mo)
Control	12	11	11
Treated	10	2	37

Results of pituitary ablation in this small retrospective study showed 11 of 12 control eyes had become blind after 11 months, whereas only 2 of 10 treated eyes had become blind after as long as 37 months follow-up. The authors concluded that pituitary ablation should be considered in young patients who had rapidly progressing florid proliferative diabetic retinopathy and who are felt to be beyond the capabilities of photocoagulation therapy.[66]

OCULAR MANAGEMENT OF THE DIABETIC PATIENT BY THE PRIMARY PHYSICIAN

Until the exact role of control of blood sugar in the development of diabetic microangiography has been elucidated, it seems reasonable for the primary physician to attempt to maintain a normal physiologic cellular environment to minimize degenerative complications.[39] If possible the primary physician should refer the patient to an ophthalmologist at the time of diagnosis of adult-onset diabetes. Juvenile-onset diabetics should have baseline examinations at time of diagnosis and at least every year thereafter.

If baseline referral to an ophthalmologist is impossible or impractical, the primary physician should serially evaluate the ocular status by visual acuity and funduscopy every visit. Referral to the ophthalmologist for evaluation and treatment is mandatory when the patient complains of subjective decrease in vision, objective evidence of decreased visual acuity is present, extensive microaneurysms and hemorrhages are present, hard exudates or cotton wool spots are present, neovascularization is present on disc or retina, and/or preretinal hemorrhage is present.

Because current treatment modalities have the capability to prevent worsening of diabetic retinopathy and worsening of vision, early referral for treatment will effect best results. For this reason, compulsive and scrupulous evaluation by the primary physician will ultimately result in a lessening of blindness in the diabetic population.

ON THE ETIOLOGY OF THE MICROANGIOPATHY OF DIABETES MELLITUS

Many factors have been evaluated and implicated in the microangiopathy of diabetes. Actually the etiology is multifactorial but an attempt will be made to examine briefly several factors that may be associated with the development of microangiopathy.

Genetic Predisposition— The HLA Alloantigens

Studies of the HLA supergene, which is located on the short arm of chromosome six, have demonstrated an association between antigens HLA-B8, Bw15, Cw3, and Dw3 and juvenile-onset diabetes.[67] Evidence suggests that genetic heterogeneity exists within insulin-dependent juvenile-onset diabetes, with at least two, and perhaps more, clearly distinct forms of juvenile-onset diabetes; one of which is associated with HLA-B8 and the other with Bw15. The HLA-B8 form may be called the autoimmune form. It is characterized by a decreased frequency of HLA-B7, an increased prevalence of pancreatic islet cell antibodies, a lack of antibody response to exogenous insulin, and an increased susceptibility to microangiopathy. The second form of juvenile-onset diabetes is associated with HLA-Bw15. It is not associated with autoimmune disease or islet-cell antibodies, and it is accompanied by an increased response to exogenous insulin.[68] Apparently, only one HLA associated diabetogenic gene is required for a susceptibility to juvenile-onset diabetes, and a person with both a B8 and Bw15 gene has an increased risk for juvenile-onset diabetes.

HLA antigen B7 has been found to be decreased in frequency in juvenile-onset diabetes. Its presence has been said to have a protective effect against microangiopathy and proliferative diabetic retinopathy. This decreased incidence of B7, however, occurs only in the B8 form of the disease.[68]

The heterogeneity that has thus been discovered may only represent the tip of the iceberg. Further studies may elucidate forms of diabetes in which complications, and the need for tight or loose control, may be factors of genetic subgroups.

A rare type of juvenile-onset diabetes has been recently documented, the maturity-onset diabetes of youth.[69] In this entity, symptoms are mild, stimulated insulin output is retained, although delayed and diminished, but ketonuria and hyperglycemia can be controlled without insulin. An autosomonal dominant type transmission seems most likely. HLA tissue typing has not been found to be associated with the hyperglycemia of this entity.[70] The classical type of maturity-onset insulin-independent diabetes has so far shown no correlation with any HLA antigens, indicating that this is a distinct genetic form.[69]

HYPOINSULINEMIA

Apart from hyperglycemia, the most prominent feature of diabetes mellitus is absolute or relative hypoinsulinemia.[71] The role of hypoinsulinemia, apart from hyperglycemia, has not been adequately studied. Intravenous injection of insulin results in a rise in pulse rate and plasma noradrenalin levels, a decrease in peripheral vessel blood flow, and a fall in glomerular filtration rate. Insulin increases the number of micropinocytotic vesicles in capillary endothelial cells, which suggests that adequate concentrations of insulin may be required for normal function of endothelial cells. Considering the close relationship between endothelial cells and capillary basement membrane, these findings may be relevant to the understanding of diabetic microangiopathy.[71]

HYPERGLYCEMIA

The role of hyperglycemia in the production of diabetic retinopathy has been discussed earlier in this chapter. Hyperglycemic diabetic dogs were found to have manifestations of diabetic retinopathy, while euglycemic diabetic dogs and control nondiabetic dogs did not.[38] In human diabetic patients control of blood sugar resulted in fewer manifestations of diabetic retinopathy than in more poorly controlled patients.[35,37] Obviously, it is not possible to accurately evaluate hyperglycemia as a single variable. However, suggestive evidence points to its implication in the formation of diabetic retinopathy.

ALTERED HORMONE LEVELS

Serum growth hormone levels may be elevated in diabetic patients. Does the diabetic state cause hypersecretion of growth hormone, or does increased growth hormone induce the diabetic state? In one study, Hansen[72] showed that following rigid control of blood sugar, the hypersecretion of growth hormone in juvenile diabetes was normalized. He concluded that abnormalities of serum growth hormone in juvenile diabetics are metabolic in origin. Other studies have shown that within three to seven days of daily injections of growth hormone, dogs develop hyperglycemia and glycosuria.[73] A strong case has been made for involvement of growth hormone in the development of diabetic microangiopathy. Growth hormone is elevated during much of the day in juvenile diabetics,[74] and hypersecretion of growth hormone in diabetic patients is accentuated with exercise.[75]

Growth hormone has an important effect on protein metabolism by activating hepatic synthesis of large proteins, including fibrinogen and alpha-2 globulins. These proteins may have an effect on red cell aggregates, sludging of the microcirculation, and increased resistance to blood flow.[75] Hypophysectomized patients given supplemental steroid, thyroid, and gonadal hormones have regression of their diabetic retinopathy without control of blood sugar, suggesting a direct beneficial effect of growth hormone deprivation.[71]

Another hormone, glucagon, has been shown to increase hepatic glucose output, stimulate production of acute-phase proteins, and to activate hepatic lysozomes.[74] Release of both growth hormone and glucagon is blocked by the recently discovered neurohumeral agent somatostatin.

RHEOLOGICAL AND RELATED FACTORS

In most disease states erythrocyte aggregation is enhanced, a change attributable to increased levels of fibrinogen and plasma globulins. Recent studies have shown an abnormality of red cell deformability in diabetics. Reduced deformability of diabetic red cells contribute to red cell aggregation.[76,77] Little,[75] has proposed that red cell aggregation in some diabetic patients causes sludging of blood flow in the microcirculation resulting in focal obstruction, local hypoxia, and accumulation of lactic acid from anerobic metabolism of the retina. Local hypoxia is associated with endothelial cell proliferation and microaneurysm formation. Little,[75] was also able to show a progressive rise in plasma levels of fibrinogen and alpha-2 globulins as one moved from controls to diabetics without retinopathy, then to diabetics with retinopathy, and finally to those with active proliferative disease. As retinopathy regressed he demonstrated a fall in fibrinogen and alpha-2 globulin levels.

By cation exchange chromatography three minor hemoglobin fractions can be eluted before the main peak. These are termed "fast hemoglobins" and are labeled HbA_{1C}, B, and C.[76] HbA_{1C} is increased to more than twice normal in diabetics, accounting for 10% of total erythrocyte hemoglobin. HbA_{1C} has glucose attached. This altered hemoglobin molecule has a greater than normal affinity for oxygen, reducing its ability to yield oxygen to tissue.[74] One means of enhancing the delivery of oxygen to tissue is the presence of 2,3-diphosphoglycerate, which is a product of the Embden-Meyerhof pathway. It acts on hemoglobin molecules during their passage through capillaries, to prevent them from taking up oxygen that has been released by other hemoglobin molecules. HbA_{1C} is insensitive to 2,3-DPG. Increased 2,3-DPG has been demonstrated in children with diabetes; this may be a response to the reduced efficiency of oxygen delivery caused by the high HbA_{1C} level.[76]

Altered platelet function was discussed earlier in this chapter. An increased sensitivity to platelet aggregation is seen in diabetics. This sensitivity correlates with elevated levels of von Willebrand factor, which, in turn, appears to be influenced by growth hormone.[41] A state of hypercoagulability associated with platelet aggregation may favor microthrombic formation leading to ischemic lesions in the retina. A correlation has been identified between the severity of retinopathy and the degree of platelet aggregation enhancing activity in the plasma of diabetic patients.[40] The increased sensitivity of diabetic platelets to aggregation can be abolished by aspirin, which is a prostaglandin synthetase inhibitor.[41]

Capillary basement membrane thickening is widely accepted as the ultrastructural hallmark of diabetic microangiopathy.[78] In juvenile diabetics, basement membranes are normal at the onset of diabetes and thicken with increasing duration of the disease. Thickening of capillary basement membrane in the diabetic, occurs in muscle, retina, and kidney. Capillary endothelial cells do not require insulin for glucose uptake, therefore, in diabetics they are subject to high levels of glucose. It appears from diverse evidence, that basement membrane thickening is a consequence of hyperglycemia. Furthermore, it has been shown that endothelial cells are capable of synthesizing basement membrane.[79] There is no evidence to implicate the sorbitol pathway in capillary basement membrane thickening, although sorbitol, a sugar alcohol derived from glucose, does accumulate in some ocular tissues, and is associated with increased intracellular water content, edema, precipitation of proteins, and cellular degeneration.[80] Capillary basement membrane thickening probably occurs as a consequence of abnormalities of synthesis, and/or degeneration, of basement membrane material by the endothelial cell, as a result of hyperglycemia. There is no evidence that thickening of capillary basement membrane interferes with vascular function, nor in any way is associated with a reduction in capillary lumen diameter. Thickening of capillary basement membrane appears to be a nonspecific manifestation of abnormal vascular function and/or injury.

INSULIN-INDUCED IMMUNOGENIC RETINOPATHY

Shabo and Maxwell sensitized monkeys with insulin and later challenged them with intravitreal injections of insulin.[81] They were able to produce proliferative tissue from the optic nerve head extending into the vitreous. Their results led them to speculate that diabetic retinopathy may result from a combination of factors including slow or intermittent leakage of blood vessel contents, including exogenous insulin, and an insulin-induced immunogenic reaction. Commercial insulin has many antigenic properties and insulin antibodies are detectable in humans after a few weeks of insulin therapy. Furthermore, Feman et al[82] have demonstrated small, but detectable, amounts of insulin in the subretinal fluid of patients undergoing retinal reattachment surgery.

SUMMARY

Diabetic retinopathy is the leading cause of vision loss in the United States. It may be manifested by nonproliferative or proliferative retinopathy. Nonproliferative diabetic retinopathy is characterized by increased vascular permeability, hemorrhages, microaneurysms, cotton wool spots, hard exudates, venous irregularities, macular edema, and generalized ischemia of the retina. Proliferative diabetic retinopathy is characterized by the growth of new blood vessels (neovascularization) from the optic disc and/or surface of the retina. With maturation, the vascular component becomes more associated with fibrous proliferation. Vision loss in nonproliferative diabetic retinopathy is caused by macular edema and ischemia of the macula and optic nerve. Vision loss in proliferative diabetic retinopathy is caused by vitreous hemorrhage, traction retinal detachment, and ischemia of the macula and optic nerve. Treatment modalities are directed toward:

- maintaining a normal biochemical milieu by diet and insulin administration
- prevention of intravascular coagulopathies by antiplatelet drugs

- focal treatment by argon laser photocoagulation for macular edema and surface retinal neovascularization
- argon laser retinal scatter treatment for disc neovasculaization
- vitrectomy for vitreous hemorrhage and traction retinal detachment
- pituitary ablation for relentlessly progressive florid proliferative diabetic retinopathy in young patients

Appropriate management by the primary physician includes:

- tight metabolic control
- measurement of visual parameters, both subjective and objective
- periodic dilated ophthalmoscopy
- referral to an ophthalmologist for baseline examination and when visual acuity drops or significant retinopathy is detected

Significant retinopathy includes large numbers of red spots (hemorrhages and microaneurysms), hard or soft exudates, macular edema, and any amount of neovascularization, either on the optic disc or on the surface of the retina.

The etiology of the microangiopathy of diabetes cannot be isolated to any single factor but is probably a result of multiple variables acting together. These include:

- genetic predisposition
- hypoinsulinemia
- hyperglycemia
- altered levels of growth hormone, glucagon, fibrinogen, alpha-2 globulin, 2,3-DPG, and HbA_{1C}
- altered platelet aggregation and abnormal red cell deformability
- changes in capillary basement membrane thickness
- altered immunogenic status to circulating and pooled insulin

Preservation of vision in the diabetic patient is predicated on early treatment. Early treatment is predicated on early diagnosis by the primary care physician who must maintain a high index of suspicion that diabetic patients harbor diabetic retinopathy. Several treatment modalities have been shown to be beneficial.

REFERENCES

1. Kahn, H.A., and Hiller, R. Blindness caused by diabetic retinopathy. *Am J Ophthalmol.* 78:58–67, 1974.

2. Cassar, J., Hamilton, A.M., and Kohner, E.M. Diabetic retinopathy in pregnancy. *Int Ophthal Clin.* 18(4):179–188, 1978.

3. Sievers, M.L. Diabetes mellitus in American Indians—standards for diagnosis and management. *J Am Diabetes Assoc.* 25:528–531, 1976.

4. The Diabetic Retinopathy Study Research Group. Preliminary report on effects of photocoagulation therapy. *Am J Ophthalmol.* 81:1–14, 1976.

5. The Diabetic Retinopathy Study Research Group. Four risk factors for severe visual loss in diabetic retinopathy. *Arch Ophthalmol.* 97:654, 1979.

6. Cunha-Vaz, J.G., Fonseca, J.R., Abreu, J.F. et al. Detection of early retinal changes in diabetes by vitreous fluorophotometry. *Diabetes* 28:16–19, 1979.

7. Waltman, S.R., Oestrich, C., Krupin, T. et al. Quantitative vitreous fluorophotometry—a sensitive technique for measuring early breakdown of the blood-retinal barrier in young diabetic patients. *Diabetes* 27:85–87, 1978.

8. Cunha-Vaz, J.G., and Lima, J.J. Studies on retinal blood flow. I. Estimation of human retinal blood flow by slit-lamp fluorophotometry. *Arch Ophthalmol.* 96:893–897, 1978.

9. Cunha-Vaz, J., Fonseca, J.R., de Abreu, J.R.F. et al. Studies on retinal blood flow. *Arch Ophthalmol.* 94:1766–1773, 1976.

10. Kohner, E.M. The evolution and natural history of diabetic retinopathy. *Int Ophthal Clin.* 18(4):1–16, 1978.

11. de Venecia, G., Davis, M., and Engerman, R. Clinicopathologic correlations in diabetic retinopathy. I. Histology and fluorescein angiography of microaneurysms. *Arch Ophthalmol.* 94:1766–1773, 1976.

12. Bresnick, G.H., Davis, M., Myers, F.L. et al. Clinicopathologic correlations in diabetic retinopathy. II. Clinical and histologic appearances of retinal capillary microaneurysms. *Arch Ophthalmol.* 95:1215–1220, 1977.

13. Bresnick, G.H., Engerman, R., Davis, M.D. et al. Patterns of ischemia in diabetic retinopathy. *Trans Am Acad Ophthalmol Otolaryngol.* 81:694–709, 1976.

14. Chester, E.M. *The Ocular Fundus in Systemic Disease.* Chicago: Year Book Medical Publisher, 1977, pp 58–69.

15. Bresnick, G.H., de Venecia, G., Meyers, F.L. et al. Retinal ischemia in diabetic retinopathy. *Arch Ophthalmol.* 93:1300–1310, 1975.

16. Spalter, H.F. Photocoagulation of circinate maculopathy in diabetic retinopathy. *Am J Ophthalmol.* 71:242–250, 1971.

17. Duke-Elder, S. (Ed.). *Diseases of the Retina,* Vol. 10 in System of Ophthalmology Series. St Louis: C.V. Mosby, 1967, pp 434–436.

18. Yanko, L., Ungar, H., and Michaelson, I.C. The exudative lesions in diabetic retinopathy with special regard to the hard exudate. *Acta Ophthalmol.* 52:150–160, 1974.

19. Patz, A., Schatz, H., Berkow, J.W. et al. Macular edema—an overlooked complication of diabetic retinopathy. *Trans Am Acad Ophthalmol Otolaryngol.* 77:34–42, 1973.

20. Ticho, U., and Patz, A. The role of capillary perfusion in the management of diabetic macular edema. *Am J Ophthalmol.* 76:880–886, 1973.

21. Rubenstein, K., and Myska, V. Pathogenesis and treatment of diabetic maculopathy. *Br J Ophthalmol.* 58:76–84, 1974.

22. Schatz, H., and Patz, A. Cystoid maculopathy in diabetics. *Arch Ophthalmol.* 94:761–768, 1976.

23. Tso, M.O.M., Cunha-Vaz, J.G.F., Shih, C.Y. et al. A clinicopathologic study of blood-retinal barrier in experimental diabetes. *Invest Ophthalmol Vis Sci [Suppl].* 18(4):169, 1979.

24. Davis, M.D. Definition, classification, and course of diabetic retinopathy. Edited by J.R. Lynn, W.B. Snyder, and A. Vaiser. In *Diabetic Retinopathy.* New York: Grune & Stratton, 1974, pp 7–34.

25. L'Esperance, F. Argon laser photo coagulation in diabetic lesions. Edited by J.R. Lynn, W.B. Snyder, and A. Vaiser. In *Diabetic Retinopathy.* New York: Grune & Stratton, 1974, pp 145-170.

26. Ramsay, W.J., Ramsay, R.C., Purple, R.L. et al. Involutional diabetic retinopathy. *Am J Ophthalmol.* 84:851–858, 1977.

27. Diabetic Source Book. Publication No. 1168, U.S. Public Health Service, 1968, p 8.

28. Gorwitz, K., Howen, G.G., and Thompson, T. Prevalence of diabetes in Michigan school-age children. *Diabetes* 25:122–127, 1976.

29. Dorf, A., Ballintine, E.J., Bennett, P.H. et al. Retinopathy in Pima Indians. *Diabetes* 25:554–560, 1976.

30. Knowler, W.C., Bennett, P.H., Hamman, R.F. et al. Diabetes incidence and prevalence in Pima Indians: a 19-fold greater incidence than in Rochester, Minnesota. *Am J Epidemiol.* 108:497–505, 1978.

31. Kini, M.M., Leibowitz, H.M., Colton, T. et al. Prevalence of senile cataract, diabetic retinopathy, senile macular degeneration, and open-angle glaucoma in the Framingham Eye Study. *Am J Ophthalmol.* 85:28–34, 1978.

32. Caird, E.I. Epidemiology of diabetic retinopathy. Edited by J.R. Lynn, W.B. Snyder, and A. Vaiser. In *Diabetic Retinopathy.* New York: Grune & Stratton, 1974, pp 35–46.

33. Keiding, N.R., Root, H.F., and Marble, A. Importance of control of diabetes in prevention of vascular complications. *JAMA.* 150:964–969, 1953.

34. Caird, F.I. Metabolic control. Edited by J.R. Lynn, W.B. Snyder, and A. Vaiser. In *Diabetic Retinopathy.* New York: Grune & Stratton, 1974, pp 65–70.

35. Job, D., Eschwege, E., Guyot-Argenton, C. et al. Effect of multiple daily insulin injections on the course of diabetic retinopathy. *Diabetes* 25:463–469, 1976.

36. Ashikaga, T., Borodic, G., and Sims, E.A.H. Multiple daily insulin injections in the treatment of diabetic retinopathy. The Job Study Revisited. *Diabetes* 27:592–596, 1977.

37. Eschwege, E., Job, D., Guyot-Argenton, C. et al. Delayed progression of diabetic retinopathy by divided insulin administration: a further follow-up. *Diabetologia* 16:13–15, 1979.

38. Engerman, R. Animal models of diabetic retinopathy. *Trans Acad Ophthalmol Otolaryngol.* 81:710–715, 1976.

39. Prout, T.E. The role of diabetic control in diabetic retinopathy. *Int Ophthal Clin.* 18(4):73–89, 1978.

40. Kwaan, H.C., Colwell, J.A., and Suwanwela, N. Disseminated intravascular coagulation in diabetes mellitus, with reference to the role of increased platelet aggregation. *Diabetes* 21:108–113, 1972.

41. Dobbie, G.J., Kwaan, H.C., Colwell, J.A. et al. The role of platelets in pathogenesis of diabetic retinopathy. *Trans Am Acad Ophthalmol Otolaryngol.* 77:43–47, 1973.

42. Colwell, J.A., Halushka, P.V., Sarji, K. et al. Altered platelet function in diabetes mellitus. *Diabetes* 25:826–831, 1976.

43. Bern, M.M. Platelet functions in diabetes mellitus. *Diabetes* 27:342–350, 1978.

44. Klimt, C.R., Doub, P.H., and Doub, N.H. Clinical trials in thrombosis: secondary prevention of myocardial infarction. *Thromb Haemost.* 35:49–56, 1976.

45. The Canadian Cooperative Study Group. A randomized trial of aspirin and sulfinpyrazone in threatened stroke. *N Engl J Med.* 299:53–59, 1978.

46. Fields, W.S., Lemak, N.A., Frankowski, R.F. et al. Controlled trial of aspirin in cerebral ischemia. *Stroke* 8:301–314, 1977.

47. Aiello, L.M., and Diabetic Retinopathy Study Research Group. Early treatment for diabetic retinopathy study design. *Invest Ophthalmol Vis Sci [Suppl].* 18(4):220–221, 1979.

48. Patz, A., and Lutty, G. Inhibitors of neovascularization in relation to diabetic and other proliferative retinopathies. *Trans Am Ophthalmol Soc.* 76:102–107, 1978.

49. Okisaka, S., and Kuwabara, T. The effects of laser photocoagulation in the retinal capillaries. *Am J Ophthalmol.* 80:591–601, 1975.

50. Bresnick, G.H. Evaluation and treatment of diabetic retinopathy. *JCE Ophthalmol.* 41:15–33, 1979.

51. Marcus, D.F., and Aaberg, T.M. Argon laser photocoagulation treatment of diabetic cystoid maculopathy. *Ann Ophthalmol.* 9:365–372, 1977.

52. Blankenship, G.W. Diabetic macular edema and argon laser photocoagulation: a prospective randomized study. *Ophthalmology* 86:69–75, 1979.

53. Merin, S., Yanko, L., and Ivry, M. Treatment of diabetic maculopathy by argon-laser. *Br J Ophthalmol.* 58:85–91, 1974.

54. Caird, F.I. Diabetic retinopathy as a cause of visual impairment. Edited by M.F. Goldberg, and S.L. Fine. In *Symposium on the Treatment of Diabetic Retinopathy*. Washington, DC: US Public Health Service, publ. no. 1890, 1968, pp 41–46.

55. Patz, A., and Berkow, J.W. Visual prognosis in advanced diabetic retinopathy. Edited by M.F. Goldberg, and S.L. Fine. In *Symposium on the Treatment of Diabetic Retinopathy*. Washington, DC: US Public Health Service, publ. no. 1890, 1968, pp 87–91.

56. Meyer-Schwickerrath, G.R.E., and Schott, M.D. Diabetic retinopathy and photocoagulation. *Am J Ophthalmol.* 66:597–603, 1968.

57. Beetham, W.P., Aiello, L.M., Balodimos, M.C. et al. Ruby laser photocoagulation of early diabetic neovascular retinopathy. *Arch Ophthalmol.* 83:261–272, 1970.

58. L'Esperance, F.A. Argon laser photocoagulation of diabetic retinal neovascularization (a five-year appraisal). *Trans Am Acad Ophthalmol Otolaryngol.* 77:6–23, 1973.

59. Machemer, R. A new concept in vitreous surgery 2. Surgical techniques and complications. *Am J Ophthalmol.* 74:1022–1033, 1972.

60. Kingham, J.D. The current use of vitrectomy instrumentation in ophthalmology. *Ariz Med.* 36:375–377, 1979.

61. Faulborn, J., Conway, B.P., and Machemer, R. Surgical complications of pars plana vitreous surgery. *Ophthalmology* 85:116–125, 1978.

62. Myers, F.L., and Bresnick, G.H. Vitrectomy in diabetic retinopathy. *Trans Am Acad Ophthalmol Otolaryngol.* 81:399–401, 1976.

63. Blankenship, G.W., and Machemer, R. Pars plana vitrectomy for the management of severe diabetic retinopathy: an analysis of results five years following surgery. *Ophthalmology* 85:553–559, 1978.

248

64. Mandelcorn, M.S., Blanksenship, G., and Machemer, R. Pars plana vitrectomy for the management of severe diabetic retinopathy. *Am J Ophthalmol.* 81:561–569, 1976.

65. Kelly, W.F., Anapliotou, M., and Joplin, G.F. Pituitary ablation and its effect on diabetic retinopathy. *Int Ophthalmol Clin.* 18(4):165–178, 1978.

66. Valone, J.A., Jr., and McMeel, J.W. Severe adolescent-onset proliferative diabetic retinopathy. *Arch Ophthalmol.* 96:1349–1353, 1978.

67. Solow, H., Hidalgo, R., and Singal, D.P. Juvenile-onset diabetes: HLA-A, -B, -C, and -DR alloantigens. *Diabetes* 28:1–4, 1979.

68. Rotter, J. I., and Rimoin, D.L. Heterogeneity in diabetes mellitus—update, 1978. *Diabetes* 27:599–608, 1978.

69. Goldstein, S., and Podolsky, S. The genetics of diabetes mellitus. *Med Clin North Am.* 62:639–654, 1978.

70. Faber, O.K., Thomsen, M., Binder, C. et al. HLA antigens in a family with maturity onset diabetes mellitus. *Acta Endocrinol.* 88:329–338, 1978.

71. Christensen, N.J., Hansen, A.P., and Lundbaek, K. Metabolic and hormonal factors in diabetic retinopathy. *Int Ophthalmol Clin.* 18(4):55–72, 1978.

72. Hansen, A.P. Normalization of growth hormone hyper-response to exercise in juvenile diabetes after "normalization" of blood sugar. *J Clin Invest.* 50:1806–1811, 1971.

73. Campbell, J., Hausler, H.R., Munroe, J.S. et al. Effects of growth hormone in dogs. *Endocrinology* 53:134–162, 1953.

74. McMillan, D.E. Deterioration of the microcirculation in diabetes. *J Am Diabetes Assoc.* 24:944–957, 1975.

75. Little, H.L. The role of abnormal hemorrheodynamics in the pathogenesis of diabetic retinopathy. *Trans Am Ophthalmol Soc.* 74:573–636, 1976.

76. McMillan, D.E. Rheological and related factors in diabetic retinopathy. *Int Ophthalmol Clin.* 18(4):35–53, 1978.

77. McMillan, D.E. Plasma protein changes, blood viscosity, and diabetic microangiopathy. *Diabetes* 25:858–864, 1976.

78. Williamson, J.R., and Kilo, C. Basement-membrane thickening and diabetic microangiopathy. *Diabetes* 25:925–927, 1976.

79. Williamson, J.R., and Kilo, C. Current status of capillary basement-membrane disease in diabetes mellitus. *J Am Diabetes Assoc.* 26:65–75, 1977.

80. Williamson, J.R., and Kilo, C. New evidence that controlling hyperglycemia in diabetes is important. *Res Staff Phys.* 4:46–52, 1979.

81. Shabo, A.L., and Maxwell, D.S. Insulin-induced immunogenic retinopathy resembling the retinitis proliferans of diabetes. *Trans Am Acad Ophthalmol Otolaryngol.* 81:497–508, 1976.

82. Feman, S.S., Turinsky, J., and Lam, K.W. The insulin concentration in human ocular fluids. *Am J Ophthalmol.* 85:387–391, 1978.

12 The Neuropathies of Diabetes Mellitus

William A. Sibley, MD

HISTORICAL CONSIDERATIONS

For more than a century physicians have recognized the frequent occurrence of nerve damage in diabetes mellitus. Late in the nineteenth century, there was some confusion clinically between tabes dorsalis and the diffuse symmetrical neuropathy of diabetes. The term diabetic "pseudotabes" was proposed; it still serves to remind us that some diabetics indeed have pains in the limbs, absent tendon reflexes, irregular poorly reactive pupils, and various trophic disturbances including Charcot joints.

Early pathologic reports suggested an ischemic origin for the neuropathy of diabetes. This was, perhaps, inevitable, since the nerves studied usually came from amputated legs, and shared in the general ischemia of the limb.[1] More detailed pathologic studies have been made in recent years, however. These, and the results of cutaneous nerve biopsies, have made it abundantly clear that a distal symmetrical neuropathy is common in diabetes and quite independent of occlusive arterial disease; indeed, it seems rather to be related to the metabolic defect, correlating best with long-term hyperglycemia.

During the past two decades, also, opportunities have arisen permitting pathologists to examine the nerves of patients with cranial mononeuropathies, limb mononeuropathies, and mononeuritis multiplex. These latter neuropathies, the clinical signs of which are usually reversible, appear to be due to microinfarcts in nerve trunks secondary to diabetic microangiopathy.

SCOPE OF THE PROBLEM AND CLASSIFICATION

Most patients who have had diabetes for more than a few years have some evidence of peripheral neuropathy.[2-4] Fortunately, in the vast majority, this nearly universal neuropathy is an asymptomatic "background" phenomenon; commonly, for example it consists only of absent Achilles reflexes and decreased vibratory perception in the toes. In still another group of diabetics, especially in the early years of the illness, evidence of neuropathy can be found only by electrodiagnostic tests. With the latter, the frequency of diagnosis of peripheral nerve involvement varies with the sensitivity of the methods used. Thus motor nerve conduction velocities are definitely abnormal in approximately 40% of unselected diabetic patients[4,5] while sural nerve sensory latency measurements are prolonged in 84% of randomly selected subjects.[4]

Bruyn and Garland[6] reviewed the extensive literature on the frequency of symptomatic neuropathy in diabetes and found that clinically significant symptomatic neuropathy occurs at some time in about 6% of patients. This may take several forms (Table 12-1), the most common of which is a diffuse symmetrical distal neuropathy, comprising about 70% of cases; the remainder of cases are manifest clinically as mononeuropathies or as mononeuritis multiplex.[5]

DIABETIC METABOLIC NEUROPATHY

As already noted the most common form of neuropathy is a chronic, chiefly sensory, symmetrical distal disorder. Occasionally it is associated with an unusually prominent autonomic neuropathy that can give rise to disturbing cardiovascular, gastrointestinal, or genitourinary symptoms. Trophic changes affecting skin, hair, muscle, ligaments, and joints occur in severe cases.

The chronic symptomatic form of this illness can be thought of as an advanced example of the background neuropathy that occurs in

Table 12-1
Classification of Diabetic Neuropathies

Metabolic neuropathy
(distal, symmetrical, chiefly sensory; autonomic features)
  Acute symptomatic
    During periods of grossly poor diabetic control
    Following correction of diabetic acidosis (?)
  Chronic
    Asymptomatic—most patients
    Symptomatic—approximately 4% of patients

Ischemic and compression neuropathies
(mononeuritis or mononeuritis multiplex)
  Nerve infarction syndromes
    Large nerve trunks—especially femoral, peroneal nerves
    Radiculopathy—any nerve root, but most commonly L3, L4
    Cranial neuropathies—especially abducens and oculomotor nerve palsies
  Nerve compression syndromes—nerves more vulnerable to trauma because
    of metabolic neuropathy (above)

---

most patients. However, a small number of acute symmetrical distal neuropathies have been described.

Acute Symmetrical Distal Neuropathies

True instances of the acute or subacute onset of distal symmetrical neuropathy are, we believe, unusual. Most acute widespread neuropathies in the legs of diabetics, in our experience, are asymmetrical and actually examples of mononeuritis multiplex (see below). A number of acute symmetrical cases were described by Rundles,[7] however, almost always in patients who had experienced recent rapid, severe weight loss; 75% of his cases had lost more than 20 lbs just before the onset of neuropathy. The outlook for recovery, with institution of adequate diabetic treatment, is good in such cases. Most patients improve within several weeks or a few months.

Even less common, in our experience, has been the paradoxical occurrence of acute distal neuropathy *after* institution of proper control with insulin. We have seen only one instance of this phenomenon in 25 years of neurologic practice, and it is seldom mentioned in the modern literature about diabetic neuropathy. Nonetheless, Rundles[7] saw the onset of neuropathy, usually about two weeks after beginning insulin, in 16% of his 125 cases. Ellenberg[8] described three patients who had onset of neuropathy shortly after starting tolbutamide therapy. One of the latter patients had a distal symmetrical neuropathy, one had mononeuritis multiplex, and the other had an acute oculomotor nerve palsy. It is difficult to be certain whether such unusual instances represent a cause-and-effect relationship or mere coincidence.

Chronic Symmetrical Distal Neuropathies

As already noted most diabetics develop a subtle asymptomatic distal neuropathy. However, in about 4% of patients this progresses and produces symptoms of pain and cramping in the feet, toes, and legs. The pain is characteristically of a burning quality, usually worse when the patient is resting and unoccupied, especially at night. Loss of sleep and depression frequently accompany this syndrome.

In severe cases the symptoms ascend to the level of the knees, at which time involvement of the hands with similar symptoms may begin. Variable degrees of motor weakness, also worse distally, occur in these severe cases. The weakness usually appears first and most prominently in the muscles that dorsiflex the feet and toes.

Physical findings, of course, depend on the severity of the disorder, but loss of Achilles reflexes and decreased or absent vibratory sense in the toes and feet are almost universal. Sensory loss to touch and pain stimuli occurs in a short-sock or long-stocking distribution, depending somewhat on the severity of the neuropathy but also on the strength of the stimulus. A light painful stimulus, for example, usually results in the finding of a larger area of sensory loss than a more strongly applied one. The ends of the nerves in the extremities become tender and easily irritated; thus the soles may become tender to pressure, and in severe cases, the palms. Tenderness may also be found on compressing the calf, and in palpating in the area of major nerve trunks. This tenderness of distal nerves may lead to exacerbation of pain with vigorous exercise in some patients.

Gait abnormalities are present in proportion to the degree of weakness or loss of position sense imposed by the neuropathy. Loss of position sense in the toes of one foot seldom produces ataxia, but when position sense is lost bilaterally, some degree of unsteadiness is common. When weakness is marked, a "steppage" gait develops in which the knee is lifted unusually high so that the tip of the shoe can clear the floor. A "slapping" type of gait may be noted either with moderate weakness of dorsiflexion of the feet, or when position sense is badly impaired.

Examination of cranial nerves is usually unremarkable in patients with this form of diabetic neuropathy, with the important exception of pupillary abnormalities. Normally the pupil decreases in size with advancing age. This occurs sooner in diabetics, who also have less hippus (rapid fluctuation in pupil size during constant illumination) than do normal subjects.[9] Smith et al[9] found some pupillary abnormality in almost all diabetics with neuropathy, but alterations in shape and light reaction occur less commonly—probably in about 25%.[7] We agree with Martin[10] that a true Argyll Robertson pupil (small, no light reaction, intact accommodation reaction, poor dilatation with atropine) is rare.

Autonomic Neuropathy

Usually evidence of autonomic neuropathy is associated with other evidence of the typical metabolic neuropathy of diabetes[7,10-12]; most reports indicate that it is usually asymptomatic. On the other hand, autonomic symptoms may occur rarely without other neuropathic symptoms.[13]

The cardiovascular system is frequently involved; Page and Watkins[12] describe 12 instances of cardiorespiratory arrest in young diabetics with autonomic neuropathy. Several of these occurred after anesthesia. A high death rate in autonomic neuropathy has been recorded by Ewing et al,[14] and some have speculated that at least part of this excess mortality can be attributed to a higher incidence of painless myocardial infarction in diabetics.[15] Faerman et al[15] found pathologic evidence of damage to autonomic nerve endings in the myocardium of five patients dying of painless infarction. Presumably some of these nerves were pain-conducting sympathetic afferent fibers.

Evidence of progressive vagal denervation of the heart can be obtained by studying the beat-to-beat variations in the length of electrocardiographic R-R intervals. These are quite marked in normals, but show little variation in advanced autonomic neuropathy, either in the resting state, or in response to standing, respiration, or the Valsalva maneuver.[16-18] Ewing et al[19] have described a simple test for cardiac autonomic neuropathy, based on their finding that tachycardia is normally maximal in response to simple standing at about the 15th beat, and bradycardia maximal at the 30th beat. If the ratio of the R-R interval at beat 30 to the R-R interval at beat 15 is 1.0 or less, they believe that a diagnosis of cardiac autonomic neuropathy can be made.

Postural hypotension may complicate most peripheral neuropathies, and is occasionally seen in relatively advanced cases due to diabetes. Symptoms include dizziness, drowsiness, and mental confusion, as well as actual syncope. Usually these symptoms do not occur unless the standing systolic blood pressure drops below 85 mm Hg. At levels higher than this, autoregulation of cerebral blood flow is apparently adequate to maintain normal flow in most patients. Full thigh length elastic hose, or an elastic leotard, may be sufficient to prevent abnormal pooling of blood in the legs in mild cases. However, often one must combine these measures with fludrocortisone (Florinef) 0.1 to 0.2 mg daily, or every other day. A responsible family member should be taught to measure supine and standing blood pressures accurately at least twice daily to ensure both that the standing blood pressure remains above the critical level, and that the supine blood pressure does not rise too high. If during this regimen, the standing blood pressure falls below 90 mm Hg extra salt may be added either as salt tablets or in the form of a well-salted bullion once or twice daily. We usually have found such methods to be adequate, as have others.[20,21] In the presence of incipient congestive heart failure, of course, salt-retaining drugs and salt loading should not be used because of the danger of precipitating pulmonary edema. Such unfortunate patients, if not helped by compressive stocking, have few alternatives, except to avoid standing. Symptoms seldom occur while seated. The sitting blood pressure is usually intermediate between supine and standing levels.

Gastrointestinal tract   Evidence of damage to the autonomic nerve supply to the gastrointestinal tract, is manifest in a few patients by delayed gastric emptying, with symptoms of nausea, vomiting, anorexia, and abdominal pain.[22] A new drug, metoclopramide (Reglan) not yet approved for use in the United States, is very effective in correcting this defect in gastric motility.[11,23]

Recurrent diarrhea, often nocturnal, was present in 27 of the 125 cases of neuropathy in Rundles' study.[7] Malins and French[24] described 28 patients with diabetic diarrhea, nocturnal in 10. All patients were poorly controlled diabetics. These authors felt that an altered transit time through the intestine and colon was responsible, but the mechanism is not certain. They found a tetracycline effective in treatment. Sumi and Finlay[25] also found antibiotics effective, and thought there might be abnormal bacterial growth in the small bowel due to decreased gastric acid secretion.

Genitourinary system   Damage to the autonomic innervation of the genitourinary system is common in diabetes. One of the most comprehensive studies is that of Frimodt-Moller[26] who did complete cystometric examinations on 124 diabetic patients who did not have bladder symptoms. Some abnormality was found in 44%. Decreased bladder sensation seems to be the primary defect, which leads, as the condition progresses, to increasing distention of the bladder. Finally, when the bladder detrusor muscle becomes critically overstretched, full voiding is no longer possible, and there is an ever-increasing volume of residual urine. This leads to frequent bladder infection. Treatment is best accomplished by teaching the patient to adhere to a regular schedule of clean nonsterile self-catheterization to prevent collection of residual urine and overdistention of the bladder wall. After a time, it may be possible to stimulate natural voiding with bethanechol 20 mg three or four times daily, combined with deep suprapubic pressure over the bladder area during the act of voiding. Periodic determination of residual urine volume should be done to determine the success of this regimen. One should be cautious about attributing urinary retention to diabetes alone, however, in patients over the age of 40 years; Frimodt-Moller[26] found 40% of such patients also had some element of obstructive uropathy, often from an enlarged prostate gland.

Sexual impotence is said to be common in diabetic men but, as in most neurologic disorders, its true incidence is difficult to determine.[27,28] Only a few studies have been concerned with sexual dysfunction in diabetic women.[29,30] Impotence should be considered to be psychogenic in men who have normal nocturnal penile erections.[31,32]

Trophic Changes

Most textbooks state that neurotrophic ulcers on the soles of the feet, and Charcot joints in the diabetic foot are chiefly due to abnormal wear and tear secondary to defective pain sensation. It is probable, however, that this view is too narrow, and represents an oversimplification. Abundant evidence exists that chemical trophic substances pass down axons by a process of axoplasmic flow. These substances seem necessary to maintain the integrity of postsynaptic cells such as muscles, skin, ligaments, bones, and joints.[33,34]

In severe diabetic symmetrical neuropathies the skin becomes thin and shiny, with an absence of hair growth, over the distal portion of the limbs. Pastan and Cohen[35] have observed roentgenographically demonstrated lysis of the distal phalanx in the feet of diabetic patients, with subsequent restoration of normal bone architecture several months later. This condition, referred to as diabetic osteopathy or osteolysis, is of unknown cause, and is said to occur in some diabetics without overt neuropathy. However, since the condition usually occurs in the distal foot, a fluctuating supply of trophic chemicals secondary to the latent or symptomatic metabolic neuropathy of diabetes, is an attractive possibility. However, a variety of other explanations have also been offered.[36,37]

Other conditions that would seem to be candidates as trophic disturbances are frozen shoulder and ankylosing hyperostosis of the spine, both of which occur with significantly greater frequency in diabetics.[38-41] At the moment, one must emphasize, however, that there is no definite proof that these conditions are related to diabetic neuropathy.

The incidence of a traditionally accepted neurotrophic disturbance in diabetes—the Charcot joint in the foot—is quite low, 0.16% in one large series.[42] The patient's chief complaint is usually that of a swollen foot, often developing rather abruptly after minor trauma.[43] The sudden onset of symptoms of neuropathic joints, commonly, was also emphasized by Charcot in tabes dorsalis.[44] The location of a neurotrophic joint in the foot is highly characteristic of the neuropathy of diabetes, as originally described by Jordan.[45]

In addition to swelling, examination usually discloses loss of the normal arch with a "rocker bottom" effect, abnormal laxity of the ligaments of the foot, and crepitus on palpation. Ellenberg[46] has likened this to a "bag of bones."

Most commonly the tarsometatarsal joints are severaly affected with lysis, fragmentation, and proliferative changes. The second tarsometatarsal joint may be the site of a fracture-dislocation (Lisfranc fracture), often with only minor trauma, before the fully developed condition is recognized.[47] The mechanical factors leading to greatest damage to these joints have been studied and described in detail by Lippmann et al.[48] A molded "atraumatic" boot has been advocated as the most suitable treatment for Charcot joints of the foot by Singleton et al.[49]

Pathophysiology of the Metabolic Neuropathy of Diabetes

On theoretical grounds the symmetry of this disorder suggests a metabolic cause. Its onset distally almost certainly represents a metabolic insult to the neuron, and that part of the cell at greatest distance from the cell body suffers first and most severely. One can speculate that its onset distally must be due to defective axoplasmic transport of proteins, transmitters, and other important substances to the periphery. It is of interest that in streptozotocin-induced diabetes in rats, defective axoplasmic transport of choline acetylase and acetylcholine esterase has been demonstrated.[50]

Clinical evidence, too, favors the concept that this form of neuropathy is related to a metabolic defect. Its occurrence correlates best with poor diabetic control, especially prolonged hyperglycemia.[7,51-53] The severity of diabetes does not seem to be an important factor, since the illness occurs in both juvenile-onset (insulin-dependent) diabetics, as well as in adult-onset (insulin- and ketoacidosis-resistant) patients. Motor nerve conduction velocities are faster in well-controlled young diabetics than in those poorly controlled,[53] and improvement in nerve conduction velocities occurs in recently diagnosed human diabetics with treatment.[54]

The mechanism whereby prolonged hyperglycemia might produce nerve damage is less certain, but has been the subject of much study and speculation. Some evidence exists that abnormal capillary leakage due to microangiopathy can be lessened or prevented by strict control of blood glucose levels.[55,56]

It should be recalled, at this point, that the endoneurial fluid within each nerve fascicle is confined by concentric layers of perineurial cells. The capillaries in the endoneurial space have endothelial tight junctions similar to those in the central nervous system. These constitute the blood-nerve barrier[57] and this barrier has been shown to break down in experimental diabetes.[58]

Asbury and Johnson[59] have proposed the possibility that a kind of toxic edema in the endoneurial space may result in axonal damage. This idea is consistent with the finding of endoneurial edema and axonal atrophy as the earliest changes in experimental diabetes.[60,61] More recently Johnson et al[62] emphasized that the most prominent electron microscopic abnormality in human diabetic neuropathy is a thickening of the basement membrane of the perineurial cell (Figure 12-1). The postulated filtration function of these cells, impaired by such thickening, might allow the accumulation of toxic substances within the nerve fascicle causing axonal damage.

Another attractive hypothesis to explain nerve dysfunction in diabetics, relates the damage to the accumulation of sorbitol and fructose in the nerves. Only a small portion of glucose is normally converted into these substances, but the fraction increases in proportion to the degree of hyperglycemia.[63] Winegrad and Greene[64] emphasized a deficiency in myoinositol concentration in the nerves in experimental diabetes, and reported one experiment in which myoinositol feeding seemed to improve nerve conduction velocities. Myoinositol levels are reduced in the cerebrospinal fluid of patients with diabetic polyneuropathy.[65] Unfortunately, however, myoinositol supplementation of the diet of diabetic patients has not been beneficial in two recently reported studies.[66,67]

The principal pathologic change in this form of neuropathy appears to be distal axonal degeneration. Hansen and Ballantyne[68] found this on the basis of quantitative electromyography (EMG) studies in 40 diabetic patients. As motor axons slowly decrease in number, there is apparently extensive collateral sprouting of the residual intact axons, with reinnervation of the orphaned muscle fibers. This process apparently limits the extent of the motor deficit, and makes the clinical neuropathy appear to be chiefly sensory. Behse et al[69] also noted quantitative EMG changes in clinically normal muscles. By sural nerve biopsy they found axonal degeneration involving both myelinated and unmyelinated fibers in all of 12 patients with neuropathy. Segmental demyelination also occurs in diabetics[70] but it is possibly secondary to axonal distress as is uremia.[71]

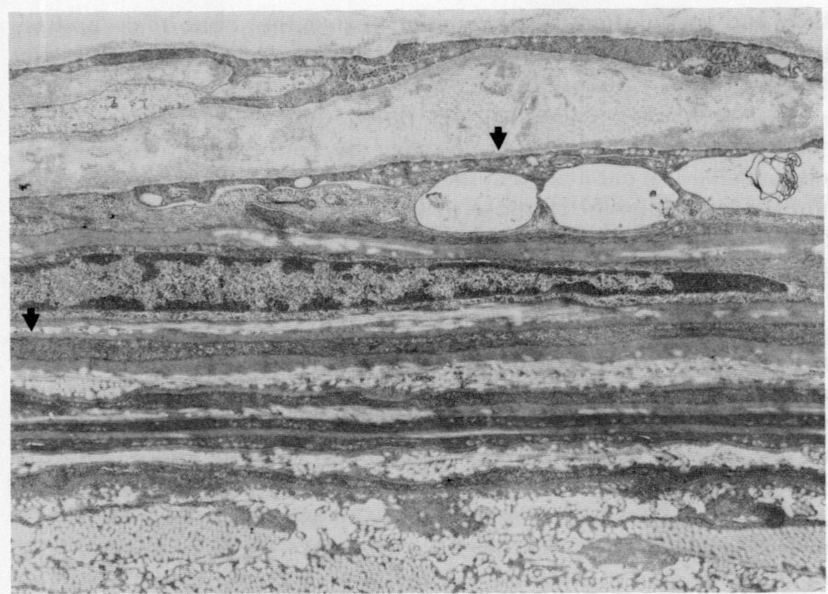

A

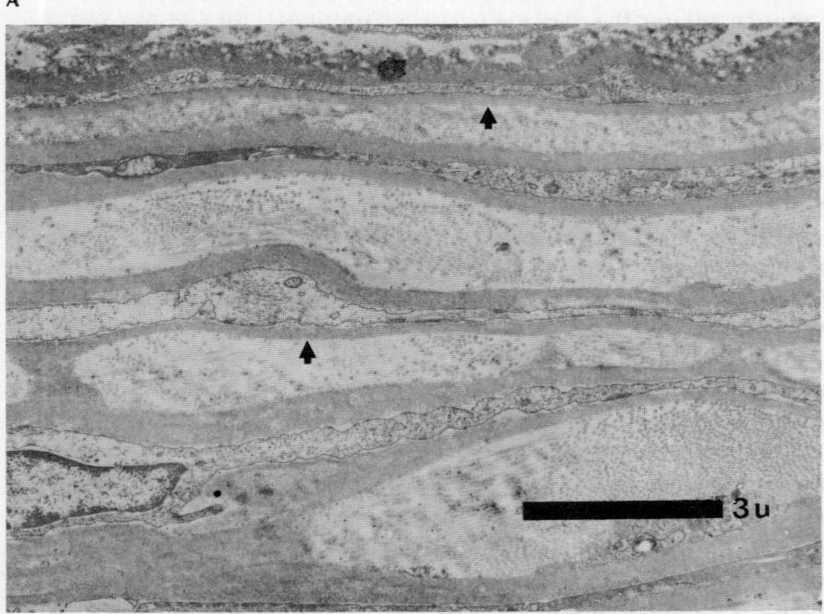

B

Figure 12-1 Electron microscopic view of concentric layers of perineurial cells **A** in a normal sural nerve and **B** in a sural nerve of a patient with diabetic neuropathy. The arrows point to the basement membranes of these cells. Note the abnormal thickening of the basement membrane in diabetic distal neuropathy. (Courtesy of Dr. P.C. Johnson.)

The concept that axonal atrophy, and eventual loss, is the primary pathology in the distal symmetrical neuropathy of diabetes has received support from the studies of Jakobsen[60] in experimental diabetes in animals.

ISCHEMIC AND COMPRESSION NEUROPATHIES— MONONEURITIS AND MONONEURITIS MULTIPLEX

As already noted, about 2% of diabetics at some time develop either a mononeuritis or mononeuritis multiplex. Most of these patients are maturity-onset, insulin-resistant diabetics; most are over 40 years of age; and many have normal fasting blood sugars (FBS). The FBS was normal in 16 of 25 patients described by Sullivan,[72] although the glucose tolerance test was very abnormal in these same patients.

In these neuropathies one or more major nerve trunks, or nerve roots, are involved. This results in an asymmetrical neurologic deficit, since the distribution of weakness, sensory loss, and reflex change depends upon the anatomic distribution of the nerves or roots affected. Weakness and muscle atrophy are usually more prominent than sensory loss. This is all in sharp contrast to the diffuse symmetrical, chiefly distal, neuropathy discussed previously.

Mononeuritis and mononeuritis multiplex are apparently most commonly the result of ischemic changes in the nerves. Collier[73] speculated that these acute chiefly motor neuropathies and radiculopathies of diabetes were probably due to nerve infarction, because of their sudden onset, and the marked tendency toward improvement. Only in recent years, however, did opportunities arise to confirm this hypothesis. Raff and Asbury[74] found myriads of scattered microinfarcts in the major nerve trunks in the legs of a patient with mononeuritis multiplex. The distribution of the lesions was appropriate to explain the patient's clinical deficit during life. Similar lesions, attributed to microangiopathy, have been described in affected cranial nerves.[75,76]

Almost any nerve trunk or nerve root may be involved, but the most common mononeuropathies involve the femoral, peroneal, oculomotor, abducens, facial, median, or ulnar nerves. The lower lumbar nerve roots are also frequently affected resulting in sciatica and neurologic changes that may simulate a herniated nucleus pulposus in the lumbosacral spine.

Femoral Neuropathy

This most common of the diabetic mononeuropathies usually is

260

manifest initially by the abrupt or subacute onset of aching pain in the hip and anterior thigh, with dysesthesias in the anterior thigh and medial aspect of the lower leg. This is accompanied almost immediately by weakness in the quadriceps muscle, resulting in buckling of the affected leg while standing or walking. Examination at that time usually discloses an absent or greatly reduced patellar reflex, and weakness of either the quadriceps muscle, or combined quadriceps and iliopsoas muscle weakness. Typically, over a period of weeks, the pain subsides, but the atrophy and weakness of the thigh recover only after many more months.

Mulder et al found mild cases of femoral neuropathy, which cause few symptoms.[5] These authors also believed that many of the cases conforming, in general, to the syndrome of acute femoral neuropathy were actually due to, or associated with, signs of involvement of the lumbar plexus or lumbar nerve roots.

Mononeuritis Multiplex

In some cases, patients may have multiple nerve trunks or nerve roots involved, in a successive manner, over a circumscribed period of time—often several weeks or months. For example, a new right femoral nerve syndrome may appear, just as improvement is beginning from a left femoral insult. In the same patient, over the next few weeks or months, there may be successive involvement of obturator, peroneal, or sciatic nerves on one or both sides. The resulting deficit is often severe and some patients may be largely bedridden for months. Usually the disability is chiefly motor, with much muscle atrophy that tends to be mostly proximal, although there are many exceptions. Pain is prominent and may occur in the low back as well as in the hip and thigh.

This syndrome was called diabetic myelopathy by Garland and Taverner,[77] however, there has been no convincing demonstration of spinal cord pathology. The later term "diabetic amyotrophy"[73] recognized the principal feature of the illness—muscle weakness and wasting—but is seldom used now. Both electric and pathologic studies indicate that the site of pathology is in the peripheral nerves.[74,79]

The reason why proximal nerves in the legs are more seriously affected is unknown. Mayer[80] suggested the term "subacute proximal diabetic neuropathy"; he and others[79] described patients who, because of the progressive nature of their proximal deficit, were suspected of having a metabolic cause for their neuropathy. We have not seen true slow progression; in our experience close observation usually reveals that worsening in this syndrome occurs in a stepwise fashion, although the increments of new deficit may be multiple and small. This method of progression is still compatible with recurring ischemic events in the nerves. There is, as yet, no pathologic evidence of a symmetrical nonischemic proximal neuropathy in diabetes.

Despite the severe incapacity and striking physical findings the many patients with mononeuritis multiplex manifest, the prognosis is good. Most patients recover after a long illness lasting 12 to 18 months or more. A number of authors note that improvement is coincident with more careful control of the underlying diabetes, especially hyperglycemia.[77,79,80] The mechanisms responsible for recovery have not been clarified; however, it seems necessary to postulate at least partial improvement in the microangiopathy in the nerves, to explain the virtually complete improvement seen in many cases.

Radiculopathy

Subacute or acute involvement of one or two nerve roots in an isolated fashion is not infrequent. The pain in such cases may simulate, in many ways, that seen with a herniated nucleus pulposus, in either the cervical or lumbosacral areas.[72,81] When a thoracic root is affected the pain may be similar to that encountered commonly in the pre-eruptive phase of herpes zoster. Back pain may be associated with these root syndromes. Clinical features that help in diagnosis are the more marked mechanical signs associated with disc disease, especially more paraspinous muscle spasm. Also, patients with disc herniations usually experience at least some relief of pain within 24 to 48 hours after beginning strict bedrest. As noted previously, by contrast, patients with diabetic neuropathy often have more pain during inactivity, especially during the night. In many cases, however, myelography is necessary to make a correct diagnosis.

Oculomotor Nerve Palsy

The third cranial nerve is a common target in diabetic neuropathy. The clinical syndrome is rather stereotyped; there is pain in and about the affected eye, followed rapidly by complete ptosis and paralysis of all of the extraocular muscles on the affected side except the external rectus and superior oblique. The pupillary light and accommodation reaction is spared in 77% to 85% of cases[82,83]; this is in contrast to the occurrence of a fixed dilated pupil in 90% of oculomotor palsies associated with congenital aneurysm and in virtually all cases due to tumor.[82] Approximately 25% of isolated oculomotor palsies are due to diabetic neuropathy,[84] about 20% are secondary to an intracranial aneurysm,[83] tumor and trauma account for about 10% and 15% respectively, and 20% to 23% remain of unknown cause after careful study.[84,85]

If the typical syndrome with pupillary sparing, and an intact corneal reflex, occurs in a diabetic patient without other neurologic symptoms or signs, extensive investigation is seldom warranted. The pain usually subsides in a few days and full recovery is the rule within eight to ten weeks. On the other hand, if the pupil is fixed and dilated, a diabetic patient with oculomotor palsy should have a full investigation to exclude other causes. If oculomotor palsy is associated with proptosis of the affected eye, orbital mucormycosis should be suspected.

Abducens Nerve Palsy

About 15% of isolated sixth-cranial-nerve palsies are secondary to diabetic neuropathy.[86] The syndrome is that of a sudden onset of a painless external rectus palsy. There is failure of ability to abduct the affected eye beyond the midline, associated with diplopia with maximal lateral displacement of images on looking toward the affected side. Other causes of an isolated abducens palsy, such as increased intracranial pressure, and multiple sclerosis must be excluded by history and associated neurologic signs. In most cases computerized tomography of the head should be done to exclude cerebral tumor.

As in oculomotor nerve palsy, the prognosis in diabetic sixth-nerve paralysis is excellent. Full recovery usually occurs in one to two months.

Facial Nerve Palsy

The seventh cranial nerve is rather frequently involved in diabetics. Although no pathologic studies are available, microinfarction of nerve must be suspected. The syndrome in diabetics is indistinguishable from ordinary Bell palsy—abrupt onset of weakness of the entire face on one side with inability to close the eye, or at least difficulty in closing the eye completely. Pain in the general region of the mastoid process on the affected side is common for the first few days of illness. Hyperacusis and loss of taste on the ipsilateral anterior two thirds of the tongue may be associated signs.

Lundgren et al[87] found that about 12% of their patients with Bell palsy had diabetes, a figure almost identical to that reported by Adour.[88] When one considers that most large surveys indicate the prevalence of diabetes in the general population to be 1.2% to 1.7%,[89,90] the increased susceptibility of diabetics to facial nerve paralysis is apparent. Diabetics with facial paralysis had a higher mean age (64 years) in comparison to all patients with Bell palsy (45 years) in the series of Lundgren et al.[87]

Nerve Compression Syndromes

The latent generalized neuropathy in most patients with diabetes renders the nerve trunks more susceptible to trauma in the form of compression and traction.[5,91] In the series of Mulder et al, among 16 patients with mononeuropathy thought to be due to compression, the peroneal nerve was involved at the fibular head in 13, the median nerve in the carpal tunnel in 9, and the ulnar nerve at the elbow in 5.

Compressive palsies of the peroneal nerve tend to occur with repetitive leg crossing, prolonged squatting, or when the nerve is compressed between the mattress and fibular head during prolonged bedrest in the supine position.

The frequency of diabetes in various reported series of carpal tunnel syndrome varies from 5% to 16%,[35] again a significantly higher rate than would be anticipated from the population prevalence of diabetes. The typical syndrome consists of pain in the hand, usually awakening the patient at night, with symptoms of pain and sensory dysesthesias in a median nerve distribution in the hand accentuated by full flexion of the wrist.[92] Weakness of the opponens and abductor pollicis brevis is present in moderately advanced cases, with atrophy of the thenar eminence in late stages. Immediate relief of pain and sensory symptoms is usually obtained by section of the transverse carpal ligament. If atrophy has not been present for more than a year, it, too, usually improves. One should be cautious about making the diagnosis of the carpal tunnel syndrome chiefly on the basis of delayed conduction velocities across the carpal tunnel in diabetic patients, since these are often delayed in asymptomatic patients also.

The ulnar nerve may be affected by repetitive minor trauma at the elbow, usually from habitually resting the elbow on a hard surface such as a table top, arm of a chair, or automobile window ledge. If the patient cannot voluntarily control such trauma, transposition of the ulnar nerve from the ulnar groove to the antecubital fossa may be necessary. With proper patient instruction about prophylaxis, and the wearing of foam rubber pads about the elbow in some cases, surgical transposition is seldom necessary in our experience.

DIAGNOSIS

Many of the syndromes described here are quite distinctive, and when they occur in a known diabetic offer little problem in differential diagnosis. However, it should be remembered that mononeuritis and mononeuritis multiplex may also occur with various other diseases of blood vessels, such as periarteritis nodosa and allergic vasculitis.

A distal symmetrical neuropathy can also occur in nutritional deficiency states, chronic alcoholism, and with exposure to various industrial solvents. Poisoning by arsenic, thallium, gold, or mercury can also cause this type of neuropathy. Certain medications, such as nitrofuran drugs (Furadantin, Macrodantin), isonicotinic acid hydrazide, hydralazine, vincristine, and disulfiram (Antabuse) may also produce a similar problem.[93] The cerebrospinal fluid (CSF) protein is more likely to be elevated, however, in diabetic neuropathy than in most of these toxic neuropathies. Fifty-eight percent of patients with diabetic neuropathy have a spinal fluid (CSF) protein content of greater than 70 mg/100 ml and 14% have protein values higher than 120 mg/100 ml.[5] The occurrence of an elevated CSF protein in neuropathy indicates involvement of nerve roots, which is common not only in diabetics but also in acute idiopathic polyneuritis (Guillain-Barré syndrome), chronic relapsing polyneuritis, amyloid polyneuropathy, and diphtheritic nerve disease. Increased CSF white-blood-cell counts occur in acute herpes zoster, especially when cranial nerves are involved, and a slight lymphocytic pleocytosis is also common in Guillain-Barré syndrome. The CSF cell count is normal in diabetic neuropathy.

The Guillain-Barré syndrome may occur in diabetics as well as others. It is distinguished from diabetic neuropathy by being an almost exclusively motor disorder symmetrically affecting both arms and legs, and often associated with facial diplegia. Paresthesias are common in the fingers and toes but sensory findings on neurologic examination are meager. Nerve conduction velocities are characteristically much slower in this demyelinating neuropathy than in the neuropathies of diabetes.

The physician should be especially cautious about making a diagnosis of diabetic neuritis when the two-hour postprandial blood sugar is only slightly elevated (eg, 120 to 160 mg/100 ml). Most cases of diabetic neuropathy occur in patients who either have overt diabetes or more markedly abnormal glucose tolerance tests.

GENERAL MANAGEMENT AND
PROGNOSIS IN DIABETIC NEUROPATHIES

The management of certain specific syndromes has already been discussed in some of the foregoing sections. One of the most difficult symptoms to treat in these neuropathies, however, is pain. Some have had good success using phenytoin,[94] or carbamazepine,[95] but in our experience and that of others[96] anticonvulsant drugs have been disappointing. Davis [97] has suggested a combination of amitriptyline and fluphenazine. The former drug will often ensure a full night's sleep. This and the drug's intrinsic mode of action help lessen the depression often associated with chronic pain. In many cases the judicious use of aspirin and codeine is as appropriate as any other treatment. Thorsteinsson et al[98] have found transcutaneous electrical nerve stimulation useful in pain control.

The prognosis in cases of diabetic neuropathy depends on several factors. In general those neuropathies, which develop acutely or subacutely, have a good outlook, and usually recover in a few months or one to two years. On the other hand, the distal symmetrical neuropathy that evolves slowly over a period of years, usually does not show spontaneous improvement; neither do those distal neuropathies that are associated with severe obliterative arterial disease in the legs.

As noted previously there is much evidence to suggest that tight control of hyperglycemia probably retards or prevents the appearance of the distal symmetrical neuropathy of diabetes. There is some indication that the microangiopathy in diabetic nerves may also be retarded or reversed by proper control of blood glucose levels. Such control usually requires the use of insulin. Tchobroutsky[99] suggests the use of multiple daily insulin injections as the most effective means of controlling hyperglycemia and its complications. One may reasonably expect that such techniques, and other new developments in insulin administration may, in time, prevent or greatly reduce the incidence of diabetic neuropathy.

REFERENCES

1. Woltman, H.W., and Wilder, R.M. Diabetes mellitus. Pathological changes in the spinal cord and peripheral nerves. *Arch Intern Med.* 44:476–603, 1929.

2. Collins, W.S., Zilensky, J.D., and Boas, L.C. Impaired vibratory sense in diabetes. *Am J Med.* 1:638–641, 1946.

3. Mirsky, I.A. Carbohydrate metabolism and diseases of the nervous system. *Assoc Res Nerv Ment Dis Proc.* 32:328–344, 1953.

4. Braddom, R.L., Hollis, J.B., and Castell, D.O. Diabetic peripheral neuropathy: a correlation of nerve conduction studies and clinical findings. *Arch Phys Med Rehabil.* 58:308–313, 1977.

5. Mulder, D.W., Lambert, E.H., Bastron, J.A. et al. The neuropathies associated with diabetes mellitus. A clinical and electromyographic study of 103 unselected diabetic patients. *Neurology* 11:275–284, 1961.

6. Bruyn, G.W., and Garland, H. Neuropathies of endocrine origin. Edited by P.J. Vinken, and G.W. Bruyn. In *Diseases of Nerves, Part II. Handbook of Clinical Neurology.* Vol. 8. New York: Elsevier North-Holland, 1970, pp 29–71.

7. Rundles, R.W. Diabetic neuropathy: general review with report of 125 cases. *Medicine* 24:111–160, 1945.

8. Ellenberg, M. Diabetic neuropathy precipitating after institution of diabetic control. *Am J Med Sci.* 236:446–471, 1958.

9. Smith, S.E., Smith, S.A., Brown, P.M. et al. Pupillary signs in diabetic autonomic neuropathy. *Br Med J.* 2(6142):924–927, 1978.

10. Martin, M.M. Diabetic neuropathy. A clinical study of 150 cases. *Brain* 76:594–624, 1953.

11. Campbell, I.W., Heading, R.C., Tothill, P. et al. Gastric emptying in diabetic neuropathy. *Gut* 18:462–467, 1977.

12. Page, M.M., and Watkins, P.J. Cardiorespiratory arrest and diabetic autonomic neuropathy. *Lancet* 1:14–16, 1978.

13. Martin, M.M. Involvement of autonomic nerve fibres in diabetic neuropathy. *Lancet* 1:560–563, 1953.

14. Ewing, D.J., Campbell, I.W., and Clarke, B.F. Mortality in diabetic autonomic neuropathy. *Lancet* 1:601, 1976

15. Faerman, I., Faccio, E., Milei, J. et al. Autonomic neuropathy and painless myocardial infarction in diabetic patients. Histological evidence of their relationship. *Diabetes* 26:1147–1158, 1977.

16. Gundersen, H.J.G., and Neubauer, B. A long-term diabetic autonomic nervous abnormality. *Diabetologia* 13:137–140, 1977.

17. Murray, A., Ewing, D.J., Campbell, I.W. et al. RR interval variations in young male diabetics. *Br Heart J.* 37:882–885, 1975.

18. Sharpey-Schafer, E.P. Absent circulatory reflexes in diabetic neuritis. *Lancet* 1:559–562, 1960.

19. Ewing, D.J., Campbell, I.W., Murray, A. et al. Immediate heart-rate response to standing: simple test for autonomic neuropathy in diabetes. *Br Med J.* 1:145–147, 1978.

20. Campbell, I.W., Ewing, D.J., and Clarke, B.F. Therapeutic experience with fludrocortisone in diabetic postural hypotension. *Br Med J.* 1:872–874, 1976.

21. Bannister, R., Ardill, L., and Fentem, P. An assessment of various methods of treatment of idiopathic orthostatic hypotension. *Q J Med.* 38:337–395, 1969.

22. Gramm, H.F., Reuter, K., and Costello, P. The radiological manifestations of diabetic gastric neuropathy and its differential diagnosis. *Gastrointest Radiol.* 3:151–153, 1978.

23. Brady, P.G., and Richardson, R. Gastric bezoar formation secondary to gastroparesis diabeticorum. *Arch Intern Med.* 137:1729, 1977.

24. Malins, J.M., and French, J.M. Diabetic diarrhea. *Am J Med.* 22:467–480, 1957.

25. Sumi, S.M., and Finlay, J.M. On the pathogenesis of diabetic steatorrhea. *Ann Intern Med.* 55:994–997, 1961.

26. Frimodt-Moller, C. Diabetic cystopathy. I. A clinical study of the frequency of bladder dysfunction in diabetics. *Dan Med Bull.* 23:267–278, 1976.

27. Rubin, A., and Babbott, D. Impotence and diabetes mellitus. *JAMA.* 168:498–500, 1958.

28. Schoffling, K., Federlin, K. Ditschuneit, H. et al. Disorders of sexual function in male diabetics. *Diabetes* 12:519–527, 1963.

29. Kolodny, R.C. Sexual dysfunction in diabetic females. *Diabetes* 20:557–559, 1971.

30. Ellenberg, M. Female sexuality in the diabetic. *Mt Sinai J Med (NY).* 44:495–500, 1977.

31. Fisher, C., Schiavi, R., Lear, H. et al. The assessment of nocturnal REM

erections in the differential diagnosis of sexual impotence and diagnosis in diabetic impotence. *J Sex Marital Ther.* 1:277–289, 1975.

32. Karacan, I., Salis, P.J., Ware, J.C. et al. Nocturnal penile tumescence and diagnosis in diabetic impotence. *Am J Psychiatry.* 135(2):191–197, 1978.

33. Drachman, D.B. Trophic functions of the neuron. *Ann NY Acad Sci.* 228:160–176, 1974.

34. Singer, M. Neurotrophic control of limb regeneration in the newt. *Ann NY Acad Sci.* 228:308–322, 1974.

35. Pastan, R.S., and Cohen, A.S. The rheumatologic manifestations of diabetes mellitus. *Med Clin North Am.* 62(4):829–839, 1978.

36. Pogonowska, M.J., Collins, L.C., and Dobson, H.L. Diabetic osteopathy. *Radiology* 89:265–271, 1967.

37. Schwarz, G.S., Berenyi, M.R., and Siegel, M.W. Atrophic arthropathy and diabetic neuritis. *Am J Roentgenol.* 106:523–529, 1969.

38. Kaklamanis, P., Rigas, A., Gianatos, J. et al. Calcification of the shoulder and diabetes mellitus. *N Engl J Med.* 293:1266–1267, 1975.

39. Bridgman, J.F. Periarthritis of the shoulder and diabetes mellitus. *Ann Rheum Dis.* 31:69–71, 1972.

40. Forestier, J., and Lagier, R. Ankylosing hyperostosis of the spine. *Clin Orthop.* 74:65–83, 1971.

41. Hajkova, Z., Streda, A., and Skrha, F. Hyperostotic spondylosis and diabetes mellitus. *Ann Rheum Dis.* 24:536–543, 1965.

42. Bailey, C.C., and Root, H.F. Neuropathic foot lesions in diabetes mellitus. *N Engl J Med.* 236:387–392, 1947.

43. Boehm, H.J. Diabetic charcot joint. *N Engl J Med.* 267:185–187, 1962.

44. Guillain, G.J.M. *Charcot, His Life–His Work.* New York: Paul B. Hoeber, 1959, p 114.

45. Jordan, W.R. Neuritic manifestations in diabetes mellitus. *Arch Intern Med.* 57:307–366, 1936.

46. Ellenberg, M. Diabetic neuropathy: clinical aspects. *Metabolism* 25:1627–1655, 1976.

47. Giesecke, S.B., Dalinka, M.K., and Kyee, G.C. Lisfranc's fracture-dislocation: a manifestation of peripheral neuropathy. *Am J Roentgenol.* 131:139–141, 1978.

48. Lippmann, H.I. Perotto, A., and Farrar, R. The neuropathic foot of the diabetic. *Bull NY Acad Med.* 52:1159–1178, 1976.

49. Singleton, E.E., Cotton, R.S., and Shelman, H.S. Another approach to the long-term management of the diabetic neurotrophic foot ulcer. *J Am Podiatry Assoc.* 68:242–244, 1978.

50. Schmidt, R.E., Matschinsky, F.M., Godfrey, D.A. et al. Fast and slow axoplasmic flow in sciatic nerve of diabetic rats. *Diabetes* 24:1081–1085, 1975.

51. Joslin, E.P., Root, H.F., White, P. et al. *The Treatment of Diabetes Mellitus.* Philadelphia: Lea & Febiger, 1952.

52. Epstein, S.H. Diabetic neuropathy and its prognosis. *Neurology* 1:228–233, 1951.

53. Gregersen, G. Diabetic neuropathy: influence of age, sex, metabolic control and duration of diabetes on motor conduction velocity. *Neurology* 17:972–980, 1967.

54. Ward, J.D., Barnes, C.G., Fisher, D.J. et al. Improvement in nerve conduction following treatment in newly diagnosed diabetics. *Lancet* 1:428–431, 1971.

55. Mogensen, C.E. Renal function changes in diabetes. *Diabetes* 25(suppl 2):872–879, 1976.

56. Parving, H.H. Increased microvascular permeability to plasma proteins

in short- and long-term juvenile diabetics. *Diabetes* 25(suppl 2):884–889, 1976.

57. Olsson, Y., and Reese, T.S. Permeability of vasa nervorum and perineurium in mouse sciatic nerve studied by fluorescence and electron microscopy. *J Neuropathol Exp Neurol.* 30:105–119, 1971.

58. Seneviratne, K.N. Permeability of blood nerve barrier in the diabetic rat. *J Neurol Neurosurg Psychiatry.* 35:156–162, 1972.

59. Asbury, A.K., and Johnson, P.C. *Pathology of Peripheral Nerve.* Philadelphia: W.B. Saunders, 1978, p 98.

60. Jakobsen, J. Axonal dwindling in early experimental diabetes. I. A study of cross sectioned nerves. *Diabetologia* 12:539–546, 1976.

61. Jakobsen, J. Peripheral nerves in early experimental diabetes: expansion of the endoneurial space as a cause of increased water content. *Diabetologia* 14:113–119, 1978.

62. Johnson, P.C., Yoshimura, M.P., and Gaines, J.A. Thickening of the perineurial cell basement membrane in diabetes and aging. *J Neuropathol Exp Neurol.* 37:637, 1978.

63. Greene, D.A., Winegrad, A.I., Carpentier, J.L. et al. Glucose metabolism and insulin effects in nerve fascicle and "endoneurial" preparations. *Clin Res.* 26:529, 1978.

64. Winegrad, A.I., and Greene, D.A. Diabetic polyneuropathy: the importance of insulin deficiency, hyperglycemia and alterations in myoinositol metabolism in its pathogenesis. *N Engl J Med.* 295:1416–1420, 1976.

65. Servo, C., Bergstrom, L., and Fogelholm, R. Cerebrospinal fluid sorbitol and myoinositol and diabetic polyneuropathy. *Acta Med Scand.* 202:301–304, 1977.

66. Clements, R.S., Vourganti, B., Kuba, T. et al. Dietary myoinositol intake and peripheral nerve function in diabetic neuropathy. *Metabolism* 28:477–483, 1979.

67. Gregersen, G., Borsting, H., Theil, P. et al. Myoinositol and function of peripheral nerves in human diabetics. *Acta Neurol Scand.* 58:241–248, 1978.

68. Hansen, S., and Ballantyne, J.P. Axonal dsyfunction in the neuropathy of diabetes mellitus: a quantitative electrophysiological study. *J Neurol Neurosurg Psychiatry.* 40:555–564, 1977.

69. Behse, F., Buchthal, F., and Carlsen, F. Nerve biopsy and conduction studies in diabetic neuropathy. *J Neurol Neursurg Psychiatry.* 40:1072–1082, 1977.

70. Thomas, P.K., and Lascelles, R.G. The pathology of diabetic neuropathy. *Q J Med.* 35:489–509, 1966.

71. Dyke, P.J., Johnson, W.J., Lambert, E.H. et al. Segmental demyelination secondary to axonal degeneration in uremic neuropathy. *Mayo Clin Proc.* 46:400–430, 1971.

72. Sullivan, J.F. The neuropathies of diabetes. *Neurology* 8:243–250, 1958.

73. Collier, J. Peripheral neuritis. Lecture III. *Edinburgh Med J.* 39:672–690, 1932.

74. Raff, M.C., and Asbury, A.K. Ischemic mononeuropathy and mononeuropathy multiplex in diabetes mellitus. *N Engl J Med.* 279:17–32, 1968.

75. Asbury, A.K., Aldredge, H., Hershberg, R. et al. Oculomotor palsy in diabetes mellitus: a clinicopathologic study. *Brain* 93:555–556, 1970.

76. Dreyfus, P.M., Hakim, S., and Adams, R.D. Diabetic ophthalmoplegia. *Arch Neurol Psychiatr.* 77:337–349, 1957.

77. Garland, H., and Taverner, D. Diabetic myelopathy. *Br Med J.* 1:1405–1408, 1953.

78. Garland, H. Diabetic amyotrophy. *Br Med J.* 2:1287–1290, 1955.

79. Chokroverty, S., Reyes, M.G., and Rubino, F.A. Bruns-Garland syndrome of diabetic amyotrophy. *Trans Am Neurol Assoc.* 102:173–175, 1977.

80. Mayer, R. Discussion of Bruns-Garland syndrome. *Trans Am Neurol Assoc.* 102:176, 1977.

81. Child, D.L., and Yates, D.A.H. Radicular pain in diabetes. *Rheumatol Rehabil.* 17:195–196, 1978.

82. Goldstein, J.E., and Cogan, D.G. Diabetic ophthalmoplegia with special reference to the pupil. *Arch Ophthalmol.* 64:592–600, 1960.

83. Rucker, C.W. Paralysis of the third, fourth and sixth cranial nerves. *Am J Ophthalmol.* 46:787–794, 1958.

84. Green, W.R., Hackett, E.R., and Schlezinger, N.S. Neuro-ophthalmologic evaluation of oculomotor nerve paralysis. *Arch Ophthalmol.* 72:154–167, 1964.

85. Rucker, C.W. The causes of paralysis of the third, fourth, and sixth cranial nerves. *Am J Ophthalmol.* 61:1293–1298, 1966.

86. Shrader, E.C., and Schlezinger, N.S. Neuro-ophthalmologic evaluation of abducens nerve paralysis. *Arch Ophthalmol.* 64:84–91, 1960.

87. Lundgren, A., Odkvist, L.M., Hendriksson, K.G. et al. Facial palsy in diabetes mellitus—not only a neuropathy? *Adv Otorhinolaryngol.* 22:182–189, 1977.

88. Adour, K.K. The bell tolls for decompression. *N Engl J Med.* 292:748–750, 1975.

89. Kenny, A.J., Chute, A.L., and Best, C.H. A study of the prevalence of diabetes in an Ontario community. *Can Med Assoc J.* 65:233–241, 1951.

90. Wilkerson, H.L.C., and Kroll, L.N. Diabetes in a New England town. *JAMA.* 135:209–216, 1947.

91. Gilliatt, R.W., and Willison, R.G. Peripheral nerve conduction in diabetic neuropathy. *J Neurol Neurosurg Psychiatry.* 25:11–18, 1962.

92. Phalen, G.S. Reflections on 21 years experience with the carpal tunnel syndrome. *JAMA.* 212:1365–1367, 1970.

93. Sibley, W.A. Polyneuritis. *Med Clin North Am.* 56:1299–1319, 1972.

94. Ellenberg, M. Treatment of diabetic neuropathy with diphenylhydantoin. *NY State J Med.* 68:2653–2655, 1968.

95. Chakrabarti, A.K., and Samantaray, S.K. Diabetic peripheral neuropathy nerve conduction studies before, during and after carbamazepine therapy. *Aust NZ J Med.* 6:565–568, 1976.

96. Saudek, C.D., Werns, S., and Reidenberg, M.M. Phenytoin in the treatment of diabetic symmetrical polyneuropathy. *Clin Pharmacol Ther.* 22(2):196–199, 1977.

97. Davis, J.L. Peripheral diabetic neuropathy treated with amitriptyline and fluphenazine. *JAMA.* 238:2291–2292, 1977.

98. Thorsteinsson, G., Stonnington, H.H., Stillwell, G.K. et al. Transcutaneous electrical stimulation: a double-blind trial of its efficacy for pain. *Arch Phys Med Rehabil.* 58:8–13, 1977.

99. Tchobroutsky, G. Relationship of diabetic control to development of microvascular complications. *Diabetologia* 15:143–152, 1978.

13 Management of Gastrointestinal Disease Associated with Diabetes Mellitus

Ian L. MacGregor, MD, and
David L. Earnest, MD

Diabetes mellitus may affect the entire gastrointestinal tract but in the majority of diabetics gastrointestinal symptoms are minor. Pathophysiologic mechanisms whereby diabetes mellitus is postulated to involve the gastrointestinal tract include diabetic autonomic neuropathy[1] and diabetic microangiopathy[2] although the correlation of such demonstrable pathology with functional changes remains less than totally convincing.

Gastrointestinal tract motility and secretions are also affected by the hormones insulin and glucagon[3,4] and by changes in blood glucose.[5,6] Blood levels of glucagon and insulin and blood glucose concentrations are abnormal in diabetes mellitus and may contribute to the described gastrointestinal tract pathophysiology.

ESOPHAGUS

The majority of patients with diabetes mellitus do not have symptoms referable to the esophagus. If present, symptoms of esophageal involvement are most likely to be those consequent upon gastrointestinal sphincter incompetence, ie, heartburn or dysphagia. However, motor disorders of the esophagus are common in diabetes mellitus. Mandelstam and Lieber[7] studied 14 patients with diabetic peripheral neuropathy and found cineradiographic abnormalities in 12, including aperistalsis, tertiary contractions, and delayed esophageal emptying. The upper esophagus was normal. Restudy of 10 patients one to three years later, including manometry in eight, showed deterioration of motor abnormalities. Pharyngeal contractions were diminished in amplitude but not in duration. The duration of upper esophageal sphincter relaxation was less in the diabetic group and primary peristalsis frequently followed swallowing. Tertiary contractions were more common in the diabetics and the lower esophageal sphincter pressure was significantly less than that of the control subjects.[8] The management of such motor disorders of the esophagus in the diabetic is the same as that recommended for the nondiabetic. However, symptoms of reflux, dysphagia, odynophagia, or spasm should not be assumed to result from motor abnormalities due to the underlying diabetes mellitus. Carcinoma should be exluded in any patient with dysphagia.

Peptic esophagitis due to lower esophageal sphincter incompetence is treated with antacids, elevation of the head of the bed, cessation of smoking and decrease in ethanol consumption, ingestion of small meals, and no food within one to two hours of going to bed. Failure to respond to this regimen will require the addition of medications such as cimetidine to decrease gastric acid secretion, and/or bethanechol or metoclopramide to increase the lower esophageal sphincter pressure. Surgical repair using a fundal wraparound procedure such as the the Nissen fundoplication may be required in patients resistant to medical management.[9] Symptoms due to esophageal spasm may respond to the smooth-muscle-relaxing effect of the slow-or long-acting nitrates.[10]

Diabetic patients with pharyngeal as well as substernal pain with swallowing should be investigated for infection with *Candida albicans*. Candida esophagitis occurs with increased frequency in diabetics and may lead to fatal systemic dissemination.[11] The fungal hyphae can be easily identified in the white plaque-like exudate on the oropharyngeal or esophageal mucosa. It is important to realize that candida may involve the esophagus without the disease being apparent in the mouth. Treatment of localized pharyngoesophageal candida with oral nystatin or 5-fluorocytosine is usually successful in limited disease.[12] The diagnosis of candida esophagitis in an immunosuppressed patient should lead to immediate systemic treatment because of the high likelihood of disseminated fungal disease.

STOMACH

Motor Abnormalities

A report of "gastroparesis diabeticorum" 20 years ago by Kassander[13] drew attention to the gastric motor abnormalities that occur in about one third of diabetic subjects. The common motor abnormalities are gastric atony and/or sluggish motility with delayed gastric emptying. Organic obstruction of the gastric outlet is absent, the gastric retention presumably resulting form the sluggish motor activity. Delayed and erratic gastric emptying contributes to difficulty in diabetic control due to the irregular delivery of ingested nutrients to intestinal absorptive sites. Gastric atony has been considered to result from diabetic autonomic neuropathy. However, the relaxing effect of glucagon on the smooth muscle of the gastrointestinal tract and the effect of hyperglycemia in delaying gastric emptying[5] may be of importance in the pathogenesis of diabetic gastric retention. Such gastric motor abnormalities occur most frequently in the presence of other complications of diabetes and typically exist in patients with a long history of severe diabetes. Most patients are asymptomatic but some have symptoms of epigastric fullness. In more severe cases there may be nausea or vomiting or both.

Management of motor abnormalities of the stomach associated with diabetes mellitus is difficult. Efforts should be made to strictly control the blood sugar. The acute gastric dilatation and retention associated with diabetic ketoacidosis should be treated with placement of a nasogastric tube and aspiration along with appropriate treatment of the diabetic ketoacidosis. Acute gastric dilatation and retention is generally a reversible process.

Management of the chronically dilated and symptomatic atonic stomach is more difficult. The response to cholinergic agents is variable. Kassander[13] found small frequent meals and carefully titrated insulin to be more effective than mecholyl or bethanechol. Others have found subcutaneous bethanechol, and to a lesser extent oral bethanechol to be useful.[14] Neostigmine has also been reported to be of benefit.[15] The cholinesterase inhibitor ambenonium chloride has been shown to produce subjective and radiologic improvement in about half of the treated group and such treatment is worthy of trial.[16]

Perhaps the most promising therapeutic agent is metoclopramide, a drug that restores sluggish upper gastrointestinal tract motility toward normal. Metoclopramide has been found to be superior to both placebo and carbachol in the treatment of postvagotomy stasis[17] and preliminary studies in gastroparesis diabeticorum have given promising results.[18] Further studies are in progress to assess the effectiveness of metoclopramide on diabetic gastric stasis. However, the drug is not yet approved for general use for this purpose.

Some patients who are refractory to medical management have been treated by surgical drainage procedures, either pyloroplasty or gastrojejunostomy. Although good results are reported in some cases,[19] no convincing evidence of improvement is evident in others.[15] The development of diabetic gastric retention is a serious prognostic sign in terms of life expectancy.[20] A large number of these patients have autonomic neuropathy, a condition that, in itself, reduces life expectancy.[21]

Gastric Secretion

Diabetics have been reported to be hypochlorhydric, the depression of acid output being related to the degree of hyperglycemia. Older literature suggests that as much as 17% of patients with diabetes mellitus are achlorhydric.[22] More recently, various authors have attempted to explain just how diabetes mellitus affects gastric acid secretion. For example, in one recent study, although the gastric acid secretory response to sham feeding was markedly decreased in a small group of diabetics, their gastric acid response to pentagastrin and to a homogenized test meal was normal. Moreover, the increment in serum gastrin in response to the test meal was greater in the diabetic subjects than in the controls. These findings were interpreted as probably resulting from "autovagotomy" occurring in the diabetics.[23]

There is also an increased incidence of histologically evident gastritis in patients with diabetes mellitus, the severity of which has been found to correlate with the degree of hypochlorhydria.[24] The degree of gastritis is related to age more than to the duration of diabetes or control of blood sugar. About one quarter of all diabetics have parietal cell antibodies compared with less than 10% of the control population.[25] Intrinsic factor antibodies are also more common in diabetics (8%) compared with controls (0%), and less intrinsic factor is secreted into the gastric lumen.[26] About 4% of patients with diabetes mellitus have pernicious anemia.[27] Whereas 95% of patients with decreased intrinsic factor secretion have normal levels of vitamin B_{12}, 8% of a large group of patients with diabetes mellitus with peripheral neuropathy were shown to have vitamin B_{12} deficiency with resultant neuropathy. Treatment by replacement of vitamin B_{12} produced a dramatic improvement in five of seven patients, emphasizing that other treatable causes of peripheral neuropathy should be sought in patients with diabetes mellitus.[28]

Gastric Ulcer

Controversy exists regarding frequency of gastric ulcer in patients with diabetes mellitus, highlighting the fact that if differences from normal do occur, they are small. However, ulcer complications may be more frequent and of greater severity. For example, the vascular changes associated with diabetes may aggravate ulcer bleeding, and gastric outlet obstruction is more likely to develop and be intractable because of the motility disturbance present. Management of gastric ulcer in the diabetic subject is generally the same as that in the non-diabetic. Once carcinoma has been excluded, treatment is based on the use of either antacids or compounds that block gastric acid secretion, such as the histamine-2 receptor blocker, cimetidine. Anticholinergic agents should be avoided due to the possibility of aggravating any problem with gastric emptying resulting from the effect of diabetes.

INTESTINAL INVOLVEMENT

Small Intestine

For reasons that are not clear, diabetics have increased rates of intestinal absorption of glucose and amino acids as demonstrated by intestinal perfusion studies. Enterocyte disaccharidase activities are normal.[29] Diabetics also have a decreased incidence of duodenal ulcer. This is possibly due to decreased gastric acid secretion.

Diabetic Diarrhea

An uncommon but difficult management problem occurring as a consequence of diabetes is diabetic diarrhea. Steatorrhea may also occur. The diagnosis of diabetic diarrhea is, to some degree, one of exclusion and such a label requires negative results of evaluation for other causes of diarrhea such as infection, parasites, chronic pancreatitis with pancreatic insufficiency, or celiac disease. An association between diabetes mellitus and celiac disease has been widely reported although the number of diabetic patients in whom the diagnosis of celiac disease has been adequately confirmed is small. Even an extensive and critical study by Walsh et al[30] did not fully resolve the question of whether or not diabetes and celiac disease coexist more frequently than would occur by chance. These authors emphasize the responsiveness of such patients to gluten withdrawal as well as the unstable nature of the diabetes mellitus with frequent hypoglycemic episodes prior to such dietary treatment. The distinction between diabetic diarrhea and celiac disease can generally be made by history and physical examination. Features such as a history of digestive symptoms prior to the diagnosis of diabetes, frequent episodes of symptomatic hypoglycemia, the absence of neuropathy, the presence of anemia, low serum folate and albumin, and a malabsorptive pattern on barium studies of the small bowel suggest the diagnosis of celiac disease. A definitive diagnosis can be made only by finding typical histologic changes on small-bowel biopsy and a favorable response to dietary gluten withdrawal.

If no obvious cause for diarrhea is present apart from the diabetes itself, then the term "diabetic diarrhea" can be applied. The incidence of diarrhea reported in diabetes has been as high as 10%. Somewhat more than half of these patients may have steatorrhea.[31] The diarrhea is usually watery and voluminous. It will often occur at night and fecal incontinence and soiling are common. The diarrhea may be precipitated by eating. In addition, it is typically episodic and may be interspersed with normal bowel habit or even constipation. Many male patients with diabetic diarrhea are also impotent.

The etiology of diarrhea associated with diabetes mellitus is unclear and probably multifactorial. Exocrine pancreatic function is usually adequate and specific mucosal absorptive defects have not been demonstrated. Small bowel histology is generally normal by light microscopy. Most studies have shown that water and electrolyte absorption are normal or exceed that in nondiabetic subjects. However, a number of unusual and unexplained phenomena have been observed. For example, in one study following oral administration of an aqueous meal containing D-xylose, the meal volume reportedly increased in the upper digestive tract and its passage through the ileum was delayed.[32]

Diabetic diarrhea is frequently related to visceral autonomic neuropathy with motor abnormalities of the gastrointestinal tract. Sluggish motor activity with stagnation of bowel contents may allow small intestinal overgrowth of colonic-type bacterial flora resulting in enterocyte damage and bile acid deconjugation leading to diarrhea and steatorrhea.[33] However, such small intestinal bacterial overgrowth occurs in only a minority of patients with diabetic diarrhea.

Diarrhea in a diabetic should be thoroughly evaluated as should any case of chronic diarrhea. Stools should be examined for volume, fat, pathogenic bacteria and ova, and parasites. A fresh stool smear should be examined microscopically for leukocytes, which are indicative of infection and inflammation. Sigmoidoscopy should be performed to rule out inflammation, ulceration, pseudomembrane, neoplasm, and local anorectal disease. Tone in the internal and external anal sphincters should be evaluated since anal incontinence may result from sphincter weakness. In such cases, further neurologic evaluation may be necessary.

The inability to find a specific cause of diabetes-associated diarrhea is not uncommon and is frequently a source of frustration to both patient and physician. Symptomatic treatment with drugs such as imodium (Loperimide®) or diphenoxylate hydrochloride plus atropine (Lomotil®) may be useful. Water-absorbing mucilages such as psyllium seed extracts (eg, Metamucil®) may make the bowel movements easier to control and prevent fecal incontinence. Successful treatment with cholestyramine in four subjects with intractable diabetic diarrhea has been reported by Condon et al.[34] These authors compare diabetic diarrhea with postvagotomy diarrhea, a condition in which some patients have been shown to excrete excessive amounts of bile acids in feces and to respond to treatment with cholestyramine.[35] It is possible that in postvagotomy diarrhea, postprandial rapid intestinal transit of luminal contents flushes bile acids past their terminal ileal absorptive sites into the colon where the unconjugated dihydroxy bile acids produce a secretory diarrhea.[36] The assumption that diabetic diarrhea may also result from a similar mechanism relating to bile acid malabsorption has not been thoroughly investigated. Some cases of diabetic diarrhea indeed do show rapid small intestinal transit of barium.[37] However, the unphysiologic nature of inert barium sulfate suspension which does not trigger normal gastric emptying and interstinal transit-controlling reflexes may give misleading information about the true rate of postprandial gastrointestinal transit.[38] Nevertheless, the possibility that such a mechanism may be operative in some cases of diabetic diarrhea justifies a therapeutic trial of cholestyramine when more conservative treatment measures have failed. It should be remembered that in addition to bile acids, cholestyramine binds other anions in the intestinal tract and may cause difficulty with absorption of various drugs. Prolonged use of large amounts of cholestyramine will diminish absorption of fat soluble vitamins and thereby may induce unwanted side effects.

COLONIC INVOLVEMENT

Many diabetic patients complain of constipation, at times so severe that it can be incapacitating.[39] The colon may be enormously dilated, containing vast quantities of stool and displaying stercoral ulcers. Intestinal obstruction may be simulated by such impaction. In addition, the massively dilated and atonic colon may predispose to sigmoid volvulus. It has been assumed that autonomic neuropathy disturbs colonic motility leading to alterations in normal propulsive activity. However, it is not certain that colonic motility disturbances actually produce the constipation. The presence of neuropathy has also been considered responsible for the fecal incontinence that occurs in some patients with diabetes mellitus. Such nerve damage interferes with efferent impulses relaying the degree of rectal distension and controlling the anal sphincter mechanisms.[40] However, constipation is common among the elderly and it is debatable whether it is actually more frequent in diabetics than in nondiabetics. The megacolon seen in some diabetic subjects often occurs in the setting of a chronically constipated patient with a history of laxative abuse.

The treatment of constipation in diabetics is the same as for nordiabetic patients. A diet of fresh vegetables, whole grain cereals and breads, increased fruit intake, and residue-forming bulk laxatives, as well as exercise and the retraining of regular bowel habits are important. This can be a difficult task and the use of stool softeners or enemas may be necessary initially. However, regular enemas and the use of irritant laxatives should be discontinued as soon as possible. Surgical resection of the massively distended and atonic segment of the colon may be required infrequently.

Diverticular disease is frequent in the diabetic. The course of diverticulitis more often is complicated and has a higher mortality rate than in the nondiabetic subject.[41]

THE EXOCRINE PANCREAS

Atrophic changes in the pancreas with fibrosis and hyalinization are histologically apparent in the majority of autopsied diabetics.[42] Exocrine secretion has also been found to be reduced in the majority of diabetics.[43] Such exocrine insufficiency is seldom severe and generally does not decline to the degree of insufficiency that results in steatorrhea.[44]

There are isolated reports of increased incidence of pancreatitis in patients with diabetes mellitus.[45] It is commonly accepted that acute pancreatitis in the diabetic is a more serious disorder than in the nondiabetic. Pancreatitis in the diabetic is treated in the usual manner with nasogastric suction, intravenous fluid replacement, pain relief, and observation for the development of a pancreatic abscess or pseudocyst. Insulin must be carefully titrated against the blood glucose with a constant awareness of the possible occurrence of sudden hypoglycemia.[46] The possibility that gallstone migration precipitated the episode of acute pancreatitis should always be suspected, as gallstones are more frequent in persons with diabetes mellitus than in normal individuals. The diseased or stone-filled gallbladder should be removed in diabetics.

Although the overall incidence of malignancy in diabetes mellitus is the same as the general population, an increase in the association of pancreatic cancer with diabetes mellitus has been shown.[47,48] However, it is probable that some cases of adult-onset diabetes occur as a consequence of undetected pancreatic cancer, rather than the diabetic state predisposing to the development of cancer. Certainly the genetically determined adult-onset diabetic does not show an unduly pronounced tendency to develop pancreatic cancer.[48] Whether or not it is associated with diabetes mellitus, the management of pancreatic cancer should be based on realization of the poor prognosis for all but periampullary tumors. Palliative surgery bypassing obstructing biliary ducts and the control of pain with skillfully titrated narcotic analgesics may allow a more superior quality of life than that resulting from heroic and usually unsuccessful surgery.

LIVER INVOLVEMENT WITH DIABETES MELLITUS

Diabetes mellitus is a metabolic disorder affecting the total body. Therefore, it is not surprising that an organ such as the liver with its varied and vital metabolic functions should be affected by this disease. The effect of diabetes mellitus on the liver recently has been extensively reviewed.[49] Hepatomegaly may occur, especially in poorly controlled diabetics during recovery from diabetic ketoacidosis. The incidence of hepatomegaly has lessened with the introduction of the longer-acting insulins but still is seen frequently, even in patients with reasonably adequate diabetic control. Fatty liver, the usual cause of hepatomegaly, certainly is seen in well-controlled diabetics, being present in about half of one group of such patients biopsied by Zimmerman et al.[50] Three of the 28 patients in this study also had liver cirrhosis.

On histologic examination of the liver in diabetes mellitus, the most characteristic feature is the presence of large intranuclear glycogen-containing vacuoles.[51] These glycogen nuclei are not, however, specific for diabetes as they are also seen in obesity, Wilson's disease, tuberculosis, and, occasionally, viral hepatitis. In addition to fat and glycogen, abnormal water accumulation in hepatic intracellular spaces may cause hepatomegaly.[52] Sudden enlargement of the liver with stretching of the capsule in such situations may cause severe pain.

The degree of liver dysfunction in patients with diabetes mellitus is variably reported, some authors claiming up to 75% of patients having abnormal liver function tests.[31,49] Other investigators claim no difference from control subjects. A reasonable conclusion is that the well-controlled and adequately nourished diabetic who is free of complications from his diabetes mellitus will have liver functions closely paralleling those of control patients who are not diabetic.

The incidence of cirrhosis in diabetes mellitus is also variably reported. There is no good evidence that diabetes mellitus leads to cirrhosis, although the association is common. About 50% of cirrhotic subjects have an abnormal glucose tolerance test and about 10% have manifest diabetes.[53] Cirrhosis has been reported to occur in patients with diabetes mellitus with an incidence of about 1%.[54] In most patients with diabetes and cirrhosis, the cirrhosis is usually first manifested by hepatomegaly and abnormal liver function tests.[55] The abnormal glucose tolerance seems to be a consequence of the liver disease and has been termed "hepatogenous diabetes."[56] The glucose tolerance test is usually only mildly impaired and blood sugar is easily controlled with diet or oral hypoglycemic agents.

The reason for abnormal glucose tolerance in cirrhotic patients remains unclear. Elevated glucagon and growth hormone levels, increased plasma nonesterified fatty acids, and impaired hepatic insulin metabolism have all been put forward as possible mechanisms. Low body potassium levels, even with normal serum potassium concentrations, have been documented in cirrhotic patients with low fasting and stimulated insulin levels.[57] This potassium deficiency is likely related to hyperaldosteronism although other potential mechanisms have not been well studied. Replacement of potassium may lead to normalization of insulin levels and glucose tolerance. Thus, potassium abnormalities may play a role in "hepatogenous diabetes" and should be considered if glucose tolerance in such patients is a concern.

BILIARY TRACT

The size of the gallbladder is increased in diabetic patients with autonomic neuropathy.[58] Poor filling of the gallbladder with oral cholecystographic dye, and poor contraction following a fatty meal may be demonstrated in such patients. In addition, many fail to concentrate dye adequately enough to allow visualization of the gallbladder at oral cholecystography.[59] Such radiologic abnormalities appear to be related to abnormal motor or contractile functions of the gallbladder wall and do not necessarily imply biliary tract inflammation or presence of stones. In the absence of cholelithiasis, surgery is not necessary. Thus, a nonvisualizing gallbladder in a diabetic with autonomic neuropathy should be investigated with ultrasonography before a diagnosis of cholecystitis with possible stones is made. Several large series of autopsied patients have shown an increased incidence of gallstones in diabetics, the occurrence of stones being about twice as common as in nondiabetics.[60,61] However, other studies have not always confirmed this finding and there is no absolutely clear evidence that diabetes mellitus predisposes to gallstones formation.

Acute cholecystitis and cholangitis are very serious in the diabetic with a mortality five times greater than that in the nondiabetic. On the other hand, elective surgery does not differ in its risks and outcome for the diabetic. Therefore, the presence of biliary tract disease or of asymptomatic gallstones is a definite indication for elective cholecystectomy as soon as conveniently possible.

SUMMARY

Diabetes mellitus can affect all parts of the human gastrointestinal tract. The majority of clinically apparent abnormalities are of disordered motor function occurring as a consequence of diabetic neuropathy. The manifestations of motor derangement include gastroesophageal reflux, esophageal spasm, delayed gastric emptying, bacterial overgrowth in the small intestine with induced malabsorption, constipation, and fecal incontinence. Diabetic diarrhea may be in part due to derangement in motor function and intestinal transit and in some cases may be worsened by bile acid malabsorption and choleretic enteropathy. Pancreatic exocrine insufficiency is seldom important clinically. Diabetes may predispose to the development of acute pancreatitis, which is often a more serious disorder in the diabetic.

The dilated and poorly contractile gallbladder seen in some diabetic subjects may predispose to the increased incidence of gallstones that is variably reported. Since acute cholecystitis and cholangitis have a much higher morbidity and mortality in diabetic than in nondiabetic individuals, be they symptomatic or not, the presence of gallstones constitutes an indication for cholecystectomy.

REFERENCES

1. Ellenberry, M. Diabetic neuropathy with special reference to visceral neuropathy. *Adv Intern Med.* 12:11–32, 1964.

2. Angervall, L., and Save-Soderbergh, J. Microangiopathy in the digestive tract in subjects with diabetes of early onset and long duration. *Diabetologia* 2:117–122, 1966.

3. Robinson, R.M., Harris, K., Hlad, C.J. et al. Effect of glucagon on gastric secretion. *Proc Soc Exp Biol Med.* 96:518–522, 1957.

4. Aylett, P. Gastric emptying and changes in blood sugar level as affected by glucagon and insulin. *Clin Sci.* 22:171–178, 1962.

5. MacGregor, I.L., Gueller, R., Watts, H.D. et al. The effect of acute hyperglycemia on gastric emptying in man. *Gastroenterology* 70:190–196, 1976.

6. MacGregor, I.L., Deveney, C., Way, L.W. et al. The effect of acute hyperglycemia on meal-stimulated gastric, biliary and pancreatic secretion and serum gastrin. *Gastroenterology* 70:197–202, 1976.

7. Mandelstam, P., and Lieber, A. Esophageal dysfunction in diabetic neuropathy-gastroenteropathy, clinical and roentgenological manifestations. *JAMA*. 201:88–92, 1967.

8. Mandelstrom, P., Siegel, C.I., Lieber, A. et al. The swallowing disorder in patients with diabetic neuropathy-gastroenteropathy. *Gastroenterology* 56:1–12, 1969.

9. Cohen, S., and Snape, W.J. The pathophysiology and treatment of gastroesophageal reflux disease. *Arch Intern Med.* 138:1398–1401, 1978.

10. Swamy, N. Esophageal spasm: clinical and monometric response to nitroglycerin and long-acting nitrates. *Gastroenterology* 72:23–27, 1977.

11. Eras, P., Goldstein, M.J., and Sherlock, P. Candida infection of the gastrointestinal tract. *Medicine* 51:367–379, 1972.

12. Edwards, J.E., Jr., Lehrer, R.I., Steihm, E.R. et al. Severe candidal infections. Clinical perspective, immune defense. *Ann Intern Med.* 89:91–106, 1978.

13. Kassander, P. Asymptomatic gastric retention in diabetes (gastroparesis diabeticorum). *Ann Intern Med.* 48:797–812, 1958.

14. Wooten, R.L., and Meriwether, T.W. Diabetic gastric atony: a clinical study. *JAMA*. 176:1082–1087, 1961.

15. Marshak, R.H., and Maklansky, D. Diabetic gastropathy. *Am J Dig Dis.* 9:366–370, 1964.

16. Zitomer, B.R., Gramm, H.F., and Kozak, G.P. Gastric neuropathy in diabetes mellitus: clinical and radiologic observations. *Metabolism* 17:199–211, 1968.

17. Stadaas, J., and Aune, S. The effect of metaclopramide on gastric motility before and after vagotomy in man. *Scand J Gastroenterol.* 6:17–23, 1971.

18. Brownlee, M., and Kroopf, S.S. Metaclopramide for gastroparesis diabeticorum. *N Engl J Med.* 291:1257–1260, 1974.

19. Roon, A.J., and Mason, G.R. Surgical management of gastroparesis diabeticorum. *Calif Med.* 116(5):58–61, 1972.

20. Izzo, J.L. *Diabetes*. Edited by R.H. Williams. New York: Paul B. Hoeber, 1960, pp 666–699.

21. Ewing, D.J., Campbell, I.W., and Clarke, B.F. Mortality in diabetic autonomic neuropathy. *Lancet* 1:601–603, 1976.

22. Dotevall, G. Gastric secretion of acid in diabetes mellitus during basal conditions and after maximal histamine stimulation. *Acta Med Scand.* 170:59–69, 1961.

23. Feldman, M., Corbett, D.B., Ramsey, F.T. et al. Abnormal gastric function in longstanding insulin dependent diabetic patients. *Gastroenterology* 77:12–17, 1979.

24. Konturek, S.J., and Urban, A. The correlation between gastric acid secretion and histology of fundic and antral gland area. *Scand J Gastroenterol.* 4:463–468, 1969.

25. Moore, J.M., and Neilson, McE. Antibodies to gastric mucosa and thyroid in diabetes mellitus. *Lancet* 2:645–647, 1963.

26. Kanaghinis, T., Iatromanolakis, N., Ikkos, D. et al. Intrinsic factor secretion in the gastric juice in diabetes mellitus. *Am J Dig Dis.* 18:85–91, 1973.

27. Ungar, R., Stacks, A.E., Martin, F.I.R. et al. Intrinsic factor antibody,

parietal cell antibody, and latent pernicious anemia in diabetes mellitus. *Lancet* 2:415–417, 1968.

28. Kahn, M.A., Wakefield, G.S., and Pugh, D.N. Vitamin B_{12} deficiency in diabetic neuropathy. *Lancet* 2:768–770, 1969.

29. Chaudhary, M.A., and Olsen, W.A. Jejunal disaccharidase activity in maturity onset diabetes. *Am J Dig Dis.* 18:199–200, 1976.

30. Walsh, C.H., Cooper, B.J., Wright, A.D. et al. Diabetes mellitus in celiac disease: a clinical study. *Q J Med.* 47:89–100, 1978.

31. Glouberman, S. Diabetes mellitus and the gastrointestinal tract. *Ariz Med.* 34:174–175, 1977.

32. Whalen, G.E., Soergel, K.H., and Geenen, J.E. Diabetic diarrhea. *Gastroenterology* 56:102–103, 1969.

33. Goldstein, F., Wirts, C.W., Kowlessar, O.D. Diabetic diarrhea and steatorrhea. *Ann Intern Med.* 72:215–218, 1970.

34. Condon, J.R., Suleman, M.I., Fan, Y.S. et al. Cholestyramine in diabetic and postvagotomy diarrhea. *Br Med J.* 4:423, 1973.

35. Condon, J.R., Robinson, V., Suleman, M.I. et al. The cause and treatment of postvagotomy diarrhea. *Br J Surg.* 62:309–312, 1975.

36. Makhjian, H.S., Phillips, S.F., and Hofmann, A.F. Colonic secretion of water and electrolytes induced by bile acids: perfusion studies in man. *J Clin Invest.* 50:1569–1577, 1971.

37. McNilly, E.F., Reinhard, A.E., and Schwartz, P.E. Small bowel motilit in diabetics. *Am J Dig Dis.* 14:163–169, 1969.

38. Wiley, Z.D., Lavigne, M.E., Liu, K.M. et al. The effect of hyperthyroidism on gastric emptying rates and pancreatic exocrine and biliary secretion in man. *Am J Dig Dis.* 23:1003–1008, 1978.

39. Mayne, N.M. Neuropathy in the diabetic and nondiabetic populations. *Lancet* 2:1313–1316, 1965.

40. Cerulli, P.R.M.A., Nikoomanesh, P., and Schuster, M.M. Progress in biofeedback conditioning for fecal incontinence. *Gastroenterology* 76:742–746, 1979

41. Schowengerdt, C.G., Hedges, G.R., Yaw, P.B. et al. Diverticulosis, diverticulitis and diabetes—a review of 740 cases. *Arch Surg.* 98:500–504, 1969.

42. Null, J., Tillman, R.L., Shelton, A.L. et al. Pancreatic changes in maturity onset diabetes mellitus. *J Natl Med Assoc.* 65:65–67, 1973.

43. Vacca, J.B., Henke, W.T., and Knight, W.A. Exocrine pancreas and diabetes mellitus. *Ann Intern Med.* 61:242–247, 1964.

44. DiMagno, E.P., Go, V.L.W., and Summerskill, W.H.J. Relations between pancreatic enzyme outputs and malabsorption in severe pancreatic insufficiency. *N Engl J Med.* 288:813–815, 1973.

45. Blumenthal, H.T., Probsein, J.G., and Berns, A.W. Interrelationship of diabetes mellitus and pancreatitis. *Arch Surg.* 87:844–850, 1963.

46. Tully, G.T., and Lowenthal, J.J. Diabetic coma and acute pancreatitis. *Ann Intern Med.* 48:310–319, 1958.

47. Bell, E.T. Carcinoma of the pancreas. I. A clinical pathologic study of 609 necropsied cases. II. The relation of carcinoma of pancreas to diabetes mellitus. *Am J Pathol.* 33:499–523, 1957.

48. Joslin, E.P., Lombart, H.L., Burrows, R.E. et al. Diabetes and cancer. *N Engl J Med.* 260:486–488, 1959.

49. Creutzfeld, W., Fredricks, H., and Sickinger, K. Liver disease and diabetes mellitus. Edited by H. Popper, and F. Schaffner, In *Progress in Liver Diseases,* Vol. 3. New York: Grune & Stratton, 1970, pp 371–407.

50. Zimmerman, H.T., MacMurray, F.G., Rappoport, H. et al. Studies of

284

liver and diabetes mellitus. II. The significance of fatty metamorphosis and its correlation with insulin sensitivity. *J Lab Clin Med.* 36:922–928, 1950.

51. Chips, H.D., and Duff, G.L. Glycogen infiltration in liver cell nuclei. *Am J Pathol.* 18:645–655, 1942.

52. Warren, S., and LeCompte, P.M. *The Pathology of Diabetes,* 3rd Edition. Philadelphia: Lea & Febiger, 1952.

53. Conn, H.O., Schreiber, W., Elkington, S.G. et al. Cirrhosis and diabetes. I. Increased incidence of diabetes in patients with Laennec's cirrhosis. *Am J Dig Dis.* 14:837–852, 1969.

54. Tachdjian, V. Metabolic disorders and the liver. Edited by H.L Brockus. In *Gastroenterology,* Vol. 3. Philadelphia: W.B. Saunders, 1976, pp 594–597.

55. Itoh, S., Tsukada, Y., Motomura, Y. et al. Five patients with non-alcoholic diabetic cirrhosis. *Acta Hepatogastroenterol.* 26:90–97, 1979.

56. Meghesi, C., Samols, E., and Marks, V. Glucose tolerance in diabetes and chronic liver disease. *Lancet* 2:1051–1055, 1967.

57. Podolsky, S., Zimmerman, H.J., and Burrows, B.A. Potassium depletion in hepatic cirrhosis. *N Engl J Med.* 288:644–648, 1973.

58. Gitelson, S., Oppenheim, D., and Schwartz, A. Size of the gallbladder in patients with diabetes mellitus. *Diabetes* 18:493–498, 1969.

59. Grodzki, M., Mazurkiewicz-Rozynska, E., and Czyzyk, A. Diabetic cholecystopathy. *Diabetologia* 4:345–348, 1968.

60. Leiber, M.M. Incidence of gallstones and their correlation with other diseases. *Ann Surg.* 135:394–405, 1952.

61. Feldman, M., Feldman, M., Jr. Incidence of cholelithiasis, cholesterosis, and liver disease in diabetes mellitus: autopsy study. *Diabetes* 3:305–307, 1954.

14 Heart Disease in Diabetes Mellitus

Jay W. Smith, MD

Cardiac disease is the most common cause of death in patients with onset of diabetes mellitus after age 20. Diabetes mellitus is now the fifth leading cause of death in the United States, accounting for at least 30,000 deaths per year, making heart disease a major health problem, certainly one of the most hazardous risks the patient with diabetes faces.[1] Although coronary artery disease is the most common form of heart disease in diabetes, diabetic cardiomyopathy is becoming a well-recognized clinical entity. Acute myocardial infarction is devastating in the diabetic patient, and the management of angina pectoris, hypertension, and congestive heart failure requires special consideration.

CORONARY ARTERY DISEASE

Data from autopsy studies and data from clinical studies reporting myocardial infarction, angina, and sudden death all document an increased prevalence of coronary artery disease in diabetes mellitus.

286

Numerous autopsy studies have reported coronary artery disease in 18% to 75% of patients with diabetes.[2] The ratio of coronary artery disease in diabetics compared to nondiabetics has varied from 1.6:1 to 6.6:1. The prevalence of coronary artery disease in living patients with diabetes depends upon the means of diagnosing coronary artery disease and has varied from 1.6% to 56%. In the Framingham study the prevalence was 1.6% and in the University Group Diabetes Program 9.5%.[3] The reasons for this marked association—a genetic defect inherited concomitantly with diabetes, a complication secondary to the metabolic defects in diabetes, an aging process accelerated by diabetes, a result of the increased incidence of uremia, hypertension, and hyperlipidemia in diabetes—are not known. Certainly the major risk factors for coronary artery disease—hypertension, hyperlipidemia, and smoking—must play a role but their relative importance in the diabetic population compared to the nondiabetic population is not known.

The role of hypertension in promoting cardiovascular disease is now appreciated and the higher prevalence of hypertension in diabetic populations has been documented.[4] Hypertension has been reported in 40% to 80% of the diabetic population and is a common manifestation of diabetic nephropathy. Lowering blood pressure will decrease cerebrovascular and renal complications in nondiabetic populations[5]; whether controlling hypertension will have a similar effect in diabetic patients has not been shown. To date no data show unequivocally that lowering blood pressure will prevent coronary artery disease.

The role of hyperlipidemia, primarily hypercholesterolemia, as an important risk factor in developing coronary artery disease has been well-documented. However, diabetic populations compared to nondiabetic populations almost always have similar serum values for cholesterol, but elevated triglyceride determinations. The serum cholesterol values in nondiabetic patients with coronary artery disease are similar to diabetic patients with coronary artery disease.[6] If kinships of patients with hyperlipoproteinemias are evaluated, the relationship of hyperlipidemia, primarily hypertriglyceridemia, and abnormal glucose tolerance is striking. In patients with hypercholesterolemia (type II) abnormal glucose tolerance is found in approximately one third of patients, while in those whose primary elevation is in triglyceride (type IV and V), abnormal glucose tolerance is found in 50% to 80%.[7] The mechanisms by which diabetes and hypertriglyceridemia are related are not known. The synthesis of triglyceride-rich very-low-density lipoproteins (VLDL) is enhanced by hyperinsulinemia, (eg, in the obese adult patient with late-onset diabetes) and the removal of VLDL is impaired in patients with insulin deficiency, presumably because the enzyme, lipoprotein lipase, is insulin-dependent. However, large populations of juvenile diabetics who are insulin-deficient do not have hypertriglyceridemia.[8] Although there is some evidence that lowering serum lipids will prevent progression of vascular disease,[9] this has not been shown in the diabetic population. However, low levels of high-density-lipoprotein cholesterol, which are associated with coronary artery disease,[10] can be increased as blood sugar levels are normalized,[11] suggesting that changing blood lipids by better controlling blood sugar might prevent the arteriosclerotic process.

Other factors, such as increased platelet aggregation,[12] renal failure and the use of oral hypoglycemic agents, may contribute to coronary artery disease in the diabetic patient. In a limited study of eleven diabetic patients with end-stage renal disease (average age was 32 years) who had no symptoms of coronary artery disease all showed multifocal atherosclerotic coronary disease on coronary angiography.[13] Eight of these patients died a mean of 19.8 months following angiography, six from coronary artery disease. Neither the presence of hyperlipidemia nor hypertension could explain the coronary artery disease. Certainly maintenance hemodialysis does not protect diabetic patients; in fact, prolonged hemodialysis probably accelerates the atherosclerotic process.[14]

Several clinical trials have suggested that the use of sulfonylureas may lead to an increase in morbidity and mortality from cardiovascular disease (Chapter 6). The University Group Diabetes Program certainly suggested an increase in cardiovascular morbidity and mortality in patients taking oral agents.[15] Animal studies with tolbutamide also suggest accelerated atherosclerosis and reduction in left ventricular function (Chapter 6).

Although the pathogenesis of coronary artery disease in diabetes is not known, it remains the most serious hazard faced by the patient with late-onset diabetes. However, there are clinical characteristics of diabetics with coronary artery disease that differ from nondiabetics with coronary artery disease, as well as special precautions that must be considered in the diabetic with myocardial infarction, angina, hypertension, and heart failure.

MYOCARDIAL INFARCTION

Acute myocardial infarction is more common in the diabetic population than the nondiabetic population. This increased prevalence is documented in autopsy studies[16] and the Framingham study. The impact of diabetes on myocardial infarction is most marked in women; diabetic women have an increase in myocardial infarction almost three times greater than nondiabetic women. Diabetic men have an increase in myocardial infarction 1.5 times that of nondiabetic men.

The course of myocardial infarction in diabetics is devastating. The in-hospital mortality is between 26% and 58%,[2] is increased in women, and approaches 85% if accompanied by ketoacidosis.[17] The in-hospital mortality for nondiabetic patients with myocardial infarction is approximately 15%. The prognosis after hospital discharge also appears grave with one study reporting a 51% one-year mortality[18] about 10% of nondiabetic patients who survive the acute episode die within one year after discharge.

A significant number of hospital deaths occurs after discharge from the coronary care unit. Approximately 50% of diabetic patients who die, succumb in the hospital after discharge from the coronary care unit; 31% within 5 to 14 days after hospital admission and another 16% between hospital day 15 and 30.[18] These data suggest that recent developments in the management of acute myocardial infarction have not altered the basic pattern of high mortality and poor prognosis among diabetics and further suggest that diabetics with acute myocardial infarction should be kept in the coronary care unit for longer periods of time. However, when the causes of death in 32 patients who died after discharge from the coronary care unit were examined deaths in 20 patients were secondary to congestive heart failure and presumably could not have been better managed in an intensive unit However, five patients died of ventricular fibrillation and might have been saved if kept under close surveillance in a unit where rapid defibrillation was possible.[19]

Also of major clinical importance is the recognition that diabetic patients with myocardial infarction frequently present to the physician with atypical symptoms for acute infarction. In one series 42% of diabetics with infarction presented with no chest pain compared to 6% of nondiabetic patients.[20] In another study, 35% of diabetics with acute myocardial infarction were admitted to the general wards, 27% without chest pain and 8% with chest pain judged to be angina pectoris, not myocardial infarction.[18] The reason for painless infarctions among diabetics is not completely known, but there is some evidence that this is secondary to diabetic neuropathy involving the autonomic nervous system; clearly abnormal morphologic findings of cardiac sympathetic and parasympathetic nerves have been described in five diabetic patients who died with painless myocardial infarctions.[21] The clinician must be aware that nausea and vomiting, increasing congestive heart failure, generalized weakness, and poorly controlled diabetes may all be manifestations of painless myocardial infarction in the diabetic. Myocardial infarction must be considered in all patients who develop ketoacidosis. Since absence of pain delays diagnosis and the opportunity for early management, the awareness of myocardial infarction in diabetic patients with symptoms unusual for myocardial infarction is the only way these seriously ill patients will receive adequate treatment early.

The diagnosis of diabetes soon after the infarction can be a problem for there are numerous studies relating glucose intolerance in the nondiabetic with acute infarction. If the nondiabetic patient has sustained hyperglycemia two weeks from the infarction, he probably has latent diabetes.[22]

Once myocardial infarction is diagnosed the management of the diabetic patient is similar to the nondiabetic patient. Hyperglycemia must be treated and hypoglycemia avoided although the myocardium is able to derive some energy from substrates such as free fatty acids regardless of the level of blood sugar. Hypoglycemia would undoubtedly precipitate a sympathetic response with an increase in heart rate, myocardial contractility, and peripheral resistance all of which demand more myocardial oxygen consumption, a situation best avoided during an acute infarction. Insulin is required to prevent the fluid and electrolyte loss attendant to hyperglycemia; ketoacidosis demands insulin therapy (Chapter 8). Most physicians give the patient the usual dose of insulin with frequent checks of blood sugar during the first 48 to 72 hours, realizing that insulin requirements may increase during an acute infarction. Others prefer to administer regular insulin in divided doses every six hours during the first day or two.

There are a few precautions the physician must keep in mind when treating the diabetic with acute myocardial infarction. T-wave changes may not reflect ischemia only, but may be secondary to shifts of potassium from the serum into cells when insulin is given and acidosis corrected. The myocardial effects of hypokalemia must always be kept in mind, especially in the potassium-deficient diabetic patient treated with insulin or bicarbonate. The earliest and most characteristic electrocardiographic manifestation of hypokalemia is the U-wave, present in 75% of patients with potassium levels below 2.7 mEq/liter. Serious arrhythmias—atrial tachycardia with block, A-V dissociation, ventricular ectopy including ventricular tachycardia, and ventricular fibrillation—can be secondary to myocardial ischemia or secondary to hypokalemia, especially if the patient is also taking a digitalis preparation.

Vasodilator therapy of acute myocardial infarction must be used cautiously. Diabetic patients with uncontrolled glycosuria are volume depleted, and vasodilator therapy may precipitate profound hypotension. The diabetic with orthostatic hypotension from autonomic neuropathy is also more susceptible to the adverse effects of vasodilators. The insertion of an aortic balloon pump is very hazardous in the diabetic with concomitant peripheral vascular disease because of the risk of further compromising peripheral circulation.

ANGINA PECTORIS

The prevalence of angina pectoris in diabetic populations has varied from 8%[23] to 38%,[24] probably because of differences in criteria for the diagnosis and differences in study populations. The prevalence of angina in the University Group Diabetes Program was 6.1% and the annual incidence was 1.6 times greater in diabetic than nondiabetic men in the Framingham Study. In diabetic women the incidence was 1.9 times greater.

The management of the diabetic patient with angina pectoris is not different from the management of nondiabetic patients. However, precautions must be taken, primarily with the use of propranolol and vasodilators.

There are three possible ways for a beta-blocking drug such as propranolol to affect glucose metabolism; only one is important clinically. Since beta-adrenergic stimulation causes insulin release from the pancreas, beta-blockade can raise blood sugar levels. Such an effect has been shown with short courses of intravenous propranolol, but hyperglycemia has not been a problem with prolonged oral use. Liver glycogen is mobilized in part by beta-adrenergic stimulation and theoretically beta-blockade could blunt glycogen mobilization following hypoglycemia. Again, this has not been shown to be a clinical problem. The most important clinical problem of diabetic patients taking propranolol is the masking of the sympathetic discharge that accompanies hypoglycemia. The warning signs that accompany hypoglycemia—anxiety, palpitations, sweating, and tremulousness—are sympathetically mediated and may be absent in patients taking propranolol. The patient may become stuporous from hypoglycemia without warning. At one time propranolol was contraindicated in the insulin-requiring patient, but now many physicians use propranolol cautiously and advise the patient that the usual symptoms of hypoglycemia may be absent.

Other effects of beta-blockers may cause adverse effects in the diabetic patient and must be kept in mind. In patients with autonomic neuropathy manifested by orthostatic hypotension, blood pressure is partially maintained by reflex sympathetic activity causing an increase in cardiac output. This reflex activity is blocked by propranolol. Therefore, patients with orthostatic hypotension must be told to rise very slowly and not to walk immediately after standing. When patients first start taking beta-blockers peripheral resistance increases because alpha-adrenergic stimulation, which causes vasoconstriction, is not balanced by beta-mediated vasodilation. The subsequent vasoconstriction may further compromise circulation in the diabetic with severe peripheral vascular disease. This is not a problem in patients taking propranolol for weeks because the long-term effect of beta-blockade is a decrease in peripheral resistance. Beta-blocking drugs also decrease adrenergic-mediated inotropic and chronotropic effects on the heart. Therefore, these drugs are contraindicated in diabetic patients with marked impairment of left ventricular function, a clinical situation not uncommon in the diabetic patient with hypertension and angina pectoris. Congestive heart failure precipitated by propranolol may be the first manifestation of diabetic cardiomyopathy.

The vasodilator drugs used in the treatment of angina, primarily the nitrites, have to be used cautiously in patients with orthostatic hypotension and patients have to be warned about standing abruptly and immediately walking after administering these drugs.

The surgical approach to coronary artery disease in the diabetic patient with angina is the same as the approach in the nondiabetic patient. Although there are no studies reporting survival results of long-term follow-up after coronary artery bypass grafting of diabetic vs nondiabetic patients, the operative mortality is about the same.[25] However, one group reported an operative mortality of 11% in the diabetic group[26] and another group reported an increased mortality (9% in diabetic vs 4% in nondiabetic) during the early years of the series.[27] In the latter series although the diabetic group had an increased prevalence of unstable angina, prior infarction, and Class IV cardiac symptoms preoperatively, the amount of obstructive coronary disease at angiography was similar in both groups. Postoperatively, blood flow through the grafts and the relief of angina were almost identical in both groups. However, the incidence of postoperative wound infections was increased in the diabetic patients (11% vs 3%).

At present the indications for surgery and the operative approach in diabetic patients with surgically correctable coronary artery disease should be the same as in the nondiabetic patients. Perhaps greater care should be taken to prevent wound infections in diabetic patients. This approach awaits results of long-term survival and morbidity studies comparing surgical results in a diabetic vs a nondiabetic population.

HYPERTENSION

As stated before, hypertension has been reported in 40% to 80% of diabetic patients and is frequently found in patients with diabetic nephropathy.[28] The consequences of hypertension in the diabetic patient are similar to those in the nondiabetic: congestive heart failure, stroke, and renal failure. There is considerable evidence that hypertension is a major determinant of accelerated atherogenesis. It seems reasonable that controlling hypertension would prevent, in part, the accelerated atherogenesis that seems to be present in diabetes. Certainly

292

lowering blood pressure has decreased the incidence of congestive heart failure, stroke, and renal failure in nondiabetic men.[5]

The causes of hypertension in diabetic patients are similar to those in nondiabetic patients except for a form of hypertension associated with diabetic glomerulosclerosis called diabetic hypertension.[4] In patients with diabetic hypertension plasma renin activity may be either low or normal suggesting that this form of hypertension is, in large part, volume-dependent. The reason for not finding elevations of renin in diabetics with renal disease is not known, for patients with ketoacidosis and volume depletion have markedly elevated plasma renin activities.[29] It has been suggested that hyalinization of the area in the glomerulus of the afferent arteriole next to the juxtaglomerular cells either replaces the juxtaglomerular cells or inhibits release of renin into the circulation. The low or normal plasma renin activity probably explains the lack of malignant hypertension in patients with diabetic renal disease.

Treatment of the diabetic patient with hypertension, although similar to that in the nondiabetic, requires some special considerations. As in the nondiabetic, diuretics constitute initial therapy. The thiazide diuretics initially decrease blood volume and later lower peripheral resistance, but also produce hypokalemia, which inhibits insulin release and further aggravates glucose intolerance. This usually is not a major clinical problem. Although potassium supplements may help in reversing this abnormality, potassium is not recommended for hypertensive patients taking thiazide diuretics unless they develop symptoms of hypokalemia or are also taking a digitalis preparation. Diabetic patients troubled by orthostatic hypotension are particularly susceptible to the vasodilating effects of hydralazine and prazosin. These patients depend upon sympathetic discharge to maintain blood pressure when standing and are particularly susceptible to the sympathetic blockers: reserpine, methyldopa, clonidine, guanethidine, and propranolol.

As in the nondiabetic patient, the diabetic patient with angina should be protected against the reflex tachycardia of hydralazine by the concomitant use of a beta-blocking drug. Likewise, diuretics should always be used with sympathetic inhibitors and vasodilators to prevent the increase in blood volume that occurs when these drugs are used as single agents. Propranolol may precipitate congestive heart failure and must be used carefully, if at all, in the diabetic patient with marginal left ventricular function.

DIABETIC CARDIOMYOPATHY

An apparent excess of congestive heart failure in diabetic patients was noted in the Framingham study in which 14% of men and 26% of women who developed congestive heart failure also had diabetes.[30] These figures represent an increased risk of 2.4 in diabetic men and 5.3 in diabetic women. The same study identified hypertension and coronary artery disease as the predominant etiologic factors for developing congestive heart failure. It is certainly logical that these factors, which occur with a greater prevalence in diabetic populations, account for the occurrence of congestive heart failure in the diabetic population. However, when patients with coronary artery disease were excluded from analysis, diabetic patients still had a fivefold increased risk of developing congestive heart failure. Likewise the association was not explained entirely by hypertension. Most of the increased risk for congestive heart failure was confined to insulin-treated diabetics, and it appeared quite unlikely that diabetes promoted congestive heart failure because of hypertension or accelerated coronary artery disease.[31] These observations suggest that diabetic patients are susceptible to a distinct type of cardiomyopathy.

There is little doubt that diabetic patients develop congestive heart failure in the absence of coronary artery disease or hypertension. Whether this cardiomyopathy is secondary to diffuse intramural small-vessel disease[32] or secondary to some extravascular metabolic abnormality is not known. Pathologically the hearts are large and heavy with scattered focal fibrosis, and show an accumulation of periodic acid-Schiff (PAS) staining in the media of the coronary arteries and the myocardium.[31] Physiologically, ventricular stiffness, decreased diastolic compliance, and abnormal systolic time intervals reflecting abnormal left ventricular performance have been described.

One study of 73 patients with cardiomyopathy, 16 who were diabetic, reported postmortem findings in three patients. All had patent large coronary arteries and all had small-vessel changes consisting of endothelial proliferation with bridging across the lumen; small-vessel disease was noted at autopsy in only one of 28 patients with cardiomyopathy who did not have diabetes.[33] In another autopsy study of four patients with diabetic glomerulosclerosis, cardiomegaly with congestive heart failure, but without hypertension or coronary artery disease, left ventricular hypertrophy with myofibrillar hypertrophy and fibrotic strands between muscle bundles were described. In one patient narrowing of the lumen of intramural arteries was noted primarily to be due to the deposition of acid mucopolysaccharide subendothially with subintimal thickening and medial hypertrophy.[34] In a more recent autopsy study of nine patients with juvenile-onset diabetes mellitus, coronary artery disease was found more extensively than in age-matched controls, and minor degrees of intimal fibrous proliferation were observed in the intramural coronary arteries of six of nine diabetic patients and in none of the controls. Although these patients had mild intimal proliferation and PAS-positive material in the media of intramural arteries, these were considered mild and of no functional or clinical significance.[35] In another autopsy study of nine diabetic patients with no obstructive disease of the coronary arteries, all nine had PAS-positive material in the interstitium and collagen accumulation in perivascular loci between myofibers. Multiple samples of myocardium had increased concentrations of cholesterol and triglycerides, but no narrowing of intramural vessels.[36] The conclusions of these authors was that perhaps a diffuse extravascular abnormality may be the basis for the cardiomyopathic features in diabetes. Thus, the question of etiology of diabetic cardiomyopathy is left unanswered by autopsy studies, some suggesting small-vessel disease and some suggesting an unknown metabolic abnormality.

Preclinical abnormalities highly suggestive of underlying cardiomyopathy have also been described in diabetic patients. Twenty-five diabetic subjects with no evidence of heart disease, no hypertension, obesity, or alcoholism were compared to 37 normal subjects and found to have shorter left ventricular ejection times (LVET), longer preejection periods (PEP), and higher ratios of PEP/LVET.[37] All of these indices reflect depressed left ventricular function in diabetics without clinical evidence of heart disease. A similar echocardiographic study was done in 23 young diabetics without clinical heart disease and was found to be abnormal in 17, 14 of whom had echocardiographic changes similar to those found in patients with other forms of cardiomyopathy.[38] These authors suggested that the abnormalities may reflect subclinical cardiomyopathy. The predictive value of these abnormalities of systolic time intervals and echocardiography await long-term follow-up. However, these physiologic studies showing subclinical depression of left ventricular function in the absence of coronary artery disease or hypertension suggest a cardiomyopathic process linked to diabetes.

CONGESTIVE HEART FAILURE

The Framingham study showed unequivocally that congestive heart failure occurred with an increased incidence in the diabetic population, especially in women.[39] Although hypertension and coronary artery disease were prominent risk factors, congestive heart failure occurred in the diabetic population even in the absence of these factors and led investigators to speculate on the cause of diabetic cardiomyopathy. Whatever the etiology of congestive heart failure, the prognosis is poor, approximately 50% of all patients surviving five years.

Management of the diabetic with congestive heart failure differs little from that of the nondiabetic, although there are two clinical situations that may become more manifest in the diabetic. Pulmonary edema has been described in six patients with coronary artery disease who did not have cardiomegaly. Five of these six patients were diabetics. This syndrome has been called the paradox of the stiff heart.[40] Compared to control patients, these patients with stiff hearts had marked increases in left ventricular end-diastolic pressures with small increases in volume. This was thought to be secondary to ischemia, which caused an increase in myocardial fibrous tissue, which reduced ventricular distensibility. Therefore, diabetics may have florid congestive heart failure in the absence of myocardial infarction and paradoxically have a normal-sized, but stiff, heart.

Rapid fluid shifts from extracellular to intracellular space have been described in a diabetic patient with uremia and congestive heart failure following correction of hyperglycemia.[41] This patient's congestive heart failure improved after hyperglycemia was corrected with insulin without the use of digitalis or diuretics. Fluid shifted from extracellular to intracellular space as the osmolality in plasma decreased. These authors concluded that although it is unwise to treat congestive heart failure with insulin alone, one should be aware that extravascular volume decreases as blood sugar decreases and this may necessitate caution in the simultaneous use of diuretics.

Drug therapy in the diabetic with congestive heart failure does not differ from the nondiabetic. One must remember that diabetic's propensity to renal failure when using digitalis preparations. Hypokalemia is frequent when ketoacidosis is corrected and must be avoided in patients taking digitalis. Hyperkalemia secondary to hypoaldosteronism from depressed renin activity has been described in diabetic patients with mild azotemia.[42] Of course, potassium supplements should not be given to these patients.

PREVENTION

Although there is no evidence that normalization of the blood sugar will prevent atherosclerotic disease in the diabetic patient, there is evidence that patients who have blood sugars brought into reasonably normal range will have fewer microvascular complications than patients who are hyperglycemic most of the time (Chapter 7). A proper diet (Chapter 3) resulting in weight loss in the obese diabetic will frequently improve hyperglycemia, hyperinsulinemia, and hypertriglyceridemia.

Since risk factors for coronary artery disease are additive, it makes sense to try to eliminate each of these factors in the high-risk diabetic patient. Evidence is now mounting that stopping cigarette smoking[4] and correcting hyperlipidemia[9] both decrease the risk of coronary artery disease. Lower blood pressure has been shown to decrease the incidence of cerebrovascular and renovascular disease.[5] Since the use of ovulation-suppressing contraceptive pills may contribute to the metabolic alterations that promote vascular disease, other forms of contraception should be prescribed to diabetic women. Since oral sulfonylureas seldom control blood sugar adequately, diet and insulin therapy should always be first line management, and oral hypoglycemics reserved for those diabetic patients in whom diet and insulin therapy are not feasible. Although the evidence is not unequivocal that correction of all of these risk factors will prevent vascular disease, it seems reasonable to try to correct a series of risk factors, each of which contributes to the atherosclerotic process.

REFERENCES

1. Scott, R.C. Diabetes and the heart. *Am Heart J.* 90:283–289, 1975.

2. Knowles, H.C. Coronary artery disease in diabetes: its development course, and response to treatment. Edited by S. Zoneraich. In *Diabetes and the Heart.* Springfield, Ill.: Charles C Thomas, 1978, pp 113–122.

3. Klent, C.R., Knatterud, G.L., Meinert, C.L. et al. The University Group Diabetes Program: a study of the effects of hypoglycemia agents on vascular complications in patients with adult-onset diabetes. I. Design, methods, and baseline results. *Diabetes* 19:747–783, 1970.

4. Christlieb, R.A. Diabetes and hypertensive vascular disease. *Am J Cardiol.* 32:592–606, 1973.

5. Veterans Administration Cooperative Study. Effects of treatment on morbidity in hypertension. II. Results in patients with diastolic blood pressure averaging 90 through 114 mm Hg. *JAMA.* 213:1143–1152, 1970.

6. Hamby, R.I., Sherman, L., Mehta, J. et al. Reappraisal of the role of the diabetic state in coronary artery disease. *Chest* 70:251–257, 1976.

7. Glueck, C.J., Levy, R.I., and Fredrickson, D.S. Immunoreactive insulin glucose tolerance, and carbohydrate inducibility in types II, III, IV, and V hyperlipoproteinemia. *Diabetes* 18:739–747, 1969.

8. Spritz, N. Diabetes, heart disease, and hyperlipidemia. Edited by S Zoneraich. In *Diabetes and the Heart.* Springfield, Ill.: Charles C Thomas, 1978 p 141.

9. Kuo, P.T., Hayase, K., Kastis, J.B. et al. Use of combined diet and colestipal in long-term (7–7½ years) treatment of patients with type II hyperlipoproteinemia. *Circulation* 59:199–211, 1979.

10. Berg, K., Hørresen, A.L., and Dahlén, G. Serum-high-density-lipoprotein and atherosclerotic heart-disease. *Lancet* 1:499–501, 1976.

11. Calvert, B.D., Marrnick, T., Graham, J.T. et al. Effects of therapy on plasma high-density-lipoprotein-cholesterol concentration in diabetes mellitus *Lancet* 2:66–68, 1978.

12. Halushka, P.V., Lurie, D., Colwell, J.A. Increased synthesis of prostaglandin-E-like material by platelets from patients with diabetes mellitus *N Engl J Med.* 297:1306–1310, 1977.

13. Bennett, W.M., Klaster, F., Rosch, J. et al. Natural history of asymptomatic coronary arteriographic lesions in diabetic patients with end-stage renal disease. *Am J Med.* 65:779–784, 1978.

14. Linder, A., Charra, B., Sherrara, D. et al. Accelerated atherosclerosis in prolonged maintenance hemodialysis. *N Engl J Med.* 290:697–701, 1974.

15. Klent, C.R., Knatterud, G.L., Meinert, C.L. et al. The University Group Diabetes Program: a study of the effect of hypoglycemic agents on vascular complications in patients with adult-onset diabetes. II. Mortality results. *Diabetes* 19:789–830, 1970.

16. Liebow, I.M., and Hellerstin, H.K., Cardiac complications of diabetes mellitus. *Am J Med.* 7:660–670, 1949.

17. Partamian, J.O., and Bradley, R.F. Acute myocardial infarction in 258 cases of diabetes — immediate mortality and five-year survival. *N Engl J Med.* 273:455–461, 1965.

18. Saler, N.G., Bennett, M.A., Pentecost, B.L. et al. Myocardial infarction in diabetes. *Aust J Med.* 44:125–132, 1975.

19. Saler, N.G., Bennett, M.A., Lamb, P. et al. Coronary care for myocardial infarction in diabetics. *Lancet* 1:475–477, 1974.

20. Bradley, R.F., and Schonfeld, A. Diminished pain in diabetic patients with acute myocardial infarction. *Geriatrics* 17:322–326, 1962.

21. Fearman, I., Faccio, E., Milec, J. et al. Autonomic neuropathy and painless myocardial infarction in diabetic patients — histologic evidence of their relationship. *Diabetes* 26:1147–1158, 1977.

22. Bradley, R.F. Heart disease and diabetes. Edited by A. Marble, P. White, R.F. Bradley, and L. Krall. In *Joslin's Diabetes Mellitus.* Philadelphia: Lea & Febiger, 1971, p 456.

23. Liebow, I.M., Newell, V.A., and Oseasoh, R. Incidence of ischemic heart disease in a group of diabetic women. *Am J Med Sci.* 248:403–407, 1964.

24. Bradley, R.F., and Bryfogle, J.W. Survival in diabetic patients after myocardial infarction. *Am J Med.* 20:207–216, 1956.

25. Chychota, M.N., Gan, G.T., Pluth, J.R. et al. Myocardial revascularization. Comparison of operability and surgical results in diabetic and non-diabetic patients. *J Thorac Cardiovasc Surg.* 65:856–862, 1973.

26. Draskoczy, S.P., Leland, O.S., and Bradley, R.F. Aorto-coronary bypass in the diabetic patient. *Kidney Int.* 65:37–40, 1974.

27. Verska, J.J., and Walker, W.J. Aorto-coronary bypass in the diabetic patient. *Am J Cardiol.* 35:774–777, 1975.

28. White, P. Natural course and prognosis of juvenile diabetes. *Diabetes* 5:445–450, 1956.

29. Christlieb, A.R., Assal, J.P., and Katsilambros, N. Plasma renin and blood volume in uncontrolled diabetes. Ketoacidosis, a state of secondary aldosteronism. *Diabetes* 24:190–193, 1975.

30. McKee, P.A., Castelli, W.P., McNamara, P.M. et al. The natural history of congestive heart failure. The Framingham Study. *N Engl J Med.* 285:1441–1446, 1971.

31. Kannel, W.B. Role of diabetes in cardiac disease: conclusions from population studies. Edited by S. Zoneraich. In *Diabetes and the Heart.* Springfield, Ill.: Charles C Thomas, 1978, pp 97–112.

32. Zoneraich, S., and Silverman, G. Myocardial small vessel disease in diabetic patients. Edited by S. Zoneraich. In *Diabetes and the Heart.* Springfield, Ill.: Charles C Thomas, 1978, pp 3–18.

33. Hamby, R.I., Zoneraich, S., and Scherman, L. Diabetic cardiomyopathy. *JAMA.* 229:1749–1754, 1974.

34. Rublec, S., Dlugash, J., Yucroglu, Y. et al. New type of cardiomyopathy associated with diabetic glomerulosclerosis. *Am J Cardiol.* 30:595–602, 1972.

35. Crall, F.V., and Roberts, W.C. The extramural and intramural coronary arteries in juvenile diabetes mellitus. *Am J Med.* 64:221–230, 1978.

36. Regan, T.J. Evidence for cardiomyopathy in familial diabetes mellitus. *J Clin Invest.* 60:885–899, 1977.

37. Ahemed, S.S., Jaferi, G.A., Narang, R.M. et al. Preclinical abnormality of left ventricular function in diabetes mellitus. *Am Heart J.* 89:153–158, 1975.

38. Sanderson, J.E., Brown, D.J., Revellese, A. et al. Diabetic cardiomyopathy: an echocardiographic study of young diabetics. *Br Med J.* 1:404–406, 1978.

39. Kannel, W.B., and McGee, D.L. Diabetes and cardiovascular disease. The Framingham Study. *JAMA.* 241:2035–2038, 1979.

40. Dodek, A., Kassebaum, D.G., and Bristow, J.D. Pulmonary edema in coronary artery disease without cardiomegaly. Paradox of the stiff heart. *N Engl J Med.* 286:1347–1350, 1972.

41. Axelrod, L. Response of congestive heart failure to correction of hyperglycemia in the presence of diabetic nephropathy. *N Engl J Med.* 293:1243–1244, 1975.

42. Goldfarb, S., Cox, M., Singer, I. et al. Acute hyperkalemia induced by hyperglycemia: hormonal mechanisms. *Ann Intern Med.* 84:426–432, 1976.

43. Wilhelmsson, C., Verdin, J., Elmfeldt, D. et al. Smoking and myocardial infarction. *Lancet* 1:415–420, 1975.